Current Topics in Pain

Mission Statement of IASP Press®

IASP brings together scientists, clinicians, health care providers, and policy makers to stimulate and support the study of pain and to translate that knowledge into improved pain relief worldwide. IASP Press publishes timely, high-quality, and reasonably priced books relating to pain research and treatment.

Current Topics in Pain:
12th World Congress on Pain

Editor

José Castro-Lopes, MD, PhD
Institute of Histology and Embryology
of the Faculty of Medicine
Institute of Molecular and Cellular Biology
University of Porto, Portugal

IASP PRESS® ◈ **SEATTLE**

Library of Congress Cataloging-in-Publication Data

World Congress on Pain (12th : 2008 : Glasgow, Scotland)
 Current topics in pain / 12th World Congress on Pain ; editor, José Castro-Lopes.
   p. ; cm.
 Includes bibliographical references and index.
 Summary: "Reviews of selected topics on pain research and management, from the neurochemistry and neurobiology of pain to the role of stress in chronic pain, are presented by leading experts who were invited to present a plenary talk or distinguished lecture at the IASP 12th World Congress on Pain in 2008"--Provided by publisher.
 ISBN 978-0-931092-76-3 (pbk. : alk. paper)
 1. Pain--Congresses. I. Castro-Lopes, José, 1959- II. International Association for the Study of Pain. III. Title.
 [DNLM: 1. Pain--physiopathology--Congresses. 2. Pain--therapy--Congresses. WL 704 W927c 2009]
 RB127.W675 2009
 616'.0472--dc22
                              2009015547

Published by:
IASP Press®
International Association for the Study of Pain
111 Queen Anne Ave N, Suite 501
Seattle, WA 98109-4955, USA
Fax: 206-283-9403
www.iasp-pain.org

Printed in the United States of America

This book is dedicated to our esteemed colleague
Mitchell Max, 1949–2008

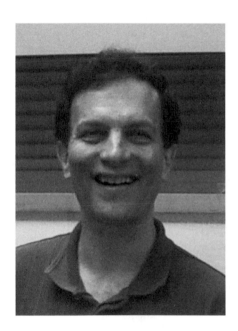

Contents

Contributing Authors

Jacob N. Ablin, MD *Institute of Rheumatology, Tel Aviv Medical Center, Israel*

Kirsty Campbell, MHA *Department of Pain Medicine and Palliative Care, The Children's Hospital at Westmead, Westmead, New South Wales, Australia*

E. Carstens, PhD *Department of Neurobiology, Physiology and Behavior, University of California-Davis, Davis, California, USA*

Daniel J. Clauw, MD *Department of Anesthesiology and Medicine, Chronic Pain and Fatigue Research Center, and Clinical and Translational Research, The University of Michigan, Ann Arbor, Michigan, USA*

John J. Collins, MBBS, PhD, FRACP *Department of Pain Medicine and Palliative Care, The Children's Hospital at Westmead, Westmead, New South Wales, Australia*

Yves De Koninck, PhD *Department of Psychiatry and Division of Cellular Neurobiology, Robert-Giffard Research Center, Laval University, Quebec, Canada*

Herta Flor, PhD *Department of Cognitive and Clinical Neuroscience, Central Institute of Mental Health, University of Heidelberg, Mannheim, Germany*

Inge Genefke, MD, DMSc *International Rehabilitation Council for Torture Victims, Copenhagen, Denmark*

Jennifer A. Haythornthwaite, PhD *Department of Psychiatry and Behavioral Sciences, Johns Hopkins University School of Medicine, Baltimore, Maryland, USA*

Satu K. Jääskeläinen, MD, PhD *Department of Clinical Neurophysiology, Turku University Hospital, Turku, Finland*

Mitchell B. Max, PhD *Departments of Anesthesiology and Medicine, University of Pittsburgh, Pittsburgh, Pennsylvania, USA*

M.R. Rajagopal, MD *Pallium India; Department of Pain and Palliative Medicine, Sree Uthradam Thirunal Academy of Medical Sciences, Pattom, Trivandrum, Kerala, India*

Peter M. Rothwell, MD, PhD, FRCP, FMedSci *Department of Clinical Neurology, John Radcliffe Hospital, Headington, Oxford, United Kingdom*

Jürgen Sandkühler, MD, PhD *Department of Neurophysiology, Center for Brain Research, Medical University of Vienna, Vienna, Austria*

Hans-Georg Schaible, Dr Med *Department of Neurophysiology, Institute of Physiology, Jena University Clinic, Jena, Germany*

Claudia Sommer, Dr Med *Department of Neurology, University of Würzburg, Würzburg, Germany*

Bent Sørensen, MD, DMSc *International Rehabilitation Council for Torture Victims, Copenhagen, Denmark*

Andrew J. Todd, MBBS, PhD *Spinal Cord Group, Faculty of Biomedical and Life Sciences, University of Glasgow, Glasgow, United Kingdom*

Suellen M. Walker, MBBS, PhD, FANZCA, FFPMANZCA *Department of Paediatric Anaesthesia and Pain Medicine, UCL Institute of Child Health and Great Ormond Street Hospital, London, United Kingdom*

C. Peter N. Watson, MD, FRCPC *Department of Medicine, University of Toronto, Toronto, Ontario, Canada*

Stephen G. Waxman, MD, PhD *Department of Neurology and Center for Neuroscience and Regeneration Research, Yale University School of Medicine, New Haven, Connecticut, USA; Neurorehabilitation Research Center, Veterans Administration Hospital, West Haven, Connecticut, USA*

Tony L. Yaksh, PhD *Department of Anesthesiology, University of California, San Diego, La Jolla, California, USA*

Preface

This book is a collection of reviews on timely topics written by the renowned experts who were invited to give a plenary or distinguished lecture at the 12th World Congress on Pain. The range of topics, from the neurobiology and neurochemistry of pain to management of pain in developing countries, mirrors the efforts of IASP to advance research on pain and translate the findings into better pain management and improved quality of life for those in pain throughout the world.

In Chapter 1, Tony L. Yaksh discusses the growing appreciation of the biological complexity of the spinal systems that process nociceptive information and describes the history and future applications of spinal drug therapy. Chapter 2 by Stephen G. Waxman explains how erythromelalgia, the first hereditary human pain disorder with a known molecular basis, may serve as a "model disorder" that will contribute to further understanding of pain mechanisms. In Chapter 3, Andrew J. Todd provides an excellent review of the neuronal circuits and receptors involved in spinal cord pain processing from both morphological and electrophysiological perspectives, and in Chapter 4, Jürgen Sandkühler describes the latest knowledge on the role of inhibition at the spinal cord level in the generation and amplification of pain, with a particular emphasis on GABAergic mechanisms.

In Chapter 5, E. Carstens describes how research on itch mechanisms will benefit greatly from the wealth of information already available regarding chronic pain mechanisms. Just as pain may be exacerbated by peripheral and central sensitization of neurons following injury, he explains that itch transmission may be enhanced by analogous mechanisms under pathological conditions.

Chapter 6, by neurologist Claudia Sommer, is an excellent review of the role of cytokines in pain. She describes recent findings in experimental nerve injury pain and evaluates how proinflammatory cytokines contribute to pain conditions including neuropathic pain, fibromyalgia, and rheumatoid arthritis. Cytokines are also discussed in Chapter 7 by Hans-Georg Schaible, who describes current knowledge on the neuronal mechanisms involved in one of the most prevalent pain conditions, joint pain derived from osteoarthritis, including the role of inflammation and the mechanisms of peripheral and central sensitization. Neuropathic pain is the focus of Chapters 8 and 9. Yves De Koninck describes signaling events and ionic mechanisms disrupting spinal inhibition in neuropathic pain, stressing the role of alterations in chloride homeostasis in the spinal cord and its modulation by glial cells. Satu K. Jääskeläinen explores issues related to the relationship between traumatic nerve injury and neuropathic pain, including potential risk factors for developing pain.

Mitchell B. Max, to whom we dedicate this volume, provides valuable insight into the potential of pain-related genome-wide association studies in Chapter 10, "Moving Pain Genetics into the Genome-Wide Association Era." He describes how such studies will contribute to the development of drugs to prevent and treat pain through better identification of analgesic targets.

In Chapter 11, Peter M. Rothwell and C. Peter N. Watson examine the importance of the external validity of randomized controlled trials. They focus on trials in neuropathic pain, but the scope of the discussion on determining the clinical usefulness of trials clearly reaches beyond the field of pain.

Herta Flor in Chapter 12 focuses on the extinction of pain memories. She reviews the contribution of memory processes to chronic pain and argues that "the extinction rather than the acquisition of aversive memory traces may be the crucial variable for pain chronicity." Further, she proposes extinction training as a new psychological approach for pain management.

Chapter 13 is a useful discussion of the relationship between stress and pain. Daniel J. Clauw and Jacob N. Ablin present evidence on the relationship between stress and pain, drawing on progress made in the field of fibromyalgia. They describe several changes found in patients with fibromyalgia and assume that a proportion of the population may be inherently vulnerable to developing such disorders, which may be triggered by a stressful event in these individuals. In Chapter 14, Jennifer A. Haythornthwaite presents valuable insights on the factors that contribute to catastrophizing, explaining how this coping strategy interacts with the nervous, endocrine, and immune systems to present a risk factor for chronic pain.

In Chapter 15, John J. Collins and coauthors present step-by-step strategies for implementing a quality improvement program in pediatric pain management and palliative care, including hospice care. They outline current research in developmental neurobiology and pharmacology, acute and chronic pediatric pain management, and palliative care.

Pain in the developing world is the topic of Chapter 16 by M.R. Rajagopal. Based on experience in Kerala, India, the author outlines a realistic action plan that includes research and development of guidelines, advocacy for governmental policy, improved opioid availability, and support for educational programs and local pain relief efforts.

Finally, in Chapter 17, Inge Genefke and Bent Sørensen of the International Rehabilitation Council for Torture Victims in Copenhagen, Denmark, describe the clinical physical and psychological aspects of pain and suffering following torture as well as the ethical and legal implications of this "worst of all traumas."

I would like to thank my colleagues on the Scientific Program Committee, who made this book possible through their selection of plenary topics and their peer review of chapters: Fernando Cervero, Beverly Collett, Carlos Mauricio de Castro Costa, G. Allen Finley, Susan Fleetwood-Walker, Herta Flor, Carmen Green, Troels Jensen, Eija Kalso, Bruce Kidd, Steven Linton, Arthur Lipman, Stephen McMahon, Jeffrey Mogil, Michael Nicholas, Koichi Noguchi, Paul Pionchon, Srinivasa Raja, Martin Schmelz, Thomas Toelle, You Wan, Judith Watt-Watson, and Harriet Wittink. Finally, I thank the IASP staff for their support, with a special acknowledgement to Elizabeth Endres, Associate Editor of IASP Press, whose professionalism, efficiency, and persistence greatly contributed to the completion of this book.

José Castro-Lopes, MD, PhD

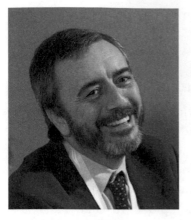

José M. Castro-Lopes, MD, PhD obtained his training at the Faculty of Medicine of the University of Porto, Portugal. He is currently full professor and chair of Histology and Embryology and coordinator of the postgraduate course on pain medicine of the same faculty. He is also coordinator of the National Program for Pain Control of the Portuguese Ministry of Health, and participated actively in the recent establishment of the Competence on Pain Medicine by the Portuguese Medical Association.

Prof. Castro-Lopes has been president of the Portuguese Association for the Study of Pain (IASP Chapter) and honorary treasurer of the European Federation of IASP Chapters (EFIC). He chaired the Scientific Program Committee of the 12th World Congress on Pain® (Glasgow, 2008) and the Local Organizing Committee of Pain in Europe VI, the 6th Congress of EFIC (Lisbon, 2009). He has also served on several other committees of IASP and EFIC.

The main research field of Prof. Castro-Lopes is the neurobiology of pain, in particular the changes induced in the central nervous system by chronic pain. He has made some contributions on the plasticity of the spinal GABAergic system in experimental pain models, as well as changes in other neurotransmitter systems at the supraspinal level. He has held positions at the Max-Planck Institute for Psychiatry in Munich, at Unit 162 of INSERM in Paris, and at the School of Pharmacy in London. He has coordinated several national and European research projects and authored over 50 original or review articles, book chapters, and books.

Theoretical and Practical Consequences of the Role Played by Spinal Systems in the Encoding of Nociceptive Information: 130 Years and Counting

John J. Bonica Distinguished Lecture

Tony L. Yaksh

Department of Anesthesiology, University of California, San Diego, La Jolla, California, USA

It is my honor to present this chapter based on the John J. Bonica lecture. John's role in furthering our interest in the understanding and management of pain is well appreciated. As a clinician he strongly fostered and supported the notion that pain was an important clinical target. As there were those whose charge was to cure cancer or prevent the destruction of the arthritic joint, others perceived the need to focus on the exceedingly complex problem of pain and its management. John's fundamental appreciation of the complexity of the pain state caused him to promote and encourage basic research into mechanisms. It is therefore in his honor that I submit my comments on spinal systems in pain and its management. This topic is quite fitting inasmuch as John was an anesthesiologist and actively employed spinal techniques in pain management.

Few concepts in neuroscience are as fundamental as the two notions that the organized response to the environment depends upon the brain (as opposed to the heart or the spleen) and that the brain organizes its response from the information that it receives about the external environment by virtue of the afferent traffic carried by sensory axons (a

Current Topics in Pain: 12th World Congress on Pain
edited by José Castro-Lopes
IASP Press, Seattle, © 2009

stimulus-response). This linkage, as regards tissue-injuring stimuli, is displayed in the Cartesian cartoon of the boy with his foot in the fire. Here the mechanisms driving the facial grimace and a likely withdrawal of the foot involve circuitry functionally connecting the site of injury to the brain though a spinal link. This iconic image reflects underlying complexities that should make us pause for thought.

Evolutionary Development of Functional Polarity in Systems Activated by Tissue Injury

The virtues of a system that facilitates survival by driving escape behavior in response to potential tissue injury seems evident, given its universal expression in the biology of all organisms. Teleologically, the most fundamental components of the system are those of chemosensitivity. The local chemical environment provides a polarity to evoke the required behaviors—approach (toward nutrition) or withdrawal (from toxic or perhaps predator markers). An effector system provides the organized response to the stimulus. This functional arrangement appears in unicellular organisms. Throughout evolutionary development, organisms have retained their exquisite chemical sensitivity with the distribution of the sensor web to all membranes that have an organ-environmental interface, whether it be the skin, the covering of the brain, the gastrointestinal lumen, or the blood vessel wall. In multicellular organisms, the membrane receptor proteins that originally communicated directly with cytosolic effector processes evolved into specialized afferent systems. These systems link these surfaces through a neural net that serves to organize elements of the response repertoire, such as the gill withdrawal response of *Aplysia* [2].

The evolving neuraxis arising from the primitive ganglionic chain receiving the afferent traffic displays increasing local circuit complexity. Unconditioned input from small-afferent systems activated by tissue-injuring stimuli initiates activity in subpopulations of spinofugally projecting dorsal horn neurons. The frequency of this activity is typically proportional to the intensity of the stimulus. This outflow evokes a hierarchy of increasingly complex responses, ranging from segmentally organized Sherringtonian somatomotor flexion reflexes to cardiovascular and hormonal responses that reflect spinal projections into brainstem and hypothalamic systems. Such systems permit optimization of the trophic response to allow the organism to appropriately respond to the polarity of the stimulus and its magnitude.

The appearance of our "higher-order functions" (self-awareness, perceptions, and emotions) doubtless reflects this encephalization and circuit complexity. At their core, these higher-order systems in their organization retain the essential nature of the negative polarity established for input generated by tissue-injuring stimuli. It is interesting to note that focal stimulation at various supraspinal sites, such as the periaqueductal gray, will robustly support escape behavior [32], which reflects the negative correlates of activity in these circuits generated by small-afferent input though spinofugal projection linkages with these regions. In humans, focal stimulation of the periaqueductal gray can evoke poorly localized, highly aversive perceptual experiences, such as generalized dread, anxiety, and a sense of foreboding [20].

Afferent traffic initiated by tissue injury broadly projects along two trajectories [24]. The first is the classical somatosensory pathway though the primary sensory thalamus to the somatosensory cortex, which retains a high level of somatotopy and is believed, using the terminology of Melzack and Casey [17], to reflect upon the sensory-discriminative aspects of a pain state ("Ouch, I hurt here, on a scale of 1–10, 3"). The second pathway comprises systems that project more medially in the diencephalon, which projects to regions that classically form part of the limbic forebrain associated with the affective-motivational aspects of the sensory experience initiated by a tissue-injuring stimulus ("Moan … The sensation reminds me that I am never going to get well"). Classical lesion studies have indeed suggested that interventions such as prefrontal lobotomies can leave the pain sensation intact, but remove or distort the affective component [26].

In short, all of these hierarchical components of the pain phenotype, from the simplest to the most complex elements, are initiated by an unconditioned high-intensity stimulus that is encoded at the level of the dorsal horn into information that travels by specific projections to a variety of brainstem and diencephalic sites. For a stimulus with which there has been previous situational experience (conditioning), afferent input may generate more complex responses that lead to an altered sensation or emotional covariate of the sensation otherwise generated by the stimulus. Moreover, higher-order systems are able to activate response circuitry. Witness the change in blood pressure evoked by a light that is conditionally linked to a noxious stimulus. These simple changes clearly indicate the ability of visual input to drive activation of bulbospinal projections to preganglionic sympathetic afferents. Moreover, such descending pathways have been shown to regulate dorsal horn excitability, providing links whereby the content of the ascending traffic may itself be modified by supraspinal processing.

Given the proposition outlined above, it is evident that the physiological, sensory, and emotional components initiated by a tissue-injuring stimulus may be inextricably linked as a result of the spinofugal connectivity established over evolutionary development. Accordingly, it is self-evident that relatively specific control over physiological and even emotional components of pain behavior initiated by tissue injury may derive from regulating the spinal encoding process.

Regulation of Spinofugal Traffic

The therapeutic utility of reversibly blocking afferent input came to be appreciated more than 130 years ago. This therapeutic advance occurred as a result of concurrent advances in pharmaceutics and technology. Research, now almost two centuries old, led to the early purification of drugs from plant product extracts that had strong and well-defined biological effects. It was a major conceptual advance heralding the development of medicinal chemistry to appreciate that the active effects could be found in a single component of the natural preparation. The separation procedures available to the early chemist were limited, but the principles of solvent extraction, distillation, precipitation, and crystallization were well-appreciated tools. The marriage of such techniques with biological testing systems (both human and animal) to screen activity permitted surprisingly sophisticated drug purification. Thus, in 1803, Frederick Serturner produced an almost pure substance from poppy resin (based on extraction by differential solubility) with a reliable potency (as defined by its effects in animal models), which he named morphine. Similarly, in 1860, Albert Niemann isolated the main alkaloid of the coca plant, which he named cocaine. The essential device for delivery into the body (under the skin, hence "hypodermic") was of course the glass syringe and the hollow needle. There were several examples, but most attribute the development to Charles Gabriel Pravaz, who invented a silver hollow needle that he combined with a glass syringe that contained about 1.5 mL. Herman Wulfing Luer in 1894 developed the connector (Leur-Lock), resulting in standardized devices that closely resemble those used today [15].

The development of soluble morphine in tablet form by Merck permitted the drug's routine formulation for parenteral delivery by a syringe, and this preparation served as an important medication in the American Civil War. Although topical application of cocaine had demonstrated efficacy in corneal surgery by Carl Koller in 1884, it was the marriage of the purified agent with the hypodermic syringe that allowed physicians such as William Halsted during 1884–1885 to undertake major surgeries with "conduction blockade." The ability of such blocks to prevent sensation from a local region led to the consideration that it might be possible—given the role of the spinal cord in transmitting information from the periphery—to produce a more significant effect by targeting that structure. James Leonard Corning, performing what turned out to be almost certainly an epidural injection, noted that "20 minims (1.3 mL) 2% cocaine ... produced hindlimb weakness and ataxia in dogs" [6]. The routine approach to the neuraxis evolved in 1891 with the work of Heinrich Quincke, who standardized lumbar puncture to remove cerebrospinal fluid for diseases associated with increased intracranial pressure. He employed a relatively sharp, beveled, hollow needle, still referred to as the Quincke needle. The therapeutic use of the intrathecal space is most commonly attributed to August Bier, who in 1899, practicing first on himself and his assistant (Hildebrand) and then in an elegant case series of six patients, reported on the utility and side-effect profile of the technique of lumbar intrathecal cocaine. He noted that the method was only useful "if dangers and inconveniences are less than with general anesthesia" [5]. Remember of course that the general anesthetics of the time were diethyl-ether and chloroform through drip masks, without intubation.

The technique of spinal anesthesia spread very rapidly after the first report by Bier. Thus, by January 1901, a *Lancet* editorial noted that there had been nearly 1,000 publications on the use of "medullary narcosis." Parenthetically, by 1910 the properties of neuraxial local anesthetic delivery were well appreciated, including the role of needle size [1] and the incidence of headaches [5], hypotension [30], ventilatory paralysis, and neurological sequelae such as the cauda equina syndrome and paraplegia [13]. Subsequent developments led to the development of other conduction-blocking agents, including procaine in 1904 and later lidocaine, and the appreciation over 50 years later that these effects were due to the role of voltage-gated sodium channels [10].

Spinal Encoding

What has been particularly intriguing in the past 40 years is the growing appreciation of the biological complexity of the spinal systems that process nociceptive information. One example is the elucidation of the actions of morphine. Consider several convergent events. William R. Martin in 1979 [14] described pivotal work that supported the existence of two opioid receptors (mu and kappa), a conclusion based in large part on work defining the pharmacology of systemically delivered drugs on spinal reflexes in spinalized animals. Hans Kosterlitz, on the basis of smooth-muscle studies, argued for a third site, the δ-opioid receptor [12]. LeBars, Besson, and colleagues [11] reported on the effects of opiates on the discharge of spinal wide-dynamic-range neurons. In an effort to define the behavioral consequences of a spinal action of opiates, Tom Rudy and I in the mid 1970s created a simple rat intrathecal catheter model [41] and demonstrated that opiates with an action limited to the spinal cord would produce a potent and functionally selective block of pain behavior in the absence of any effect on motor function [40]. This specificity was particularly surprising given the effects of opiates on spinal motor systems. The role of the spinal opioid receptor in this analgesic action was confirmed by the pharmacology of the spinal drug effect.

Subsequent work emphasized that the sensory selectivity reflected upon the differential association of the μ-opioid receptor with small, high-threshold primary afferents [9] and that opiates could diminish transmitter release from populations of such afferents [38]. The clinical relevance of the preclinical findings was confirmed 2 years later by demonstration of a potent analgesic effect after intrathecal delivery by Wang et al. [34] at the Mayo Clinic and after epidural delivery by Behar et al. [4] in Israel.

Management of chronic pain with implanted spinal systems soon followed [22]. Subsequent work revealed a role for other spinal receptor systems in regulating acute pain behavior in animals, such as the δ-opioid receptor [31] and α-adrenergic receptor [25]. Importantly, these preclinical results were also mirrored in human studies [21,29].

An important development that has arisen from the investigation of the pharmacology of spinal nociceptive processing is the elucidation of the enormous regulation characterizing the input-output function of the dorsal horn. Human and animal psychophysics emphasizes that local injury yields an enhanced response to otherwise innocuous or moderately noxious stimuli (e.g., hyperalgesia or allodynia) and that often these pain states involve dermatomes that are not injured. It has long been appreciated that many therapeutic agents, such as nonsteroidal anti-inflammatory drugs, have little effect upon normal thresholds, but appear to normalize the hyperpathic state. Work dating from the early 1930s through the 1970s suggested that local injury may lead to sensitization of the peripheral afferent terminals by local tissue injury products [19]. However, speculations embodied in the gate control theory of Melzack and Wall [16] and represented by the schematic of the first-order synapse in the spinal dorsal horn reflect an enhanced response to small-afferent input, a regulation consistent with the physiological phenomena of C-fiber-mediated "wind-up" as described by Mendell and Wall [18]. This physiological observation indicated that the spinal input-output algorithm was subject to enormous modification, both upward (as in wind-up and increased receptive field size) and downward. These changes were in tandem with the alterations in behavioral thresholds observed following tissue injury, where high levels of traffic in small afferents were commonly noted.

Studies undertaking the spinal delivery of pharmacological agents have revealed that the behaviorally defined hyperpathia occurring after tissue injury and inflammation is mediated by an extraordinarily complex spinal biology that includes glutamate, purines, peptides, monoamines, chemokines, and cytokines released from primary afferent terminals, local neurons, bulbospinal pathways, and non-neuronal cells [23,27,36]. Even lipid mediators, long thought to exert their primary hyperalgesic effect on the peripheral terminal, clearly have a primary spinal site of action, as do agents that block their synthetic enzymes [28]. Moreover, after tissue and nerve injury, dorsal horn systems can show significant reactive changes over time, including altered expression and distribution of many receptor and channel proteins, kinases, and cytokines, along with the activation of non-neuronal cells [42]. Again, the importance of these spinal systems to the conscious state initiated by such peripheral injury is reflected by the potent effects of pharmacologically manipulating these spinal systems on the hyperpathic behavior of the intact and unanesthetized animal. The fact that these changes after spinal drugs can occur without altering motor function or the response to otherwise innocuous stimuli emphasizes the uniqueness of the systems to the hyperpathic state, the function of which is altered after peripheral tissue and nerve injury.

Significance of Spinal Encoding to the Pain Phenotype

While it is clear that the eventual expression of the pain experience arises from forebrain functions, the above comments reflect the theme that many of the properties that we ascribe to the psychophysics of tissue and nerve injury pain—such as primary and secondary hyperpathia, the onset of large-afferent tactile allodynia, and referred pain—result from alterations in spinal processing. Changes in the input-output algorithm of the spinal dorsal horn can lead to spinofugal outflow that corresponds to the information content generated by stimuli that initiate the pain experience. To return to the initial theme of this chapter, these projections have connections to supraspinal regions, which throughout evolution have retained their role in regulating the phenotype of the response process, whether it be changes in cardiovascular function, hormone release, or the affective response initiated by a painful experience. It is to be expected that more sophisticated behavioral techniques and the coupling of non-invasive imaging with spinal drug delivery will reveal specific linkages between components of the outflow and supraspinal components that reflect upon this polarity of organization. These components include those arising from superficially nociceptive-specific versus deep dorsal horn convergent neurons, ipsilateral versus contralateral neurons, and opioid- or neurokinin-1-receptor positive versus negative projection neurons. Given the potent analgesic effect of spinal opiates and the limited distribution of the systems with which dorsal horn opioid receptors are associated, it may be expected that after administration of spinal opiates, activation of forebrain systems such as the anterior insula or the inferior insula may be selectively reduced.

The Future of Spinal Drug Therapy

Given the role of spinal encoding in generating anomalous pain states and the richness of the biology of spinal systems that regulate the content of spinal outflow, there are many potential pharmacological targets. Some have found their way into human spinal canals [33]. It must be emphasized here that movement of novel agents into the human spinal canal must occur with specific attention to the spinal safety of the agent [7]. This is true even for agents with which there is significant experience with systemic delivery in humans. The proximity of neural tissue, the modest circulation of the intrathecal space, and the invariably high concentrations of the drugs delivered in that space pose specific concerns for spinal agents. Appropriate development steps require specific validated models with robust histological analyses. It might be argued that if a given drug candidate has been widely examined in preclinical studies, that evidence will suffice for introduction into humans. However, pharmacological studies do not often concern themselves with systematic exposure to higher or extended doses such as may be used in patients [8]. Moreover, such studies rarely assess the presence of histological changes. Such histological examination is a key component to any safety assessment paradigm because morphological changes may occur with minimal effects upon the functions being examined [37,39].

It is interesting to note that potential issues of spinal drug safety have been appreciated from the very beginning. Barker [3] reported on cerebrospinal fluid pleocytosis after local anesthetics, and Wossidlo [35] reported on changes in Nissl substance in the dorsal root ganglia of a dog after 5% procaine. In spinal drug delivery, given the high concentrations and poor distribution, robust assessments of spinal safety are invariably required, even for drugs with which there is significant experience with other routes of delivery. Perhaps a more sophisticated reminder is provided by the 15th-century father of medicinal chemistry,

Paracelsus, who, loosely translated, noted that there are no safe drugs, only safe doses.

Acknowledgments

I would like to thank those for whom I have had the greatest respect and from whom I have learned much: Patrick Wall at University College London, Frederick Kerr at Mayo, Tom Rudy at Wisconsin, Jim Eisenach at Wake Forrest, and my colleagues at San Diego, Linda Sorkin, Xiao Ying Hua, and Camilla Svensson, as well as the National Institutes of Health and the many study sections that have largely provided the wherewithal for my career.

References

[1] Babcock WW. The technique of spinal anesthesia. NY J Med 1914;50:637–702.
[2] Bailey CH, Kandel ER. Synaptic remodeling, synaptic growth and the storage of long-term memory in Aplysia. Prog Brain Res 2008;169:179–98.
[3] Barker AE. Elimination of stovaine after spinal analgesia. BMJ 1904;2:789–91.
[4] Behar M, Magora F, Olshwang D, Davidson JT. Epidural morphine in treatment of pain. Lancet 1979;8115:527–9.
[5] Bier A. Versuche über Cocainisirung des Rückenmarkes. Dtsh Z Chir 1899;51:361–9.
[6] Corning JL. Spinal anaesthesia and local medication of the cord. NY Med J 1885;42:483–5.
[7] Eisenach JC, Gordh T Jr, Yaksh TL. New epidural drugs: primum non nocere. Anesth Analg 1998;87:1211–2.
[8] Eisenach JC, Yaksh TL. Safety in numbers: how do we study toxicity of spinal analgesics? Anesthesiology 2002;97:1047–9.
[9] Fields HL, Emson PC, Leigh BK, Gilbert RF, Iversen LL. Multiple opiate receptor sites on primary afferent fibres. Nature 1980;284:351–3.
[10] Hodgkin AL, Huxley AF. A quantitative description of membrane current and its application to conduction and excitation in the nerve. J Physiol (Lond) 1952;117:500–44.
[11] Le Bars D, Ménétrey D, Conseiller C, Besson JM. Depressive effects of morphine upon lamina V cells activities in the dorsal horn of the spinal cat. Brain Res 1975;98:261–77.
[12] Lord JA, Waterfield AA, Hughes J, Kosterlitz HW. Endogenous opioid peptides: multiple agonists and receptors. Nature 1977;267:495–9.
[13] Lusk WC. The anatomy of spinal puncture with some considerations on technique and paralytic sequelae. Ann Surg 1911;54:449–83.
[14] Martin WR. History and development of mixed opioid agonists, partial agonists and antagonists. Br J Clin Pharmacol 1979;7(Suppl 3):273–9S.
[15] McAuley JE. The hypodermic syringe. Dent Hist 1997;40–1.
[16] Melzack R, Wall PD. Pain mechanisms: a new theory. Science 1965;150:971–9.
[17] Melzack R, Casey KL. Sensory, motivational, and central control determinants of pain. In: Kenshalo D, editor. The skin senses. Springfield, IL: Thomas; 1968. p. 423–39.
[18] Mendell LM, Wall PD. Responses of single dorsal cord cells to peripheral cutaneous fibres. Nature 1965;206:97–9.
[19] Moncada S, Ferreira SH, Vane JR. Inhibition of prostaglandin biosynthesis as the mechanism of analgesia of aspirin-like drugs in the dog knee joint. Eur J Pharmacol 1975;31:250–60.
[20] Nashold BS Jr, Wilson WP, Slaughter DG. Sensations evoked by stimulation in the midbrain of man. J Neurosurg 1969;1:14–24.

[21] Onofrio BM, Yaksh TL. Intrathecal delta-receptor ligand produces analgesia in man. Lancet 1983;8338:1386–7.
[22] Onofrio BM, Yaksh TL, Arnold PG. Continuous low-dose intrathecal morphine administration in the treatment of chronic pain of malignant origin. Mayo Clin Proc 1981;56:516–20.
[23] Pezet S, McMahon SB. Neurotrophins: mediators and modulators of pain. Annu Rev Neurosci 2006;29:507–38.
[24] Price DD. Psychological and neural mechanisms of the affective dimension of pain. Science 2000;288:1769–72.
[25] Reddy SV, Yaksh TL. Spinal noradrenergic terminal system mediates antinociception. Brain Res 1980;189:391–401.
[26] Rubins JL, Friedman ED. Asymbolia for pain. Arch Neurol Psychiatry 1948;60:554–73.
[27] Scholz J, Woolf CJ. The neuropathic pain triad: neurons, immune cells and glia. Nat Neurosci 2007;10:1361–8.
[28] Svensson CI, Yaksh TL. The spinal phospholipase-cyclooxygenase-prostanoid cascade in nociceptive processing. Annu Rev Pharmacol Toxicol 2002;42:553–83.
[29] Tamsen A, Gordh T. Epidural clonidine produces analgesia. Lancet 1984;8396:231–2.
[30] Tuffier, Hallion. Effects circulatoires des injections sous-aracho de coca dans la region lombaire. Comptes Rendus 1900;52:897–9.
[31] Tung AS, Yaksh TL. In vivo evidence for multiple opiate receptors mediating analgesia in the rat spinal cord. Brain Res 1982;247:75–83.
[32] Vianna DM, Brandão ML. Anatomical connections of the periaqueductal gray: specific neural substrates for different kinds of fear. Braz J Med Biol Res 2003;36:557–66.
[33] Wallace M, Yaksh TL. Long-term spinal analgesic delivery: a review of the preclinical and clinical literature. Reg Anesth Pain Med 2000;25:117–57.
[34] Wang JK, Nauss LA, Thomas JE. Pain relief by intrathecally applied morphine in man. Anesthesiology 1979;50:149–51.
[35] Wossidlo E. Experimentelle Untersuchungen über Veränderungen Nissl'schen Granuloma bei der Lumbaranasthesie. Arch Klin Chir 1908;86:1017–53.
[36] Yaksh TL. Central pharmacology of nociceptive transmission. In: McMahon S, Koltzenburg M, editors. Wall and Melzack's textbook of pain. Edinburgh: Churchill Livingstone; 2007.
[37] Yaksh TL, Allen JW. The use of intrathecal midazolam in humans: a case study of process. Anesth Analg 2004;98:1536–45.
[38] Yaksh TL, Jessell TM, Gamse R, Mudge AW, Leeman SE. Intrathecal morphine inhibits substance P release from mammalian spinal cord in vivo. Nature 1980;286:155–6.
[39] Yaksh TL, Rathbun ML, Provencher JC. Preclinical safety evaluation for spinal drugs. In: Yaksh TL, editor. Spinal drug delivery. Amsterdam: Elsevier; 1999. p. 417–37.
[40] Yaksh TL, Rudy TA. Analgesia mediated by a direct spinal action of narcotics. Science 1976;192:1357–8.
[41] Yaksh TL, Rudy TA. Chronic catheterization of the spinal sub-arachnoid space. Physiol. Behav 1976;17:1031–6.
[42] Yaksh TL, Sorkin LS. Mechanisms of neuropathic pain. Curr Med Chem 2005;5:129–40.

Correspondence to: Tony L. Yaksh, PhD, Anesthesiology 0818, University of California, San Diego, 9500 Gilman Drive, La Jolla, CA 92093-0818, USA. Email: tyaksh@ucsd.edu.

2

Lessons from Men on Fire: What Erythromelalgia Can Teach Us about Pain-Signaling Neurons

Stephen G. Waxman

Department of Neurology and Center for Neuroscience and Regeneration Research, Yale University School of Medicine, New Haven, Connecticut, USA; Neurorehabilitation Research Center, Veterans Administration Hospital, West Haven, Connecticut, USA

In this age of molecular medicine, it is becoming increasingly clear that inherited diseases, even rare ones, can teach us important lessons that are applicable to large numbers of patients with more common disorders. This certainly appears to be the case for erythromelalgia, the first hereditary human pain disorder for which a molecular basis has been delineated. Looking back, it is clear that erythromelalgia has already taught us some important lessons over the past few years. Looking forward, it seems likely that some of the unanswered questions posed by erythromelalgia will soon be answered, and some of the speculations arising from consideration of this disorder, as outlined in this chapter, will soon be tested. In this regard, erythromelalgia may emerge as a "model disorder" that will continue to teach us important lessons about pain.

Largely on the basis of observations in human subjects with inherited pain syndromes, the $Na_V1.7$ voltage-gated sodium channel has, over the past few years, emerged as a major player in pain signaling, and in at least some forms of chronic pain. The first disorder to be associated with a locus on chromosome 2q31–32, and then with mutations in $Na_V1.7$, was

erythromelalgia, also termed erythermalgia [16,45]. Nearly a dozen mutations in $Na_v1.7$, each producing a gain-of-function at the channel level that
enhances activation, and in most cases enhancing the response to slow
small stimuli (termed the "ramp response"), have now been identified in
patients with inherited erythromelalgia and have been characterized at
the biophysical level [6,8,11,14,25,26,28,37]. These mutations, their functional effects on the $Na_v1.7$ channel, and the link between channel gain-
of-function and disease have been discussed in detail in several recent reviews [15,17]. Rather than reiterating the growing list of $Na_v1.7$ mutations
that have been linked to inherited erythromelalgia to date, this chapter
will discuss some lessons that derive from the growing list of mutations
linked to erythromelalgia, and from consideration of the clinical aspects
of this previously enigmatic and complex disorder. This chapter will also
consider some recently described aspects of $Na_v1.7$ function that illustrate
important points and raise new questions about $Na_v1.7$ and its function in
human pain-signaling pathways.

Erythromelalgia is clinically characterized by episodes of severe
pain, in many cases triggered by mild warmth (e.g., putting on a pair of
socks, entering a warm room, or engaging in exercise) and often ameliorated by cooling [20,32,41]. Ingestion of alcoholic beverages, caffeine,
spicy foods, or other specific foods, or stress can precipitate symptoms
in some patients with inherited erythromelalgia, via mechanisms that are
not yet clear [32]. Notably, the pain of erythromelalgia has a characteristic
topographical distribution, usually manifesting itself first in the feet and
then in the hands. Later, the upper leg, earlobes, nose tip, and chin can be
involved. Marked redness of the skin accompanies the pain, and there is
evidence for defective sympathetic vasoregulation [12,29,30]. Inheritance
is autosomal dominant, and penetrance is usually 100%. Age of onset varies from family to family, with patients in most families manifesting disease early in childhood, while in some families the onset occurs later, during adolescence or early adulthood. Occasional sporadic juvenile-onset
cases have been found to arise from de novo mutations [25,26].

The physiological effects of $Na_v1.7$ mutations associated with
erythromelalgia include a hyperpolarizing shift in the voltage dependence
of activation, which makes it easier to activate the channel; slowed deactivation, which keeps the channel open longer, once it is activated; and an

increase in the size of the "ramp" response that is evoked by small depolarizations close to resting potential [11]. Some erythromelalgia mutations shift the voltage dependence of inactivation in a depolarized direction, which increases the availability of the channels at any given potential close to resting potential. As a result of altered voltage dependence, there is increased overlap between activation and steady-state inactivation, which is predicted to produce a "window current," thus depolarizing the cell by several millivolts [11,26,34] at rest; as discussed below, this can have a significant effect on excitability of nociceptors.

Thus far, the story appears clear and simple: a mutation of a sodium channel that is preferentially expressed within nociceptors produces a gain-of-function at the channel level. As a result, nociceptors become hyperexcitable; this, in turn, produces pain. Despite the apparent linearity of the story, however, erythromelalgia also illustrates some complexities of channel mutations and the disorders that they can cause, and raises some important questions. These will be the focus of this chapter.

A Single Mutation Can Have Opposing Effects in Different Types of Neurons

$Na_V1.7$ is preferentially expressed in two types of neurons: dorsal root ganglion (DRG) neurons, particularly nociceptive cells, and sympathetic ganglion neurons [34,38]. The role of this channel in setting the gain in nociceptors is reflected by increased thermal and mechanical pain thresholds, as well as by reduced inflammatory pain responses in nociceptor-specific $Na_V1.7$ knockout mice [31] and by the profound insensitivity to pain that has been reported in humans with loss-of-function mutations in $Na_V1.7$ [1,9,21].

Nociceptive DRG neurons, and some sympathetic ganglion neurons, display aberrant behavior in erythromelalgia, with hyperexcitability of nociceptive DRG neurons producing pain [14,26] and impaired sympathetic vasomotor control producing redness of the skin [12,29,30]. Rush et al. [34] recently studied the functional effects of L858H, one of the first $Na_V1.7$ mutations to be found in erythromelalgia, in nociceptive DRG neurons and sympathetic ganglion neurons. This study showed that a single sodium channel mutation can have strikingly different effects on neuronal excitability in these two different cell types, producing hyperexcitability in one cell type and hypoexcitability in another.

As predicted from its large window current [11], the L858H mutant Na$_V$1.7 channel depolarizes resting potential by approximately 5 mV in both DRG and sympathetic ganglion neurons [34]. Within DRG neurons, the 5-mV depolarization of the resting potential is accompanied by a lowering of action potential threshold and by an increase in the rate of action potential firing in response to long-lasting depolarizing stimuli. For example, the firing frequency evoked by 50- and 100-pA stimuli is increased by 550% and 280%, respectively, in DRG neurons expressing the L858 mutant Na$_V$1.7 channel, compared to similar cells expressing the wild-type channel.

The same L858H mutant Na$_V$1.7 channel has an opposite effect on the excitability of sympathetic ganglion neurons [34]. Resting potential in superior sympathetic ganglion neurons expressing this mutant channel is depolarized by about 5 mV, similar to the depolarizing shift produced by the mutant channel in DRG neurons. Sympathetic ganglion neurons expressing the mutant channel, however, display an increased action potential threshold, and when they fire, they generate attenuated action potentials with markedly reduced amplitudes. Sympathetic ganglion neurons expressing the L858H mutant channel also display attenuated responses to sustained depolarizing stimuli, for example, displaying action potential frequencies that are decreased by 88% and 72% in response to 30- and 40-pA stimuli.

These observations illustrate an important general point: an ion channel mutation does not necessarily have the same functional effect on all cells in which it is expressed. On the contrary, a single ion channel mutation can have different, and even opposing, functional effects in different types of neurons in which it is expressed. In the extreme case, as illustrated above, a single sodium channel mutation can produce hyperexcitability in some types of neurons, while producing hypoexcitability in other types of neurons. This principle, derived from observations on an erythromelalgia mutation, may apply to other disorders associated with inherited channelopathies, including other genetically determined pain disorders, inherited forms of epilepsy, and possibly inherited forms of migraine.

$Na_V1.7$ and $Na_V1.8$ Collaborate to Produce Spiking in Nociceptors

Why does the L858H $Na_V1.7$ mutation produce hyperexcitability within nociceptors and hypoexcitability within sympathetic ganglion neurons? $Na_V1.7$ displays slow closed-state inactivation, a property that, along with its voltage dependence, enables $Na_V1.7$ to produce a depolarizing response to small, slow, ramp-like depolarizations close to resting potential [10]. $Na_V1.7$ also, however, recovers slowly from inactivation and, as a result, cannot contribute to the upstroke of closely spaced action potentials during high-frequency firing [10]. Rather, $Na_V1.7$ acts within the subthreshold range (with respect to all-or-none action potential generation), amplifying subthreshold inputs so as to set the gain on nociceptors [43].

Rush et al. [34] showed that the divergent effects of the L858H mutation can be explained on the basis of different electrogenic backgrounds in DRG neurons and sympathetic ganglion neurons. In particular, most nociceptive DRG neurons that express $Na_V1.7$ also express the sensory-neuron-specific $Na_V1.8$ sodium channel, while other types of neurons, including sympathetic ganglion neurons, do not [2,4,36]. The $Na_V1.8$ sodium channel displays a relatively depolarized voltage dependence of inactivation, which is shifted by more than 20 mV compared with other sodium channels [2,4,36]. Thus, $Na_V1.8$ channels remain available for activation even when cells are depolarized to levels that inactivate other sodium channels. The activation threshold of $Na_V1.8$ is also relatively depolarized, i.e., the channel requires a high level of depolarization for activation. In sympathetic ganglion neurons, which do not contain $Na_V1.8$, the depolarization imposed by erythromelalgia mutations such as L858H inactivates the sodium channels that are necessary for action potential electrogenesis. As a result, the $Na_V1.7$ mutation renders the cells hypoexcitable. In contrast, the mutation-induced depolarization does not decrease the availability of the $Na_V1.8$ channels that are present within DRG neurons because their inactivation is relatively insensitive to depolarization. The mutation-induced depolarization in fact brings DRG neurons closer to the threshold for activation of $Na_V1.8$ channels. This property is functionally important because $Na_V1.8$ channels produce about 80% of the current underlying the depolarizing phase of the action potential, and support repetitive firing, in DRG neurons where they are expressed [3,33]. Depolarization thus contributes to a lower threshold (although it is not the only factor leading to hyperexcitability [26]) in DRG neurons expressing erythromelalgia mutations such as L858H.

Coexpression studies have demonstrated definitively that the absence or presence of $Na_V1.8$ acts as a switch, determining the response of the cell to L858H-induced depolarization in sympathetic ganglion neurons that lack $Na_V1.8$ (hypoexcitability) and in DRG neurons that express $Na_V1.8$ (hyperexcitability). In these studies mutant L858H $Na_V1.7$channels were expressed in sympathetic ganglion neurons, thus depolarizing these cells, and the effect of the mutant Na_V channel on excitability was measured in the absence or presence of $Na_V1.8$ channels [34]. When $Na_V1.8$ was coexpressed, together with L858H $Na_V1.7$ mutant channels within sympathetic ganglion neurons, action potential threshold was reduced so that excitability was increased, even though the $Na_V1.7$ mutation produced a depolarizing shift in resting potential. This finding teaches us that the electrogenic milieu in which an ion channel is expressed, i.e., the ensemble of other electrogenic channels and receptors in the cell, can influence the functional effect of the mutant channel.

Nociceptors of a Single Class Are Not All the Same

Sensory abnormalities in the feet, and later in the hands, are a characteristic of many of the distal symmetric polyneuropathies, including those associated with diabetes, alcoholism, and vincristine. In these disorders, the distance from the proximal border of sensory loss to the level of the corresponding DRG within the spinal column is often the same for all four limbs [35]. The remarkable length-dependent pattern of sensory loss in these disorders has been attributed to dying-back axonopathies that affect the longest fibers first, or to randomly scattered injuries to individual Schwann cells, which are more likely to affect longer fibers at early stages of the disease [44]. This schema does not, however, explain why a channelopathy would affect neurons giving rise to the longest fibers first. Thus it is not clear, a priori, why pain is felt in the feet and hands, and not over the trunk, in erythromelalgia. A similar enigma surrounds the topographic pattern of discomfort in paroxysmal extreme pain disorder (PEPD), in which pain is experienced in perirectal, periorbital, and perimandibular regions [19], as a result of mutations that impair inactivation of $Na_V1.7$ [18]. In both erythromelalgia and PEPD, mutations affecting $Na_V1.7$ channels might be predicted to affect all DRG neurons, producing pain over the entire body, but in fact, the pain is highly localized. If DRG neurons at all spinal levels and trigeminal neurons were all the same, in terms of their electrogenic makeup, this highly localized pattern of sensory abnormality would not occur. In what ways, then, might primary sensory neurons innervating different parts of the body differ so as to explain the regional nature of the pain that patients experience in erythromelalgia? While the answer is not known, we can speculate about a number of possibilities.

One possibility is that the density of $Na_V1.7$ channels may be different in primary sensory neurons innervating different parts of the body. There is precedent for this, not only in neurons, but also in other cell types such as astrocytes, which express different densities of sodium channels in different parts of the central nervous system [39]. The different levels of channel expression could be due, for example, to differences in expression of transcription factors, of other regulators of channel gene expression, of neurotrophic molecules that regulate channel expression, or of molecules that traffic the channels to or from the cell membrane or anchor the channels within it. Another possibility is that the electrogenic background, in which $Na_V1.7$ channels are expressed and act, is different in primary sensory neurons innervating different parts of the body. For example, differences in the levels of expression of $Na_V1.8$ could endow DRG and trigeminal neurons innervating different parts of the body with different responses to $Na_V1.7$ mutations.

Alternatively, different levels of expression of potassium channels, transient receptor potential channels, or other channels might endow primary sensory neurons, at different levels within the neuraxis, with different functional responses to the expression of $Na_V1.7$ mutant channels. In addition, it is clear that calmodulin and protein kinases such as protein kinase A (PKA), protein kinase C (PKC), extracellular regulated kinase (ERK), and p38 mitogen-activated protein (MAP) kinase, can modulate $Na_V1.7$ and $Na_V1.8$ [7,27,40,42]. Thus, $Na_V1.7$ channels, or other molecules with which they interact, may be differentially modulated by kinases or other modulators in sensory neurons innervating different parts of the body. It is also possible that there are differences in energetic supply needed for fueling of Na/K ATPase in long, as opposed to short, nociceptor axons, with resultant differences in resting potential, and thus differences in the availability of sodium channels within primary sensory neurons with long, as opposed to short, axons.

Finally, it is possible that there are dynamic interactions between the neurogenic component of inherited erythromelalgia (enhanced action potential activity in nociceptors) and a component of sympathetic dysfunction (with abnormal vasomotor control leading to vascular pooling or microvascular shunting or even increased vascular permeability [29,30]). Or perhaps enhanced firing in nociceptors activates axon reflexes, with a resultant release of vasodilators and/or proinflammatory cytokines within peripheral tissues [15]. Differences in ambient temperature, or in mechanisms of vasomotor control in different parts of the body, might also contribute, at least in part, to the localization of pain and erythema to the distal limbs, and sometimes the nose and ears, in erythromelalgia. In this regard, inherited erythromelalgia may hold some lessons that are applicable to complex regional pain syndrome (reflex sympathetic dystrophy).

Irrespective of the mechanism, the clinical observations in erythromelalgia suggest that there is no "canonical" nociceptor. On the contrary, it appears possible there are molecular differences in the primary sensory neurons innervating different parts of the body, which endow these neurons with functional differences. Whether these differences can be utilized for the design of a new generation of regionally effective pain medications is not yet known.

Channelopathies Can Manifest Themselves in a Time-Dependent Manner

Mutant $Na_V1.7$ channels are present within affected individuals during later stages of embryogenesis, and at birth. Yet the pain of erythromelalgia begins to occur in some families in childhood, and in others in adulthood [6]. We do not yet understand the molecular basis for this time-dependent aspect of erythromelalgia, or for the different time dependence in different families. In this regard, we may speculate about several potential explanations.

Most sodium channels, including $Na_V1.7$, are expressed in various forms, including neonatal and adult splice variants, with the possibility of other splice variants [5]. It is possible that the transition from a pain-free state early in life to a painful condition at later ages may be the result of a change in the level of expression of the various variants of $Na_V1.7$. Similar considerations could apply to $Na_V1.8$.

It is also possible that, with maturation, changes occur in the cellular milieu, within the DRG and sympathetic ganglion neurons, within which mutated $Na_V1.7$ channels are expressed. As noted above, it is clear that $Na_V1.7$ and $Na_V1.8$ can be modulated, although in different ways, by protein kinases such as PKA, PKC, ERK, and p38 MAP kinase [7,27,40,42]. Changing levels within DRG neurons of protein kinases, modulatory factors such as fibroblast growth factor homologous factors (FHF factors), and/or calmodulin, for example, could result in expression, after birth, of symptoms of erythromelalgia.

Finally, it is possible that erythromelalgia mutations enhance excitability of DRG neurons and reduce excitability in sympathetic ganglion neurons throughout life (from the time of birth), so that there is a barrage of activity, beginning very early in life, arising within peripheral nociceptors. These impulses, of course, are relayed via the dorsal horn to higher levels in the neuraxis. It is plausible that a gating mechanism, within the spinal cord or higher in the neuraxis, attenuates the rostral transmission of pain messages originating in hyperexcitable peripheral nociceptors early in life. With increasing age, this mechanism may be overcome (perhaps by secondary changes that increase the excitability of second- or third-order neurons within the pain-signaling chain [22–24]), so that, after a critical age, pain messages reach the brain, where they are consciously appreciated. Although there is, at present, no direct evidence for a central component of the pain that erythromelalgia patients experience, such a mechanism might explain the transient response that some patients exhibit during treatment with sodium channel blockers such as lidocaine, with pain being ameliorated at first, followed by breakthrough pain after a period of weeks or months.

Do Genetics and Environment Converge in Inherited Erythromelalgia?

As noted above, via mechanisms that remain unexplained, symptomatic episodes are precipitated by ingestion of certain foods, alcohol, or caffeine in some patients with erythromelalgia [32]. Stress, also, appears to play a role in some patients. Interestingly, some patients report that symptomatic episodes tend not to be triggered during "quiet periods" but are easier to trigger at other times. One possibility is that this finding reflects differences in ambient vasomotor status at different times [29,30]. It is also possible, however, that environmental factors, via mechanisms that are not understood at this time, trigger changes in expression of critical molecules such as protein kinases and calmodulin within DRG neurons and/or sympathetic ganglion neurons. Irrespective of the precise mechanism, it seems likely that inherited erythromelalgia may teach us lessons about the convergence of genetics and environmental factors in the triggering of pain. Thus, this familial disorder may teach us some lessons about acquired disorders such as acquired inflammatory pain, neuropathic pain, and complex regional pain syndrome.

Acknowledgments

Work in the author's laboratory has been supported in part by grants from the Medical Research Service and the Rehabilitation Research Service, Department of Veterans Affairs, and the Erythromelalgia Association. The Center for Neuroscience and Regeneration Research is a collaboration between the Paralyzed Veterans of America and Yale University.

References

[1]   Ahmad S, Dahllund L, Eriksson AB, Hellgren D, Karlsson U, Lund P-E, Meijer IA, Meury L, Mills T, Moody A, et al. A stop codon mutation in SCN9A causes a lack of pain sensation. Hum Mol Genet 2007;16:2114–21.

[2]   Akopian AN, Sivilotti L, Wood JN. A tetrodotoxin-resistant voltage-gated sodium channel expressed by sensory neurons. Nature 1996;379:257–62.

[3]   Blair NT, Bean BP. Roles of tetrodotoxin (TTX)-sensitive Na$^+$ current, TTX-resistant Na$^+$ current and Ca^{2+} current in the action potentials of nociceptive sensory neurons. J Neurosci 2002;22:10277–90.

[4]   Catterall WA, Goldin AL, Waxman SG. International Union of Pharmacology. XLVII. Nomenclature and structure-function relationships of voltage-gated sodium channels. Pharmacol Rev 2005;57:397–410.

[5] Chatelier A, Dahllund L, Eriksson A, Krupp J, Chahine M. Biophysical properties of human Na$_v$1.7 splice variants and their regulation by protein. J Neurophysiol 2008;99:2241–50.

[6] Cheng X, Dib-Hajj SD, Tyrrell L, Waxman SG. Mutation I136V alters electrophysiological properties of the Na$_v$1.7 channel in a family with onset of erythromelalgia in the second decade. Mol Pain 2008;4:1.

[7] Choi JS, Hudmon A, Waxman SG, Dib-Hajj SD. Calmodulin regulates current density and frequency-dependent inhibition of sodium channel Na$_v$1.8 in DRG neurons. J Neurophysiol 2006;96:97–108.

[8] Choi J, Dib-Hajj SD, Waxman SG. Inherited erythermalgia: limb pain from an S4 charge-neutral Na channelopathy. Neurology 2006;67:1563–8.

[9] Cox JJ, Reimann F, Nicholas AK, Thornton G, Roberts E, Springell K, Karbani G, Jafri H, Mannan J, Raashid Y, et al. An SCN9A channelopathy causes congenital inability to experience pain. Nature 2006;444:894–8.

[10] Cummins TR, Howe JR, Waxman SG. Slow closed-state inactivation: a novel mechanism underlying ramp currents in cells expressing the hNE/PN1 sodium channel. J Neurosci 1998;18:9606–19.

[11] Cummins TR, Dib-Hajj SD, Waxman SG. Electrophysiological properties of mutant Na$_v$1.7 sodium channels in a painful inherited neuropathy. J Neurosci 2004;24:8232–6.

[12] Davis MD, Sandroni P, Rooke TW, Low PA. Erythromelalgia; vasculopathy, neuropathy, or both? A prospective study of vascular and neurophysiologic studies in erythromelalgia. Arch Dermatol 2003;139:1337–43.

[13] Dib-Hajj SD, Cummins TR, Black JA, Waxman SG. From genes to pain: Na$_v$1.7 and human pain disorders. Trends Neurosci 2007;30:555–64.

[14] Dib-Hajj SD, Rush AM, Cummins TR, Hisama FM, Novella S, Tyrrell L, Marshall L, Waxman SG. Gain-of-function mutation in Na$_v$1.7 in familial erythromelalgia induces bursting of sensory neurons. Brain 2005;128:1847–54.

[15] Dib-Hajj SD, Rush AM, Cummins TR, Waxman SG. Mutations of the Na$_v$1.7 sodium channel underlie inherited erythromelalgia. Drug Discov Today Dis Mech 2006;3:343–50.

[16] Drenth JP, Finley WH, Breedveld GJ, Testers L, Michiels JJ, Guillet G, Taieb A, Kirby L, Heutink P. The primary erythermalgia-susceptibility gene is located on chromosome 2q31–32. Am J Hum Genet 2001;68:1277–82.

[17] Drenth J, Waxman SG. Mutations in sodium channel gene SCN9A cause a spectrum of human genetic pain disorders. J Clin Invest 2007;177:3603–9.

[18] Fertleman CR, Baker MD, Parker KA, Moffatt S, Elmslie FV, Abrahamsen B, Ostman J, Klugbauer N, Wood JN, Gardiner RM, Rees M. SCN9A mutations in paroxysmal extreme pain disorder: allelic variants underlie distinct channel defects and phenotypes. Neuron 2006;52:767–74.

[19] Fertleman CR, Ferrie CD, Aicardi NAF, Bednarek O, Eeg-Olofsson FV, Elmslie D, Griesemer A, Goutières M, Kirkpatrick INO, Malmros M, et al. Paroxysmal extreme pain disorder (previously familial rectal pain syndrome). Neurology 2007;69:586–95.

[20] Finley WH, Lindsey JR Jr, Fine JD, Dixon GA, Burbank MK. Autosomal dominant erythromelalgia. Am J Med Genet 1992;42:310–5.

[21] Goldberg YP, MacFarlane J, MacDonald ML, Thompson J, Dube M-P, Mattice M, Fraser R, Young C, Hossain S, Pape T, et al. Loss-of-function mutations in the Na$_v$1.7 gene underlie congenital indifference to pain in multiple human populations. Clin Genet 2007;71:311–9.

[22] Hains BC, Klein JP, Saab CY, Craner MJ, Black JA, Waxman SG. Upregulation of sodium channel Na$_v$1.3 and functional involvement in neuronal hyperexcitability associated with central neuropathic pain after spinal cord injury. J Neurosci 2003;23:8881–92.

[23] Hains BC, Saab CY, Klein JP, Craner MJ, Waxman SG. Altered sodium channel expression in second-order spinal sensory neurons contributes to pain after peripheral nerve injury. J Neurosci 2004;24:4832–40.

[24] Hains BC, Saab CY, Waxman SG. Changes in electrophysiologic properties and sodium channel Na$_v$1.3 expression in thalamic neurons after spinal cord injury. Brain 2005;128:2359–71.

[25] Han C, Rush AM, Dib-Hajj SD, Li S, Xu Z, Wang Y, Tyrrell L,Wang X, Yang Y, Waxman SG. Sporadic onset of erythermalgia: a gain-of-function mutation in Na$_v$1.7. Ann Neurol 2006;59:553–8.

[26] Harty TP, Dib-Hajj SD, Tyrrell L, Blackman R, Hisama FM, Rose JB, Waxman SG. Na$_v$1.7 mutant A863P in erythromelalgia: effects of altered activation and steady-state inactivation on excitability of nociceptive DRG neurons. J Neurosci 2006;26:12566–75.

[27] Hudmon A, Choi JS, Tyrrell L, Black JA, Rush AM, Waxman SG, Dib-Hajj SD. Phosphorylation of Sodium channel Na$_v$1.8 by p38 mitogen-activated protein kinase increases current density in dorsal root ganglion neurons. J Neurosci 2008;28:3190–201.

[28] Lampert A, Dib-Hajj SD, Tyrell L, Waxman SG. Size matters: erythromelalgia mutation S241T in Na$_v$1.7 alters channel gating. J Biol Chem 2006;281:36029–36.

[29] Mork C, Asker A, Salerud EG, Kvernebo K. Microvascular arteriovenous shunting is a probable pathogenic mechanism in erythromelalgia. J Invest Dermatol 2000;114:643–6.

[30] Mork C, Kalgaard OM, Kvernebo K. Impaired neurogenic control of skin perfusion in erythromelalgia. J Invest Dermatol 2002;118:699–703.

[31] Nassar MA, Stirling C, Forlani G, Baker MD, Matthews EA, Dickenson AH, Wood JN. Nociceptor-specific gene deletion reveals a major role for Na$_v$1.7 (PN1) in acute and inflammatory pain. Proc Natl Acad Sci USA 2004;101:12706–11.

[32] Novella SN, Hisama FM, Dib-Hajj SD, Waxman SG. A case of inherited erythromelalgia. Nat Clin Pract Neurol 2007;4:229–35.

[33] Renganathan M, Cummins TR, Waxman SG. Contribution of Na$_v$1.8 sodium channels to action potential electrogenesis in DRG neurons. J Neurophysiol 2001;86:629–40.

[34] Rush AM, Dib-Hajj SD, Liu S, Cummins TR, Black JA, Waxman SG. A single sodium channel mutation produces hyper-or hypoexcitability in different types of neurons. Proc Natl Acad Sci USA 2006;103:8245–50.

[35] Sabin TD, Geschwind N, Waxman SG. Patterns of clinical deficits in peripheral nerve disease. In: Waxman SG, editor. Physiology and pathobiology of axons. New York: Raven Press; 1978. p. 431–9.

[36] Sangameswaran L. Structure and function of a novel voltage-gated, tetrodotoxin-resistant sodium channel specific to sensory neurons. J Biol Chem 1996;271:5953–6.

[37] Sheets PL, Jackson JO, Waxman SG, Dib-Hajj S, Cummins TR. A Na$_v$1.7 channel mutation associated with hereditary erythromelalgia contributes to neuronal hyperexcitability and displays reduced lidocaine sensitivity. J Physiol 2007;581:1019–31.

[38] Toledo-Aral JJ, Moss BL, Zhi-Jun H, Koszowski AG, Whisenand T, Levinson SR, Wolf JJ, Silos-Santiago I, Halegoua S, Mandel G. Identification of PN1, a predominant voltage-dependent sodium channel expressed principally in peripheral neurons. Proc Natl Acad Sci USA 1997;94:1527–32.

[39] Sontheimer H, Waxman SG. Ion channels in spinal cord astrocytes in vitro: II. Biophysical and pharmacological analysis of two Na$^+$ current types. J. Neurophysiol 1992;68:1000–11.

[40] Stamboulian S, Choi J-S, Tyrrell L, Waxman SG, Dib-Hajj SD. The sodium channel Na$_v$1.7 is a substrate and is modulated by the MAP kinase ERK. Soc Neurosci Abstr 2007;466:20/I6.

[41] van Genderen PJ, Michiels JJ, Drenth JP. Hereditary erythermalgia and acquired erythromelalgia. Am J Med Genet 1993;45:530–2.

[42] Vijayaragavan K, Boutjdir M, Chahine M. Modulation of Na$_v$1.7 and Na$_v$1.8 peripheral nerve sodium channels by protein kinase A and protein kinase C. J Neurophysiol 2004;91:1556–69.

[43] Waxman SG. A channel sets the gain on pain. Nature 2006;444:831–2.

[44] Waxman SG, Brill MH, Geschwind N, Sabin TD, Lettvin JY. Probability of conduction deficit as related to fiber length in random-distribution models of peripheral neuropathies. J Neurol Sci 1976;29:39–53.

[45] Yang Y, Wang Y, Li S, Xu Z, Li H, Ma L, Fan J, Bu D, Liu B, Fan Z, et al. Mutations in SCN9A, encoding a sodium channel α subunit, in patients with primary erythermalgia. J Med Genet 2004;41:171–4.

Correspondence to: Stephen G. Waxman, MD, PhD, Department of Neurology, LCI 708, P.O. Box 208018, Yale Medical School, New Haven, CT 06520-8018, USA. Tel: 1-203-785-6351; fax: 1-203-785-2238; email: stephen.waxman@yale.edu.

Neuronal Circuits and Receptors Involved in Spinal Cord Pain Processing

Andrew J. Todd

Spinal Cord Group, Faculty of Biomedical and Life Sciences,
University of Glasgow, Glasgow, United Kingdom

Anatomical Organization of the Dorsal Horn

The dorsal horn receives inputs from primary afferents that are arranged in a modality-specific manner, with nociceptive afferents terminating mainly in the superficial part (laminae I and II). It contains a mixed population of neurons, including projection cells, which transmit information to the brain, and interneurons, which are involved in local circuits.

Rexed [72] divided the dorsal horn of the cat spinal cord into six parallel laminae, based on variations in neuronal size and packing density, and this scheme has since been applied to several other mammalian species. Lamina I (also known as the marginal zone) and lamina II (the substantia gelatinosa) are often referred to as the superficial dorsal horn and have been extensively studied, since they represent the main target for the central projections of nociceptive primary afferents and contain many neurons that respond to noxious stimulation. Although the primary afferent input to the deeper laminae (III–VI) is mainly from low-threshold (tactile, hair, and proprioceptive) afferents, this region is also important in pain mechanisms because it contains many neurons that are activated by noxious stimuli and because these low-threshold inputs may contribute to the tactile allodynia that is a feature of neuropathic pain states.

Apart from the primary afferent input to the dorsal horn, the other neuronal constituents include descending axons, which originate in various parts of the brain and are involved in modulating sensory transmission, and dorsal horn neurons. The latter can be divided into two broad classes based on their axonal projections: (a) neurons with axons that remain within the spinal cord (interneurons) and (b) projection neurons, whose axons travel to the brain and form a major output from the dorsal horn. The interneurons include cells with short axons that are involved only in local circuits, as well as neurons with axons that travel between spinal segments (propriospinal neurons). Interneurons can be either inhibitory (using γ-aminobutyric acid [GABA] and/or glycine as transmitters) or excitatory (glutamatergic) cells, while most projection neurons are thought to be glutamatergic [7,84].

The neuronal circuitry within the dorsal horn is complex and still poorly understood. At least in part, this complexity results from the diversity of dorsal horn neurons, which has made it difficult to identify discrete neuronal populations and examine their functions and synaptic connections. This chapter will describe some of the circuits involving projection neurons in laminae I, III, and IV, with emphasis on substance P and the neurokinin-1 (NK1) receptor and on the anatomical aspects of glutamatergic transmission. This account is based on findings in the rat (unless otherwise stated), because most anatomical data have been obtained in this species.

Anatomy and Neurochemistry of Primary Afferents

All primary afferents use glutamate as their main fast excitatory neurotransmitter. Most of the nociceptive afferents have unmyelinated (C) axons, and these can be divided into two major groups: those that contain neuropeptides (e.g., substance P) and those that do not. These differ in their central projections and in the types of synaptic circuit in which they are involved.

Most fine myelinated (Aδ) and unmyelinated (C) primary afferents terminate in the periphery as free nerve endings and function as nociceptors or thermoreceptors, although some Aδ afferents innervate down hairs (D-hair afferents). In contrast, the majority of large myelinated (Aβ) cutaneous primary afferents are low-threshold mechanoreceptors that are associated with specialized endings in the dermis (tactile or hair-follicle afferents). However, some myelinated nociceptors have conduction velocities in the Aβ range [23,84], and so the traditional distinction between small nociceptive/thermoreceptive and large tactile/hair afferents should be treated with caution.

C fibers can be divided into two major groups that differ in both their neurochemistry and central termination patterns: those that contain neuropeptides—such as calcitonin gene-related peptide (CGRP), substance P, galanin, and somatostatin—and those that do not. The peptidergic C afferents express the high-affinity nerve growth factor receptor TrkA, while most of the nonpeptidergic ones are sensitive to glial-derived neurotrophic factor and bind the lectin IB4 (obtained from *Bandeiraea simplicifolia*). All peptidergic primary afferents in the rat appear to contain CGRP [43], and because this peptide is not present in any other types of axon in the dorsal horn, it provides a marker for these afferents. For example, central terminals of substance P-containing primary afferents can be differentiated from those of substance P-containing spinal neurons by the presence of CGRP [60,86]. It should be noted that a significant proportion of peptidergic afferents have myelinated axons [45], and at present it is not possible to distinguish between these and peptidergic C fibers. Although some peptidergic afferents bind IB4, the nonpeptidergic C fibers can be recognized in anatomical studies by combining IB4 binding with CGRP immunostaining [76].

Although most C fibers will be labeled with anti-CGRP and/or IB4, a population of nonpeptidergic unmyelinated afferents that do not bind IB4 has recently been identified in the mouse. These afferents are sensitive to innocuous cooling, express the cold sensor transient receptor potential melastatin 8 (TRPM8), and have central terminals that are restricted to lamina I [22].

The nonpeptidergic C fibers that bind IB4 terminate in a narrow band that occupies the central part of lamina II, where they form central axons of type I synaptic glomeruli [73,74]. These axons are frequently postsynaptic to GABAergic boutons at axo-axonic synapses, and they are therefore subject to classical presynaptic inhibition [73,82]. The central arborizations of peptidergic primary afferents are concentrated in lamina I and the outer half of lamina II (IIo), although some of these afferents extend ventrally into deeper parts of the dorsal horn. In the rat, these axons generally form simple (nonglomerular) endings, which seldom receive axo-axonic synapses [75].

Central terminals of most myelinated primary afferents can be identified in anatomical studies by their ability to transport cholera toxin B subunit (CTb) that has been injected into a peripheral nerve. This is because the GM1 ganglioside (to which CTb binds) is expressed by most myelinated afferents, but not by intact C fibers. Transganglionic labeling with CTb is seen in lamina I and in a region extending ventrally from the inner part of lamina II (IIi). The labeling in lamina I is presumed to be contained in terminals of Aδ nociceptors, which are known to arborize in this region [46]. We have found that primary afferent terminals in lamina I that are transganglionically labeled with CTb are seldom CGRP- or substance P-immunoreactive (A.J. Todd and R.C. Spike, unpublished observations), and this finding suggests that peptidergic Aδ afferents do not normally express the GM1 ganglioside. The CTb labeling in the deeper region of the dorsal horn includes central terminals of Aδ D-hair afferents (laminae IIi/III) and low-threshold Aβ mechanoreceptors (laminae IIi–V) [9,46].

All primary afferents are thought to use glutamate as their principal transmitter. Until recently it was difficult to identify glutamatergic axons in anatomical studies, and the development of antibodies against the vesicular glutamate transporters was therefore extremely important for our understanding of circuits involving these axons. Both VGLUT1 and VGLUT2 are highly expressed in the dorsal horn, but with differing distributions [91]. VGLUT1 is relatively sparse in laminae I and IIo, but is present in numerous axon terminals elsewhere in the gray matter, whereas VGLUT2 has a more uniform distribution throughout the gray matter. Immunocytochemical and in situ hybridization studies have suggested the following pattern of expression for the vesicular glutamate transporters in the spinal cord [3,63,83]: VGLUT1 is expressed by all of the low-threshold mechanoreceptive (Aβ/Aδ) and proprioceptive myelinated afferents and is present at high levels in their central terminals in the deeper part of the dorsal horn (laminae IIi–VI) and ventral horn. It is also expressed by some descending axons. VGLUT2 is present in the central terminals of most of the (nonpeptidergic) Aδ nociceptors in lamina I that are transganglionically labeled with CTb, and it is also expressed by axons of most glutamatergic spinal neurons. Surprisingly, even though C fibers are known to be glutamatergic [7,19] and have strong VGLUT2 labeling in their cell bodies in the mouse [11], their central terminals show weak or undetectable labeling with VGLUT2 antibodies and do not express VGLUT1. VGLUT3-containing terminals are relatively sparse in the spinal gray matter, and all of these terminals appear to be of supraspinal origin.

Substance P and the NK1 Receptor

All substance P-containing primary afferents are nociceptors, and the main target for the peptide is the NK1 receptor (NK1r), which is expressed by certain neurons throughout the dorsal horn. Although substance P-containing primary afferents and NK1r-expressing dorsal horn neurons play an important role in pain and hyperalgesia, this may involve signaling pathways other than the NK1 receptor itself.

Axons that contain substance P form a dense plexus in the superficial part of the dorsal horn (laminae I and IIo) (Fig. 1c). Much of this plexus consists of primary afferents, although some of it is derived from axons of spinal neurons. Substance P acts principally on the NK1 receptor. This receptor shows a restricted distribution in the dorsal horn: it is present at high density in lamina I, is largely absent from lamina II, and is expressed by some neurons in deeper laminae (III–V) [10,54] (Fig. 1a). We have estimated that ~45% of lamina I neurons express the NK1 receptor [87], and it has been reported that these cells show a bimodal size distribution, with a population of small neurons that are weakly immunostained for the receptor and a group of large cells that generally show strong NK1r immunostaining [17]. Among the NK1r-immunoreactive neurons in laminae III–IV, there is a population of strongly stained neurons with prominent dorsal dendrites that enter the superficial dorsal horn [10,54,55].

Several lines of evidence suggest a significant role for substance P and the NK1 receptor in nociception: (1) All substance P-containing primary afferents in the guinea-pig are nociceptors (although many

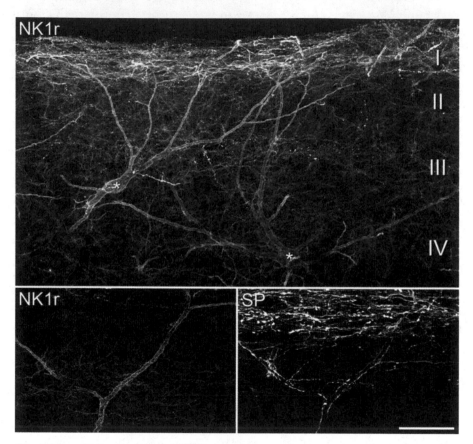

Fig. 1. Neurokinin-1 receptor (NK1r) and substance P immunoreactivity in sagittal sections of the rat spinal dorsal horn. (a) NK1r immunostaining in laminae I–IV. Lamina I contains a dense plexus of immunoreactive dendrites and cell bodies, whereas there are few labeled cells in lamina II. Scattered large neurons with prominent dorsal dendrites are present in deeper laminae (III–IV), and the cell bodies of two of these are marked with asterisks. Parts (b) and (c) show immunostaining for NK1r and substance P (SP) in a single field that includes part of laminae II and III. A NK1r-immunoreactive dorsal dendrite (that belongs to a neuron in lamina III) is associated with substance P-immunoreactive axons. These axons have many boutons that contact the dendrite and are so numerous that they outline it. Note the plexus of substance P-immunoreactive axons in the upper half of the image (which corresponds to the outer part of lamina II). Scale bar for all images = 50 μm. Part (a) is reproduced from Todd and Koerber [84], with the permission of Elsevier. Parts (b) and (c) are adapted and reproduced, with the permission of Blackwell Publishing, from Polgár et al. [68].

nociceptors lack substance P) [45]. (2) In the cat dorsal horn, NK1 receptors are apparently only associated with neurons that respond to noxious stimuli [77]. (3) NK1r antagonists block a slow excitatory postsynaptic potential that is evoked by noxious stimulation in cat dorsal horn neurons [21]. (4) Noxious stimulation causes internalization of NK1 receptors on neurons in the superficial dorsal horn, presumably as a result of substance P released from nociceptive afferents binding to the receptor [55]. (5) Selective ablation of NK1r-expressing neurons in the superficial dorsal horn leads to a dramatic reduction in hyperalgesia in both inflammatory and neuropathic models [56,61]. However, deletion of genes coding for either substance P [15] or the NK1 receptor [20] in mice results in a relatively modest alteration in pain responses, and NK1r antagonists have proved disappointing as analgesics in humans [34]. Taken together, these findings suggest that substance P-containing primary afferents and NK1r-expressing dorsal horn neurons are of considerable importance in pain and hyperalgesia, but that other types of signaling used by these neurons may be more significant than those involving the NK1 receptor itself.

Projection Neurons in Laminae I–IV

Projection neurons are found throughout the gray matter, but they are particularly numerous in lamina I. Their axons travel to several targets in the brainstem and thalamus, and in many cases a single cell sends axon collaterals to more than one of these targets. Most lamina I projection neurons express the NK1 receptor, although there is a population of very large neurons that lack this receptor. There is also a group of very distinctive NK1r-expressing projection neurons in laminae III and IV that have dendrites extending through the superficial dorsal horn.

The laminar locations of the cell bodies of projection neurons can be identified by the retrograde transport of tracer substances from the region where their axons terminate. Studies of this type in which tracers have been injected into all known supraspinal targets have shown that projection neurons in the mid-lumbar spinal cord of the rat are not uniformly distributed throughout the gray matter, but are concentrated in lamina I, largely absent from lamina II, and scattered throughout the remainder of the dorsal horn, ventral horn, and lateral spinal nucleus. An example of retrograde labeling seen after injection of tracer into the caudal part of the ventrolateral medulla (CVLM) is shown in Fig. 2. Projection neurons with cell bodies in lamina I, together with many of those located in deeper laminae, have axons that cross the midline and ascend in the contralateral white matter to arborize in various regions of the brainstem and thalamus

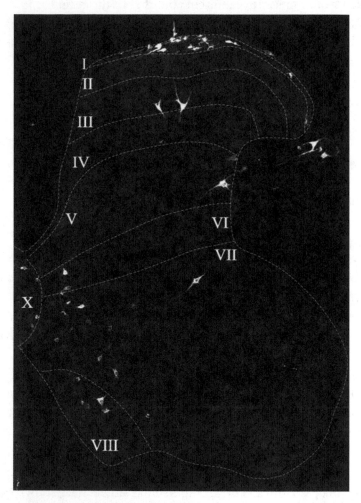

Fig. 2. Projection neurons labeled in a transverse section through the L4 segment of the rat spinal cord. These cells have transported cholera toxin B subunit (CTb) from an injection site in the caudal ventrolateral medulla; they have been stained with antibody against CTb. Many labeled cells are present in lamina I, and scattered cells are seen throughout laminae III–X and in the lateral spinal nucleus. Approximate positions of laminar boundaries are indicated. Reproduced with the permission of Elsevier from Todd [82a].

[18,84,92]. The brainstem targets of lamina I neurons include the CVLM, the dorsal reticular nucleus (DRt), the nucleus tractus solitarius (NTS), the lateral parabrachial area (LPb), and the periaqueductal gray matter (PAG) [16,37,52,53,57,78,85]. Lamina I spinothalamic neurons in the rat are known to project mainly to the lateral parts of the thalamus (ventral posterolateral and posterior nuclei), providing only a modest input to the medial part [29,31,44]. Recent studies have shown that many (if not all) of the lamina I spinothalamic neurons innervate the triangular part of the posterior nuclear group (PoT), which is located at the extreme caudal end of the thalamus [1,29,99].

We have performed quantitative studies of projection neurons in the mid-lumbar spinal cord of the rat by injecting different tracers into various combinations of their supraspinal targets [1,78,8]. Our results suggest that there are approximately 400 lamina I projection neurons on each side in the L4 segment (corresponding to approximately 5–10% of the neuronal population in this lamina). The great majority (85%) of these neurons send their axons to the contralateral LPb, with approximately 30% projecting to the PAG and 20% to the dorsal medulla (DRt and/or NTS), while only about 4% (15 cells) have axons that continue as far as the thalamus [1]. The finding that few lamina I neurons from the lumbar en-largement belong to the spinothalamic tract is consistent with the results of quantitative studies carried out in other laboratories [13,51]. Although spinothalamic lamina I neurons are relatively infrequent in the mid-lum-bar cord, they are much more numerous in the cervical enlargement (~90 per side in C7), with most (or all) of these having axonal arborizations in the PoT nucleus [1,13]. Most lamina I projection neurons can be labeled from the CVLM, but since the injection sites in these experiments are close to the main ascending bundle of axons that pass up from the spinal cord, it is difficult to rule out the possibility that some of the retrograde labeling from the CVLM is through uptake by ascending axons. Given that virtually all of the lamina I cells that project to either the thalamus or PAG can also be retrogradely labeled from the LPb [37,78] (K.M. Al-Khater and A.J. Todd, unpublished observations), it is clear that many projec-tion neurons in this lamina must send axon collaterals to more than one supraspinal target, After tracer injections into the brainstem, most retro-gradely labeled lamina I neurons are on the contralateral side, although a significant number are ipsilateral. We have given symmetrical injections of two different tracers into the LPb or the CVLM of both sides, and found that virtually all cells labeled ipsilateral to an injection site are also labeled from the contralateral side, indicating that they have bilaterally projecting axons; these cells make up around 25% of the lamina I projection neurons in the L4 segment [78].

Lima and Coimbra [50] classified lamina I neurons into fusiform, pyramidal, flattened, and multipolar types, based on their somatodendritic morphology. This scheme has subsequently been modified for lamina I projection neurons to include three types: fusiform, pyramidal, and multipolar [32,78,98]. However, it should be noted that the "multipolar" neurons in this latter scheme correspond to the "flattened" cells of Lima and Coimbra. Although it has been reported that particular morphological types of lamina I neuron project to specific brain regions [51–53], we have found that proportions of lamina I cells belonging to each of these three morphological types did not differ among the neuronal populations that were retrogradely labeled from the PAG, LPb, or CVLM [78]. Our finding suggests that there is no correlation between morphology and projection target, a view that is consistent with other recent reports [2,96].

Given that the NK1 receptor is present on a relatively high proportion of neurons in lamina I [87], we have examined the expression of the receptor on projection cells in this lamina [1,78,85]. We found that the great majority (~80%) of neurons that could be retrogradely labeled from the thalamus, PAG, LPb, DRt/NTS, or CVLM were NK1r immunoreactive. The sizes of cell bodies of these retrogradely labeled NK1r-immunoreactive neurons closely match those of the large NK1r-positive lamina I cells identified by Cheunsuang and Morris [17,66], and it is likely that all of the latter are projection neurons. The small, less intensely stained NK1r-positive cells observed by Cheunsuang and Morris are likely to be interneurons.

Among the lamina I projection neurons that lack the NK1 receptor, we have identified a population of very large cells that are characterized by the high density of inhibitory synapses on their cell bodies and proximal dendrites [71]. These synapses express the glycine-receptor-associated protein gephyrin, and they are so numerous that the cells are coated with gephyrin-immunoreactive puncta, which outline their cell bodies and proximal dendrites. These large, gephyrin-coated lamina I cells have been shown to project (often bilaterally) to the LPb, but little is known about other potential supraspinal targets. Although these cells are readily identified in horizontal sections, there are only approximately 10 of them per side in the L4 segment [63a], and so they constitute around 2–3% of the projection neurons in this lamina.

As described above, immunostaining with NK1r antibodies reveals a population of large neurons with cell bodies in lamina III or IV. These cells have dendrites that can travel for some distance along both dorsoventral and rostrocaudal axes, but invariably extend dorsally into the superficial laminae, where they arborize profusely (Fig. 1a). They are present in all segments [10], but they are not numerous at any level: we have estimated that there are 20–25 of the large NK1r-positive cells on either side in the L4 segment, and slightly fewer (15–20) in C7 [1]. All of them are projection neurons, as they can be labeled from injections of retrograde tracer into the CVLM, while many project to other brainstem targets (LPb and DRt/NTS) [85]. Approximately 20% of those in the lumbar cord and 85% in the cervical enlargement are spinothalamic neurons and project to the PoT nucleus, although apparently not to other thalamic targets [1]. Since there are approximately 20,000 neurons in lamina III on each side in the L4 segment [65], the large NK1r-positive neurons presumably make up approximately 0.1% of the neuronal population in this lamina. Nonetheless, since the vast majority of neurons in this region are interneurons, these cells provide a significant part of its output.

Synaptic Circuits Involving Projection Neurons in Laminae I, III, and IV

Although the synaptic circuits in the dorsal horn are complex and still poorly understood, emerging evidence indicates that they are arranged in an orderly way. Substance P-containing primary afferents densely innervate projection neurons in laminae I, III, and IV that express the NK1 receptor, and these cells appear to receive little direct input from other types of C fiber. There is also some evidence that different types of excitatory and inhibitory interneuron selectively innervate various types of projection neuron.

As stated above, the central terminals of substance P-containing primary afferents can be identified in anatomical studies by immunoreactivity to both substance P and CGRP. We have used this approach to show that these afferents densely innervate NK1r-expressing projection neurons in lamina I, as well as those in laminae III–IV. This input is selective, in that the peptidergic afferents make far more numerous contacts on these neurons than on other types of dorsal horn neuron, including lamina I projection cells that lack the NK1 receptor [60,86]. Although the lamina I neurons lie almost entirely within the plexus of substance P axons that occupies laminae I–IIo, the cell bodies and proximal dendrites of the lamina III/IV NK1r-expressing projection neurons are below this plexus. However, these parts of the lamina III/IV cells are often densely innervated by substance P-containing primary afferents, which appear to run ventrally along their dorsal dendrites [60] (Fig. 1b,c). Given that neuropeptides are thought to act through nonsynaptic "volume" transmission, the proximity of substance P-containing axons to the NK1r-expressing projection cells would presumably be sufficient to allow activation of the receptor following release of substance P from axonal boutons, without the need for synaptic specializations. However, substance P-containing afferents are also glutamatergic [19], and we have found asymmetrical synapses at more than 80% of the contacts between substance P-containing primary afferents and NK1r-expressing projection neurons belonging to these two populations. These synapses presumably underlie monosynaptic glutamatergic transmission between the afferents and the projection neurons.

Unlike the lamina I cells, lamina III/IV NK1r-expressing projection neurons have dendrites that extend through several laminae, and they could potentially receive synapses from various types of primary afferent. We have found that although they do have a moderate synaptic input from presumed low-threshold mechanoreceptive myelinated afferents in laminae IIi–IV [59], they receive very few contacts from either nonpeptidergic C fibers (identified by binding of IB4 and the lack of CGRP immunoreactivity) or from the somatostatin-containing population of peptidergic primary afferents [76]. This finding indicates that the primary afferent input to these neurons is highly selective, and could not be predicted solely from knowing the laminar location of their dendritic trees.

There is evidence for selective innervation of projection neurons by specific populations of dorsal horn interneurons. NK1r-expressing projection neurons in laminae I, III, and IV receive a significant synaptic input from glutamatergic axons that express the α_{2C} adrenoceptor and are thought to originate from local excitatory interneurons [62]. The lamina III/IV NK1r-positive cells are selectively innervated by axons that contain GABA and neuropeptide Y, and these are likely to originate from inhibitory interneurons in laminae I–III [67]. Many of the GABAergic synapses onto the cell bodies and dendrites of the large gephyrin-coated lamina I projection neurons contain neuronal nitric oxide synthase (nNOS), which is expressed by a subset of GABAergic neurons in the dorsal horn [71]. We have recently found that these large cells also receive a very dense synaptic input from boutons with high levels of VGLUT2 that are likely to originate from local excitatory interneurons, with relatively few contacts from peptidergic primary afferents [63a].

Both the lamina I and lamina III/IV NK1r-expressing projection neurons are innervated by serotoninergic axons originating from the raphe nuclei [66,79], and so their activity is likely to be modulated directly by descending monoaminergic input. A diagram summarizing these inputs to projection neurons is shown in Fig. 3.

Functions of Projection Neurons in Laminae I, III, and IV

Functions of projection neurons have been investigated in electrophysiological studies, and also in anatomical studies with activity-dependent markers. Both approaches have shown that most projection neurons in the upper dorsal horn respond to noxious stimuli, with some responding to other modalities. There appears to be a link between neuronal morphology and responses to different types of stimulus, although the details are still controversial. Selective ablation of NK1r-expressing neurons (including projection cells) leads to a reduction in chronic pain (of inflammatory and neuropathic origin).

Electrophysiological recordings have been obtained from lamina I neurons that project to various supraspinal targets in primates, cats, and rats. Recorded neurons have generally had small receptive fields, and the majority responded exclusively to noxious stimuli, with varying numbers being activated by low-threshold mechanical, innocuous thermal, or pruritic stimuli [4,5,26,32,47].

Based on intracellular recordings in the cat, Han et al. [32] proposed that there is a correlation between neuronal morphology and function for lamina I neurons, with multipolar and fusiform cells responding to noxious stimuli, and pyramidal cells responding only to innocuous cooling. Consistent with this finding is the suggestion that projection neurons with pyramidal morphology in both monkeys [97] and rats [2,96] are seldom NK1r-immunoreactive, unlike multipolar and fusiform cells. However, in our studies of the rat spinal cord we have found that the great majority (80%) of pyramidal projection neurons in lamina I (retrogradely labeled from the CVLM, LPb, or PAG) are NK1r-immunoreactive [78,86], and that among the NK1r-immunoreactive projection neurons in this lamina the pyramidal cells had the same intensity of NK1r immunostaining [78] and had the same density of contacts from substance P-containing primary afferents as did multipolar and fusiform cells [86].

An alternative approach to investigating the function of projection neurons involves the use of anatomical markers of activation, such as Fos protein [36] or the phosphorylation of extracellular signal-regulated kinases (ERKs) [41]. This approach has the advantage that large numbers of neurons can be sampled, and it is straightforward to examine the morphology and neurochemistry of Fos or phospho-ERK (pERK)-positive neurons. However, it also has important limitations, including the problem of false-negatives (i.e., not all cells activated by a noxious stimulus are necessarily detected) and the inability to test responses to more than one type of noxious stimulus, or to innocuous stimuli. With this technique we have shown that among the NK1r-positive lamina I projection neurons,

Fig. 3. A diagram summarizing the known inputs to three different types of projection ⟶ neuron. The three types of projection neuron (PN) are those in lamina I and lamina III that express neurokinin-1 (NK1) receptors, and the large lamina I cells that lack the NK1 receptor but have a high density of gephyrin puncta (large non-NK1r PN). Inputs from primary afferents, from various types of interneuron, and from descending axons that contain serotonin (5-HT) are shown. CGRP: calcitonin gene-related peptide, GLU α_{2c} IN: glutamatergic interneurons with axons that express the adrenergic α_{2c} receptor, GABA/ NOS IN: GABAergic interneurons that contain neuronal nitric oxide synthase, GABA/ NPY IN: GABAergic interneurons that contain neuropeptide Y, LTM: low-threshold mechanoreceptive, SP: substance P.

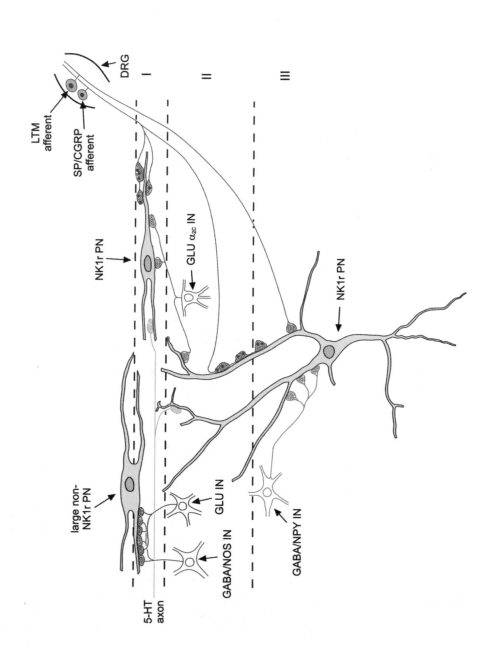

pyramidal cells had the same likelihood of upregulating Fos as did multipolar or fusiform cells after subcutaneous injection of formalin or noxious heating [78,88]. However, after noxious cooling, more multipolar cells
than fusiform or pyramidal cells were Fos-positive.

Little is known about the functions of lamina I projection neurons
that do not express the NK1 receptor. Neurons that respond to innocuous
cooling but not to noxious stimuli have been identified in lamina I in the
rat [48], and if any of these are projection neurons, they would presumably
be included among the cells that are not NK1r-immunoreactive [77]. Approximately 35% of the non-NK1r-immunoreactive projection neurons,
including virtually all of the large gephyrin-coated cells, express Fos after
subcutaneous injection of formalin [71,86]. Thus, at least some of the projection neurons that lack NK1 receptors respond to noxious stimuli. Taken
together, these observations suggest that while there may be a relationship
between somatodendritic morphology and function for lamina I projection neurons, it is likely to be complex. For example, the large gephyrin-
coated neurons that we have identified are nearly all multipolar cells, but
so are many of the NK1r-expressing projection neurons. Although cells
in both of these groups are activated by noxious stimuli [71,86], they differ not only in receptor expression but also in synaptic inputs, with the
NK1r-expressing neurons receiving numerous synapses from substance
P-containing primary afferents, and the gephyrin-coated cells having fewer contacts from peptidergic afferents but a much denser excitatory input
from VGLUT2-immunoreactive axons, which are probably derived from
glutamatergic interneurons. This finding suggests that sensory inputs to
the latter cells are predominantly polysynaptic.

We also know little about the response properties of lamina III/
IV NK1r-expressing projection neurons. All of these cells are densely innervated by substance P-containing (nociceptive) afferents, and they have
a modest input from low-threshold myelinated afferents, and so would be
expected to have wide-dynamic-range receptive fields. Doyle and Hunt
[24] reported that some cells of this type expressed Fos following noxious
stimulation, with subcutaneous injection of formalin being a particularly effective stimulus. We have shown that virtually all of these neurons
phosphorylate ERK (and are therefore presumably activated) after noxious
thermal, mechanical, or chemical stimuli [64]. We have recently identified

another population of neurons with cell bodies in lamina III and dorsally directed dendrites that enter the superficial laminae. These neurons closely resemble the NK1r-expressing cells in terms of dendritic morphology, but they differ in that they lack the NK1 receptor, have few contacts from substance P-containing primary afferents, and are apparently not projection neurons [68]. These findings provide further evidence that morphology alone cannot be used to classify functional types of neuron within the dorsal horn.

The roles of projection neurons in laminae I–IV will also be determined by their projection targets. However, interpretation is difficult for two reasons: first, because many of these neurons project to more than one supraspinal target, and second, because many neurons in deeper laminae have similar supraspinal projections. The targets of projection neurons in laminae I, III, and IV include structures that are involved in sensory-discriminative aspects of pain, such as the lateral thalamus, which is reciprocally connected to the somatosensory cortex. The PoT nucleus has recently been identified as a major thalamic target for superficial dorsal horn neurons [1,29], and cells in this nucleus project to secondary somatosensory and insular cortices [30] (equivalent to areas that are activated in human pain imaging studies [14]). Lamina I, III, and IV neurons also send their axons to structures that play a role in affective/motivational/autonomic responses, such as the NTS and the lateral parabrachial area (which projects to the hypothalamus and amygdala). In addition, there are projections to brainstem regions that send axons back to the dorsal horn (CVLM, DRt, and PAG), forming supraspinal loops that may have pro- or antinociceptive effects [35,49,81].

The functions of NK1r-expressing neurons in the superficial laminae have been investigated after intrathecal administration of the ribosome-inactivating protein saporin, conjugated to substance P (SP-SAP), which results in a selective loss of NK1r-immunoreactive neurons from laminae I and III [56,61]. Rats that have received SP-SAP show normal withdrawal thresholds to noxious thermal stimuli, but significant reductions in (1) capsaicin-induced pain behavior, (2) the second phase in the formalin test, and (3) thermal and mechanical hyperalgesia, in both inflammatory and nerve-injury models. These results indicate that the cells that have been destroyed with this technique are involved in the development of hyperalgesia, but they are apparently not required for detection of acute noxious stimuli. Many of the lamina I and III neurons that strongly express NK1 receptor are projection neurons, and researchers have assumed that the changes seen after application of SP-SAP reflect the functions of these pathways. However, it must be remembered that not all of the projection neurons in lamina I possess NK1 receptors, and the NK1r-lacking cells (some of which respond to noxious stimuli) will presumably remain intact following SP-SAP treatment. In addition, it is likely that a significant number of NK1r-expressing neurons survive the treatment, particularly those cells with a low level of receptor expression. We have reported that the strength of NK1r immunoreactivity varies considerably among lamina I projection neurons and that this variability is related to projection target, because cells retrogradely labeled from the PAG generally had low or medium levels of immunoreactivity, whereas cells that were strongly NK1r-immunoreactive were more likely to be labeled from the LPb or CVLM [78]. SP-SAP may therefore cause relatively less destruction of spino-PAG neurons than of other populations. For these reasons, it is difficult to interpret the function of projection neurons in laminae I, III, and IV simply on the basis of results obtained with SP-SAP.

Glutamatergic Synapses and AMPA Receptors

Glutamate released by primary afferents, local interneurons and descending axons acts on various receptors, with AMPA (α-amino-3-hydroxy-5-methyl-4-isoxazole propionate) receptors being particularly important for perception of both acute and chronic pain. AMPA receptors are made from four subunits (GluR1–4), and subunit composition influences receptor function. It appears that different types of projection neuron and interneuron each have characteristic receptor composition.

Sources of glutamatergic boutons in the dorsal horn include all classes of primary afferent [7], axons of excitatory interneurons [83], collateral axons of glutamatergic spinal projection neurons [47], and certain descending axons that originate in the brain. Glutamate released from axon terminals acts on both ionotropic and metabotropic receptors, and these receptors are widely expressed throughout the spinal gray matter. Ionotropic receptors of the AMPA type are located at the postsynaptic aspect of glutamatergic synapses, and they underlie fast excitatory synaptic transmission [94,95]. These receptors are thought to be responsible for the perception of both acute and chronic pain [28]. AMPA receptors (AMPArs) are tetrameric structures that are made up of four different subunits (GluR1–4, also known as GluRA–D). Each subunit is a membrane-spanning structure, with an extracellular N-terminus and an intracellular C-terminus. It is thought that both homomeric and heteromeric arrangements of these subunits can form functional receptors, and subunit composition is important in determining properties of the receptor. For example, receptors that lack the GluR2 subunit are permeable to Ca^{2+}, while those that contain this subunit are not [12]. Ca^{2+}-permeable AMPArs are present in the dorsal horn [25,33] and appear to be responsible for the development of certain forms of inflammatory pain [33,42].

Messenger RNAs for all four AMPAr subunits have been identified in the dorsal horn [27,40,89], and antibodies have been used to reveal the presence of different subunits in spinal cord neurons with immunocytochemistry [39,70,80]. However, immunocytochemical detection of synaptic AMPAr subunits in fixed tissue is normally impossible, because the fixation-induced cross-linking of proteins in the synaptic cleft and the postsynaptic density prevents access of antibodies to either C- or N-terminal regions of the receptor subunits [93]. An antigen-retrieval method, in which sections are treated briefly with pepsin, will allow immunocytochemical detection of AMPAr subunits at synapses [93], and we have used this approach to investigate the distribution of synaptic AMPAr subunits in the dorsal horn [58,69]. We have confirmed the validity of the method by showing that there is no staining with antibodies against the GluR1, GluR2, or GluR3 subunits in spinal cord tissue from mice in which these subunits have been knocked out [69]. In addition, we have demonstrated with electron microscopy that following pepsin treatment, immunostaining with antibodies directed against the C-terminal of either GluR1 or GluR2 is associated with the postsynaptic aspect of synaptic active zones [58].

By comparing the distribution of staining with antibodies against each of the four subunits to that obtained with an antibody that recognizes all four subunits (pan-AMPAr antibody), we have recently mapped the expression of each AMPAr subunit at synapses in laminae I–III of the rat dorsal horn [69] (Fig. 4). We found that virtually all pan-AMPAr-positive puncta (99%) were immunostained with GluR2 antibody. This finding is consistent with our previous discovery that about 96% of glutamatergic boutons in the spinal cord (identified either with antibodies against VGLUT1, VGLUT2, or CGRP, or by the binding of IB4) were associated with GluR2-immunoreactive puncta [58]. Our results suggest that nearly all glutamatergic synapses in laminae I–III contain GluR2. Ca^{2+}-permeable (GluR2-lacking) AMPArs at these synapses must therefore be intermingled with GluR2-containing (Ca^{2+}-impermeable) receptors, which is consistent with electrophysiological data indicating that glutamatergic synapses in this region contain a mixture of Ca^{2+}-permeable and Ca^{2+}-impermeable receptors [90] (T. Yasaka., A.J. Todd, and J.S. Riddell, unpublished observations).

We found that 60–65% of AMPAr-puncta in lamina I–II were immunoreactive with GluR1 or GluR3 antibodies, and only about 10%

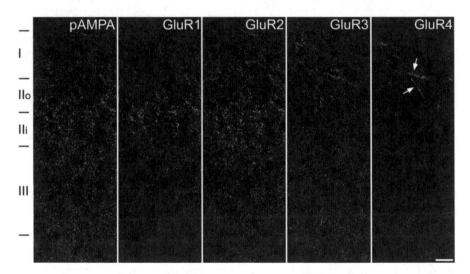

Fig 4. Immunostaining for AMPA-receptor (AMPAr) subunits in laminae I–III of the rat dorsal horn following antigen retrieval with pepsin. Each image shows staining obtained with a pan-AMPAr (pAMPA) or subunit-specific antibody, and the puncta represent receptors at glutamatergic synapses. The images are obtained from the central part of the dorsal horn, where lamina I is relatively thick. GluR1 puncta are most numerous in laminae I–II, while GluR2 and GluR3 puncta are present throughout the dorsal horn. GluR4 puncta are sparse in laminae I–III, and those that are present are arranged in clusters that appear to outline dendrites of individual neurons (arrows). Scale bar = 20 μm. Reproduced from Polgár et al. [69] with permission from BioMed Central.

lacked either of these subunits [69]. In contrast, GluR4-immunoreactivity was only found at 23% of AMPAr puncta in lamina I, and at less than 10% of those in lamina II. Although GluR1 and GluR3 were often colocalized in this region, puncta with strong GluR1-immunostaining were usually weakly positive for GluR3 and vice versa. GluR4 showed little colocalization with GluR1, but it was sometimes colocalized with GluR3. These results suggest wide variation in the subunit composition of individual AMPArs at synapses in the superficial dorsal horn, but they indicate that the predominant arrangement consists of GluR2 together with GluR1 and/or GluR3, but not GluR4. Since interneurons make up the great majority of the neuronal population in the superficial dorsal horn, this combination of subunits is likely to be expressed by most of these cells.

A relatively small number of synapses in the superficial dorsal horn (less than 25% of those in lamina I and less than 10% of those in lamina II) contain GluR2 and GluR4, with some also containing GluR3. In deeper parts of the spinal gray matter, the percentage of pan-AMPAr puncta that contain GluR1 decreases, while the percentage with GluR4 increases [69], and the majority of synapses below lamina III have the combination GluR2/GluR3/GluR4 [58]. The GluR4-immunoreactive puncta that were seen in the superficial dorsal horn were often in the form of clusters that appeared to outline dendrites of individual neurons [69]. The clusters in lamina I were generally arranged in the horizontal plane, while those in lamina II were often orientated along the dorsoventral axis [69]. We have recently found that numerous GluR4 puncta are present on the dendrites of the large gephyrin-coated lamina I neurons, as well as on certain lamina I NK1r-immunoreactive cells and on all of the lamina III/IV NK1r-expressing projection neurons (A.J. Todd and E. Polgár, unpublished observations). This finding indicates that some, if not all, of the GluR4 subunits seen in the superficial dorsal horn are located at synapses on projection neurons. Ikeda et al. [38] have demonstrated that NK1r-expressing spinoparabrachial neurons in lamina I show long-term potentiation (LTP) in response to high-frequency stimulation of C fibers. Both GluR1- and GluR4-containing AMPArs can undergo activity-dependent insertion, leading to LTP in the hippocampus [6], so it will be of interest to determine whether either of these types of AMPAr is involved in LTP in spinal projection neurons.

The GluR1 subunit is thought to play a particularly important role in the receptor trafficking that underlies LTP in the hippocampus [6]. GluR1 has phosphorylation sites near its C-terminal end, including a serine residue at position 845 (S845). Phosphorylation of GluR1 S845 in synaptic receptors leads to greater current flow by increasing peak open probability of the channel. Phosphorylation at this site is also thought to be necessary for the insertion of new AMPArs into glutamatergic synapses during LTP [6]. We have found that the basal level of phosphorylation of GluR1 at S845 is very low at synapses in the superficial dorsal horn, but that 10 minutes after noxious stimulation with subcutaneous capsaicin, there is a significant increase in the level of GluR1 phosphorylated at S845 in lamina I and II in a somatotopically appropriate part of the ipsilateral dorsal horn [58] (Fig. 5). More recently, we have found that this phosphorylation can also be induced by application of a noxious heat stimulus, and that the phosphorylation starts within 5 minutes and lasts for at least 2 hours (E. Polgár and A.J. Todd, unpublished observations). Although we do not yet know whether this finding represents newly inserted receptors that have remained phosphorylated, or results from the phosphorylation of GluR1-containing receptors that were already in the synapse, our study provides direct anatomical evidence for a form of synaptic plasticity that presumably contributes to central sensitization of dorsal horn neurons.

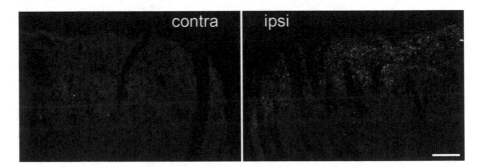

Fig. 5. Immunostaining for phosphorylated GluR1 subunits in the rat dorsal horn following noxious stimulation. These images show parts of the contralateral (contra) and ipsilateral (ipsi) dorsal horn from a rat that had received a subcutaneous injection of capsaicin under terminal anesthesia 10 minutes before perfusion fixation. The sections were processed for antigen retrieval and immunostained with an antibody that recognizes GluR1 subunits that are phosphorylated at the serine 845 residue. There is little labeling in the contralateral dorsal horn, but a prominent band of labeling in laminae I and II can be seen on the ipsilateral side. Scale bar = 50 μm.

Acknowledgments

This work was supported by grants from the Wellcome Trust and the BBSRC. I am grateful to David Maxwell, John Riddell, Erika Polgár, David Hughes, Toshi Yasaka, Gergely Nagy, and Khulood Al-Khater for helpful discussion and advice, and to Robert Kerr and Christine Watt for expert technical assistance.

References

[1]   Al-Khater KM, Kerr R, Todd AJ. A quantitative study of spinothalamic neurons in laminae I, III and IV in lumbar and cervical segments of the rat spinal cord. J Comp Neurol 2008;511:1–18.

[2]   Almarestani L, Waters SM, Krause JE, Bennett GJ, Ribeiro-da-Silva A. Morphological characterization of spinal cord dorsal horn lamina I neurons projecting to the parabrachial nucleus in the rat. J Comp Neurol 2007;504:287–97.

[3]   Alvarez FJ, Villalba RM, Zerda R, Schneider SP. Vesicular glutamate transporters in the spinal cord, with special reference to sensory primary afferent synapses. J Comp Neurol 2004;472:257–80.

[4]   Andrew D, Craig AD. Spinothalamic lamina I neurons selectively sensitive to histamine: a central neural pathway for itch. Nat Neurosci 2001;4:72–7.

[5]   Bester H, Chapman V, Besson JM, Bernard JF. Physiological properties of the lamina I spinoparabrachial neurons in the rat. J Neurophysiol 2000;83:2239–59.

[6]   Bredt DS, Nicoll RA. AMPA receptor trafficking at excitatory synapses. Neuron 2003;40:361–79.

[7]   Broman J, Anderson S, Ottersen OP. Enrichment of glutamate-like immunoreactivity in primary afferent terminals throughout the spinal cord dorsal horn. Eur J Neurosci 1993;5:1050–61.

[8]   Broman J. Neurotransmitters in subcortical somatosensory pathways. Anat Embryol (Berl) 1994;189:181–214.

[9]   Brown AG. Organization in the spinal cord: the anatomy and physiology of identified neurones. Berlin: Springer; 1981.

[10] Brown JL, Liu H, Maggio JE, Vigna SR, Mantyh PW, Basbaum AI. Morphological characterization of substance P receptor-immunoreactive neurons in the rat spinal cord and trigeminal nucleus caudalis. J Comp Neurol 1995;356:327–44.

[11] Brumovsky P, Watanabe M, Hokfelt T. Expression of the vesicular glutamate transporters-1 and -2 in adult mouse dorsal root ganglia and spinal cord and their regulation by nerve injury. Neuroscience 2007;147:469–90.

[12] Burnashev N, Monyer H, Seeburg PH, Sakmann B. Divalent ion permeability of AMPA receptor channels is dominated by the edited form of a single subunit. Neuron 1992;8:189–98.

[13] Burstein R, Dado RJ, Giesler GJ Jr. The cells of origin of the spinothalamic tract of the rat: a quantitative reexamination. Brain Res 1990;511:329–37.

[14] Bushnell MC, Apkarian AV. Representation of pain in the brain. In: McMahon S, Koltzenburg M, editors. Melzack and Wall's textbook of pain. Edinburgh: Churchill Livingstone; 2006. p. 107–24.

[15] Cao YQ, Mantyh PW, Carlson EJ, Gillespie AM, Epstein CJ, Basbaum AI. Primary afferent tachykinins are required to experience moderate to intense pain. Nature 1998;392:390–4.

[16] Cechetto DF, Standaert DG, Saper CB. Spinal and trigeminal dorsal horn projections to the parabrachial nucleus in the rat. J Comp Neurol 1985;240:153–60.

[17] Cheunsuang O, Morris R. Spinal lamina I neurons that express neurokinin 1 receptors: morphological analysis. Neuroscience 2000;97:335–45.

[18] Craig AD. Distribution of brainstem projections from spinal lamina I neurons in the cat and the monkey. J Comp Neurol 1995;361:225–48.

[19] De Biasi S, Rustioni A. Glutamate and substance P coexist in primary afferent terminals in the superficial laminae of spinal cord. Proc Natl Acad Sci USA 1988;85:7820–4.

[20] De Felipe C, Herrero JF, O'Brien JA, Palmer JA, Doyle CA, Smith AJ, Laird JM, Belmonte C, Cervero F, Hunt SP. Altered nociception, analgesia and aggression in mice lacking the receptor for substance P. Nature 1998;392:394–7.

[21] De Koninck Y, Henry JL. Substance P-mediated slow excitatory postsynaptic potential elicited in dorsal horn neurons in vivo by noxious stimulation. Proc Natl Acad Sci USA 1991;88:11344–8.

[22] Dhaka A, Earley TJ, Watson J, Patapoutian A. Visualizing cold spots: TRPM8-expressing sensory neurons and their projections. J Neurosci 2008;28:566–75.

[23] Djouhri L, Lawson SN. Abeta-fiber nociceptive primary afferent neurons: a review of incidence and properties in relation to other afferent A-fiber neurons in mammals. Brain Res Brain Res Rev 2004;46:131–45.

[24] Doyle CA, Hunt SP. Substance P receptor (neurokinin-1)-expressing neurons in lamina I of the spinal cord encode for the intensity of noxious stimulation: a c-Fos study in rat. Neuroscience 1999;89:17–28.

[25] Engelman HS, Allen TB, MacDermott AB. The distribution of neurons expressing calcium-permeable AMPA receptors in the superficial laminae of the spinal cord dorsal horn. J Neurosci 1999;19:2081–9.

[26] Ferrington DG, Sorkin LS, Willis WD, Jr. Responses of spinothalamic tract cells in the superficial dorsal horn of the primate lumbar spinal cord. J Physiol 1987;388:681–703.

[27] Furuyama T, Kiyama H, Sato K, Park HT, Maeno H, Takagi H, Tohyama M. Region-specific expression of subunits of ionotropic glutamate receptors (AMPA-type, KA-type and NMDA receptors) in the rat spinal cord with special reference to nociception. Brain Res Mol Brain Res 1993;18:141–51.

[28] Garry EM, Fleetwood-Walker SM. A new view on how AMPA receptors and their interacting proteins mediate neuropathic pain. Pain 2004;109:210–3.

[29] Gauriau C, Bernard JF. A comparative reappraisal of projections from the superficial laminae of the dorsal horn in the rat: the forebrain. J Comp Neurol 2004;468:24–56.

[30] Gauriau C, Bernard JF. Posterior triangular thalamic neurons convey nociceptive messages to the secondary somatosensory and insular cortices in the rat. J Neurosci 2004;24:752–61.

[31] Giesler GJ, Jr., Menetrey D, Basbaum AI. Differential origins of spinothalamic tract projections to medial and lateral thalamus in the rat. J Comp Neurol 1979;184:107–26.

[32] Han ZS, Zhang ET, Craig AD. Nociceptive and thermoreceptive lamina I neurons are anatomically distinct. Nat Neurosci 1998;1:218–25.

[33] Hartmann B, Ahmadi S, Heppenstall PA, Lewin GR, Schott C, Borchardt T, Seeburg PH, Zeilhofer HU, Sprengel R, Kuner R. The AMPA receptor subunits GluR-A and GluR-B reciprocally modulate spinal synaptic plasticity and inflammatory pain. Neuron 2004;44:637–50.

[34] Hill R. NK1 (substance P) receptor antagonists: why are they not analgesic in humans? Trends Pharmacol Sci 2000;21:244–6.

[35] Hunt SP, Bester H. The ascending pain pathways. In: Hunt SP, Koltzenburg M, editors. The neurobiology of pain. Oxford: Oxford University Press; 2005. p. 165–84.

[36] Hunt SP, Pini A, Evan G. Induction of c-fos-like protein in spinal cord neurons following sensory stimulation. Nature 1987;328:632–4.

[37] Hylden JL, Anton F, Nahin RL. Spinal lamina I projection neurons in the rat: collateral innervation of parabrachial area and thalamus. Neuroscience 1989;28:27–37.

[38] Ikeda H, Heinke B, Ruscheweyh R, Sandkuhler J. Synaptic plasticity in spinal lamina I projection neurons that mediate hyperalgesia. Science 2003;299:1237–40.

[39] Jakowec MW, Fox AJ, Martin LJ, Kalb RG. Quantitative and qualitative changes in AMPA receptor expression during spinal cord development. Neuroscience 1995;67:893–907.

[40] Jakowec MW, Yen L, Kalb RG. In situ hybridization analysis of AMPA receptor subunit gene expression in the developing rat spinal cord. Neuroscience 1995;67:909–20.

[41] Ji RR, Baba H, Brenner GJ, Woolf CJ. Nociceptive-specific activation of ERK in spinal neurons contributes to pain hypersensitivity. Nat Neurosci 1999;2:1114–9.

[42] Jones TL, Sorkin LS. Calcium-permeable alpha-amino-3-hydroxy-5-methyl-4-isoxazolepropionic acid/kainate receptors mediate development, but not maintenance, of secondary allodynia evoked by first-degree burn in the rat. J Pharmacol Exp Ther 2004;310:223–9.

[43] Ju G, Hokfelt T, Brodin E, Fahrenkrug J, Fischer JA, Frey P, Elde RP, Brown JC. Primary sensory neurons of the rat showing calcitonin gene-related peptide immunoreactivity and their relation to substance P-, somatostatin-, galanin-, vasoactive intestinal polypeptide- and cholecystokinin-immunoreactive ganglion cells. Cell Tissue Res 1987;247:417–31.

[44] Kobayashi Y. Distribution and morphology of spinothalamic tract neurons in the rat. Anat Embryol (Berl) 1998;197:51–67.

[45] Lawson SN, Crepps BA, Perl ER. Relationship of substance P to afferent characteristics of dorsal root ganglion neurones in guinea-pig. J Physiol 1997;505(Pt 1):177–91.

[46] Light AR, Perl ER. Spinal termination of functionally identified primary afferent neurons with slowly conducting myelinated fibers. J Comp Neurol 1979;186:133–50.

[47] Light AR, Sedivec MJ, Casale EJ, Jones SL. Physiological and morphological characteristics of spinal neurons projecting to the parabrachial region of the cat. Somatosens Mot Res 1993;10:309–25.

[48] Light AR, Willcockson HH. Spinal laminae I–II neurons in rat recorded in vivo in whole cell, tight seal configuration: properties and opioid responses. J Neurophysiol 1999;82:3316–26.

[49] Lima D, Almeida A. The medullary dorsal reticular nucleus as a pronociceptive centre of the pain control system. Prog Neurobiol 2002;66:81–108.

[50] Lima D, Coimbra A. A Golgi study of the neuronal population of the marginal zone (lamina I) of the rat spinal cord. J Comp Neurol 1986;244:53–71.

[51] Lima D, Coimbra A. The spinothalamic system of the rat: structural types of retrogradely labelled neurons in the marginal zone (lamina I). Neuroscience 1988;27:215–30.

[52] Lima D, Coimbra A. Morphological types of spinomesencephalic neurons in the marginal zone (lamina I) of the rat spinal cord, as shown after retrograde labelling with cholera toxin subunit B. J Comp Neurol 1989;279:327–39.

[53] Lima D, Mendes-Ribeiro JA, Coimbra A. The spino-latero-reticular system of the rat: projections from the superficial dorsal horn and structural characterization of marginal neurons involved. Neuroscience 1991;45:137–52.

[54] Littlewood NK, Todd AJ, Spike RC, Watt C, Shehab SA. The types of neuron in spinal dorsal horn which possess neurokinin-1 receptors. Neuroscience 1995;66:597–608.

[55] Mantyh PW, DeMaster E, Malhotra A, Ghilardi JR, Rogers SD, Mantyh CR, Liu H, Basbaum AI, Vigna SR, Maggio JE. Receptor endocytosis and dendrite reshaping in spinal neurons after somatosensory stimulation. Science 1995;268:1629–32.

[56] Mantyh PW, Rogers SD, Honore P, Allen BJ, Ghilardi JR, Li J, Daughters RS, Lappi DA, Wiley RG, Simone DA. Inhibition of hyperalgesia by ablation of lamina I spinal neurons expressing the substance P receptor. Science 1997;278:275–9.

[57] Menetrey D, Chaouch A, Binder D, Besson JM. The origin of the spinomesencephalic tract in the rat: an anatomical study using the retrograde transport of horseradish peroxidase. J Comp Neurol 1982;206:193–207.

[58] Nagy GG, Al Ayyan M, Andrew D, Fukaya M, Watanabe M, Todd AJ. Widespread expression of the AMPA receptor GluR2 subunit at glutamatergic synapses in the rat spinal cord and phosphorylation of GluR1 in response to noxious stimulation revealed with an antigen-unmasking method. J Neurosci 2004;24:5766–77.

[59] Naim MM, Shehab SA, Todd AJ. Cells in laminae III and IV of the rat spinal cord which possess the neurokinin-1 receptor receive monosynaptic input from myelinated primary afferents. Eur J Neurosci 1998;10:3012–9.

[60] Naim M, Spike RC, Watt C, Shehab SA, Todd AJ. Cells in laminae III and IV of the rat spinal cord that possess the neurokinin-1 receptor and have dorsally directed dendrites receive a major synaptic input from tachykinin-containing primary afferents. J Neurosci 1997;17:5536–48.

[61] Nichols ML, Allen BJ, Rogers SD, Ghilardi JR, Honore P, Luger NM, Finke MP, Li J, Lappi DA, Simone DA, Mantyh PW. Transmission of chronic nociception by spinal neurons expressing the substance P receptor. Science 1999;286:1558–61.

[62] Olave MJ, Maxwell DJ. Neurokinin-1 projection cells in the rat dorsal horn receive synaptic contacts from axons that possess alpha2C-adrenergic receptors. J Neurosci 2003;23:6837–46.

[63] Oliveira AL, Hydling F, Olsson E, Shi T, Edwards RH, Fujiyama F, Kaneko T, Hokfelt T, Cullheim S, Meister B. Cellular localization of three vesicular glutamate transporter mRNAs and proteins in rat spinal cord and dorsal root ganglia. Synapse 2003;50:117–29.

[63a] Polgár E, Al-Khater KM, Shehab S, Watanabe M, Todd AJ. Large projection neurons in lamina I of the rat spinal cord that lack the neurokinin 1 receptor are densely innervated by VGLUT2-containing axons and possess GluR4-containing AMPA receptors. J Neurosci 2008;28:13150–60.

[64] Polgár E, Campbell AD, MacIntyre LM, Watanabe M, Todd AJ. Phosphorylation of ERK in neurokinin 1 receptor-expressing neurons in laminae III and IV of the rat spinal dorsal horn following noxious stimulation. Mol Pain 2007;3:4.

[65] Polgár E, Gray S, Riddell JS, Todd AJ. Lack of evidence for significant neuronal loss in laminae I–III of the spinal dorsal horn of the rat in the chronic constriction injury model. Pain 2004;111:144–50.

[66] Polgár E, Puskar Z, Watt C, Matesz C, Todd AJ. Selective innervation of lamina I projection neurones that possess the neurokinin 1 receptor by serotonin-containing axons in the rat spinal cord. Neuroscience 2002;109:799–809.

[67] Polgár E, Shehab SA, Watt C, Todd AJ. GABAergic neurons that contain neuropeptide Y selectively target cells with the neurokinin 1 receptor in laminae III and IV of the rat spinal cord. J Neurosci 1999;19:2637–46.

[68] Polgár E, Thomson S, Maxwell DJ, Al Khater K, Todd AJ. A population of large neurons in laminae III and IV of the rat spinal cord that have long dorsal dendrites and lack the neurokinin 1 receptor. Eur J Neurosci 2007;26:1587–98.

[69] Polgár E, Watanabe M, Hartmann B, Grant SG, Todd AJ. Expression of AMPA receptor subunits at synapses in laminae I–III of the rodent spinal dorsal horn. Mol Pain 2008;4:5.

[70] Popratiloff A, Weinberg RJ, Rustioni A. AMPA receptor subunits underlying terminals of fine-caliber primary afferent fibers. J Neurosci 1996;16:3363–72.

[71] Puskar Z, Polgar E, Todd AJ. A population of large lamina I projection neurons with selective inhibitory input in rat spinal cord. Neuroscience 2001;102:167–76.

[72] Rexed B. A cytoarchitectonic atlas of the spinal cord in the cat. J Comp Neurol 1954;100:297–379.

[73] Ribeiro-da-Silva A, Coimbra A. Two types of synaptic glomeruli and their distribution in laminae I–III of the rat spinal cord. J Comp Neurol 1982;209:176–86.

[74] Ribeiro-da-Silva A, de Koninck Y. Morphological and neurochemical organization of the spinal dorsal horn. In: Bushnell MC, Basbaum AI, editors. Pain. San Diego: Academic Press; 2008. p. 279–310.

[75] Ribeiro-da-Silva A, Tagari P, Cuello AC. Morphological characterization of substance P-like immunoreactive glomeruli in the superficial dorsal horn of the rat spinal cord and trigeminal subnucleus caudalis: a quantitative study. J Comp Neurol 1989;281:497–15.

[76] Sakamoto H, Spike RC, Todd AJ. Neurons in laminae III and IV of the rat spinal cord with the neurokinin-1 receptor receive few contacts from unmyelinated primary afferents which do not contain substance P. Neuroscience 1999;94:903–8.

[77] Salter MW, Henry JL. Responses of functionally identified neurones in the dorsal horn of the cat spinal cord to substance P, neurokinin A and physalaemin. Neuroscience 1991;43:601–10.

[78] Spike RC, Puskar Z, Andrew D, Todd AJ. A quantitative and morphological study of projection neurons in lamina I of the rat lumbar spinal cord. Eur J Neurosci 2003;18:2433–48.

[79] Stewart W, Maxwell DJ. Morphological evidence for selective modulation by serotonin of a subpopulation of dorsal horn cells which possess the neurokinin-1 receptor. Eur J Neurosci 2000;12:4583–8.

[80] Tachibana M, Wenthold RJ, Morioka H, Petralia RS. Light and electron microscopic immunocytochemical localization of AMPA-selective glutamate receptors in the rat spinal cord. J Comp Neurol 1994;344:431–54.

[81] Tavares I, Lima D. The caudal ventrolateral medulla as an important inhibitory modulator of pain transmission in the spinal cord. J Pain 2002;3:337–46.

[82] Todd AJ. GABA and glycine in synaptic glomeruli of the rat spinal dorsal horn. Eur J Neurosci 1996;8:2492–8.

[82a] Todd AJ. Anatomy and neurochemistry of the dorsal horn. In: Cervero F, Jensen TS. Handbook of clinical neurology, vol. 81. Amsterdam: Elsevier; 2006. p. 61–76.

[83] Todd AJ, Hughes DI, Polgar E, Nagy GG, Mackie M, Ottersen OP, Maxwell DJ. The expression of vesicular glutamate transporters VGLUT1 and VGLUT2 in neurochemically defined axonal populations in the rat spinal cord with emphasis on the dorsal horn. Eur J Neurosci 2003;17:13–27.

[84] Todd AJ, Koerber R. Neuroanatomical substrates of spinal nociception. In: McMahon S, Koltzenburg M, editors. Melzack and Wall's textbook of pain. Edinburgh: Churchill Livingstone; 2006. p. 73–90.

[85] Todd AJ, McGill MM, Shehab SA. Neurokinin 1 receptor expression by neurons in laminae I, III and IV of the rat spinal dorsal horn that project to the brainstem. Eur J Neurosci 2000;12:689–700.

[86] Todd AJ, Puskar Z, Spike RC, Hughes C, Watt C, Forrest L. Projection neurons in lamina I of rat spinal cord with the neurokinin 1 receptor are selectively innervated by substance p-containing afferents and respond to noxious stimulation. J Neurosci 2002;22:4103–13.

[87] Todd AJ, Spike RC, Polgar E. A quantitative study of neurons which express neurokinin-1 or somatostatin sst2a receptor in rat spinal dorsal horn. Neuroscience 1998;85:459–73.

[88] Todd AJ, Spike RC, Young S, Puskar Z. Fos induction in lamina I projection neurons in response to noxious thermal stimuli. Neuroscience 2005;131:209–17.

[89] Tolle TR, Berthele A, Zieglgansberger W, Seeburg PH, Wisden W. The differential expression of 16 NMDA and non-NMDA receptor subunits in the rat spinal cord and in periaqueductal gray. J Neurosci 1993;13:5009–28.

[90] Tong CK, MacDermott AB. Both Ca^{2+}-permeable and -impermeable AMPA receptors contribute to primary synaptic drive onto rat dorsal horn neurons. J Physiol 2006;575:133–44.

[91] Varoqui H, Schafer MK, Zhu H, Weihe E, Erickson JD. Identification of the differentiation-associated Na^+/PI transporter as a novel vesicular glutamate transporter expressed in a distinct set of glutamatergic synapses. J Neurosci 2002;22:142–55.

[92] Villanueva L, Bernard JF. The multiplicity of ascending pain pathways. In: Lydic R, Baghdoyan H, editors. Handbook of behavioral state control: cellular and molecular mechanisms. Boca Raton, FL: CRC Press; 1999. p. 569–85.

[93] Watanabe M, Fukaya M, Sakimura K, Manabe T, Mishina M, Inoue Y. Selective scarcity of NMDA receptor channel subunits in the stratum lucidum (mossy fibre-recipient layer) of the mouse hippocampal CA3 subfield. Eur J Neurosci 1998;10:478–87.

[94] Yoshimura M, Jessell T. Amino acid-mediated EPSPs at primary afferent synapses with substantia gelatinosa neurones in the rat spinal cord. J Physiol 1990;430:315–35.

[95] Yoshimura M, Nishi S. Excitatory amino acid receptors involved in primary afferent-evoked polysynaptic EPSPs of substantia gelatinosa neurons in the adult rat spinal cord slice. Neurosci Lett 1992;143:131–4.

[96] Yu XH, Ribeiro-da-Silva A, De Koninck Y. Morphology and neurokinin 1 receptor expression of spinothalamic lamina I neurons in the rat spinal cord. J Comp Neurol 2005;491:56–68.

[97] Yu XH, Zhang ET, Craig AD, Shigemoto R, Ribeiro-da-Silva A, De Koninck Y. NK-1 receptor immunoreactivity in distinct morphological types of lamina I neurons of the primate spinal cord. J Neurosci 1999;19:3545–55.

[98] Zhang ET, Han ZS, Craig AD. Morphological classes of spinothalamic lamina I neurons in the cat. J Comp Neurol 1996;367:537–49.

[99] Zhang X, Giesler GJ, Jr. Response characteristics of spinothalamic tract neurons that project to the posterior thalamus in rats. J Neurophysiol 2005;93:2552–64.

Correspondence to: Andrew J. Todd, MB BS, PhD, Spinal Cord Group, Spinal Cord Group, West Medical Building, University of Glasgow, Glasgow G12 8QQ, UK, Tel.: 44-141-330-5868, Fax: 44-141-330-2868, Email: a.todd@bio.gla.ac.uk.

The Role of Inhibition in the Generation and Amplification of Pain

Jürgen Sandkühler

Department of Neurophysiology, Center for Brain Research,
Medical University of Vienna, Vienna, Austria

It is a general rule that in the nervous system, all forms of activation are balanced by some kind of inactivation or inhibition. This principle also applies, of course, to all levels of the nociceptive system, from the activation of nociceptive Aδ or C fibers to the excitation of nociceptive neurons in the spinal dorsal horn and the brain. This chapter focuses on spinal mechanisms of inhibition, but it is likely that similar findings also apply to the processing of nociceptive information in the trigeminal system and to supraspinal nociception. In the dorsal horn of the spinal cord, about 30–40% of all neurons are inhibitory [51], using γ-aminobutyric acid (GABA) as their fast inhibitory neurotransmitter, which acts on ionotropic $GABA_A$ or G-protein-coupled metabotropic $GABA_B$ receptors. A significant proportion of these neurons use glycine as a cotransmitter, which acts on ionotropic glycine receptors (see also Chapter 3 by Todd, this volume). Inhibitory spinal interneurons may also use endogenous opioids, and supraspinal descending fiber systems may further use monoamines as neurotransmitters to modulate spinal nociception [30,42]. The peptidergic and monoaminergic systems are not considered here. Spinal inhibition may be impaired under conditions of neuropathy and inflammation, and the available evidence suggests that disinhibition in the spinal dorsal horn may lead to characteristic symptoms of neuropathic pain such as hyperalgesia, dynamic mechanical allodynia, and spontaneous paroxysmal pain (see the new definitions of technical terms by the International Association for the Study of Pain from 2008 and comments and illustrations in Sandkühler [42a]).

Mechanisms of Impaired Inhibition in the Spinal Dorsal Horn

The properties and functions of inhibition in the spinal dorsal horn have attracted much attention, and considerable progress has been made in understanding the role of inhibitory systems in nociception. These systems could be impaired at all sites, from the input to inhibitory neurons to their transfer functions and their output. Potential changes of spinal inhibition include (1) a reduced afferent drive to inhibitory neurons, (2) apoptotic or necrotic cell death of inhibitory spinal neurons, (3) reduced excitability or changes in discharge properties of inhibitory neurons, (4) reduced levels of inhibitory neurotransmitters due to lower rates of synthesis or reuptake, (5) reduced efficacy of receptors for inhibitory neurotransmitters, and (6) a reduced or inverted driving force for chloride ions (see Fig. 1).

Reduced Drive of Spinal GABAergic Neurons

Transgenic mice are now available that selectively express green fluorescent protein (GFP) in GABAergic neurons under the promoter of GAD67, one of the GABA-synthesizing enzymes [19,44]. Another mouse line expressing GFP in glycinergic neurons has also been developed [57]. This advance facilitates research on the electrophysiological properties of identified neurons in slice preparations of the spinal dorsal horn. In mice with a chronic constriction injury (CCI) of the sciatic nerve and mechanical hyperalgesia, the global excitatory drive to GABAergic neurons in the superficial lumbar spinal dorsal horn is greatly reduced. This conclusion is evident from the lower rate and reduced amplitude of miniature excitatory postsynaptic currents in these neurons [26]. Our recent data suggest that the primary afferent drive from Aδ and C fibers is reduced in these animals (J. Leitner et al., unpublished observations).

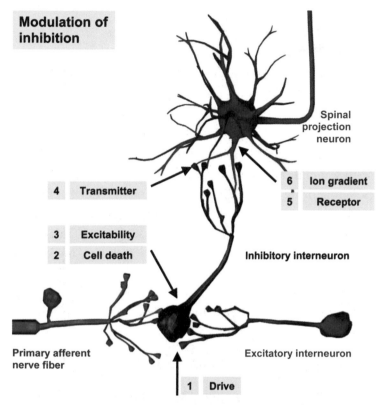

Fig. 1. Inhibition of a nociceptive spinal dorsal horn projection neuron (in red) by an inhibitory interneuron (in black), which in turn receives excitatory inputs (in blue and red). Six sites are shown where inhibition may be altered. (1) Reduced afferent drive to the inhibitory neuron, either from primary afferents (in blue), from excitatory spinal interneurons (in red), or from supraspinal descending pathways (not shown). (2) Apoptotic or necrotic cell death of inhibitory spinal neurons. (3) Reduced excitability or changes in discharge properties of inhibitory neurons. (4) Reduced levels of inhibitory neurotransmitters due to lower rates of synthesis or reuptake. (5) Reduced efficacy of receptors for inhibitory neurotransmitters. (6) Reduced or inverted driving force for chloride ions.

Cell Death of Inhibitory Interneurons?

Some studies have provided evidence for a programmed cell death of GABAergic neurons in animals with a spared nerve injury [31]. Others, however, have challenged this conclusion by determining the number of neurons—including identified GABAergic neurons—in the spinal dorsal horn of control rats and rats with a spared nerve injury [33,34]. In neuropathic animals with mechanical hyperalgesia, neither the number of neurons nor that of GABAergic profiles was any different from controls.

Stable Membrane and Discharge Properties of GABAergic Neurons

Inhibition would be impaired if membrane excitability were to decrease in inhibitory neurons or if their discharge patterns were to switch to low activity patterns. We assessed the membrane properties of GABAergic neurons. Recordings were made from GFP-labeled GABAergic neurons in lamina II [44] or lamina III [16] in transverse slices from the lumbar spinal cord. Resting membrane potentials, input resistance, and thresholds for action potential firing were unchanged in neurons recorded from animals with a CCI of the sciatic nerve. The distribution of typical discharge patterns also did not differ in neuropathic animals [16,44]. This finding suggests that (1) these GABAergic neurons do not change membrane excitability in the course of an injury of the sciatic nerve, and (2) the reduced excitatory input to these neurons faithfully translates into a reduced inhibitory output, because the transfer function of these GABAergic neurons remains stable.

GABA Synthesis, Reuptake, and Release

There is evidence that after a peripheral nerve lesion, levels of GABA may be reduced in the spinal dorsal horn. GABA immunoreactivity decreases 2–4 weeks after a transection or a CCI of the sciatic nerve [5,14]. This decrease could be caused by a loss of GABAergic neurons. However, GABA immunoreactivity recovers 8 weeks after nerve lesion [14], which suggests that it is not the number of neurons but rather the content of GABA within the neurons that might be changed. And indeed, levels of GAD65 (one of the two GABA-synthesizing enzymes) are reduced in the spinal dorsal horn ipsilateral to a CCI, and to a lesser extent, levels of GAD67 decrease as well [14,31]. Furthermore, reuptake of GABA after its release may also be impaired in neuropathic animals, given that the GABA transporter GAT-1 is downregulated bilaterally to about 40% 7 days after a CCI of the sciatic nerve as compared to controls [29,46]. In line with this finding, potassium-induced GABA release in spinal cord slices taken from rats with spinal nerve ligation is reduced as compared to slices from sham-operated controls [27]. However, a recent study found no changes in the level of GABA or of the vesicular GABA transporter in animals with a spared nerve injury [34]. Other studies have reported that the synaptosomal level of GABA is unchanged in animals with a CCI of the sciatic nerve [49]. Some authors found that the spinal content of GABA is even enhanced bilaterally 1–30 days after a unilateral CCI of sciatic nerve in the rat, as measured by high-performance liquid chromatography (HPLC) with electrochemical detection [43]. The reasons for these discrepant results are presently unknown.

Altered Functions of Inhibitory Neurotransmitter Receptors

The inhibitory effects of GABA or glycine depend on a variety of factors, all of which could change during neuropathy or inflammation. These include the number, subunit composition, and sensitivity of postsynaptic receptors and the driving force for Cl^-. Ipsilateral to a CCI of the sciatic nerve, the number of dorsal root ganglion (DRG) cells that express the γ_2 subunit of the $GABA_A$ receptor is reduced [32]. This finding suggests that $GABA_A$ receptors may be downregulated at the central terminals of primary afferent nerve fibers. If so, the sensitivity of these terminals to GABA should be diminished. And indeed, the mean depolarization elicited by GABA on dorsal roots is significantly reduced after chronic sciatic axotomy, dorsal root axotomy, or crush injury. In contrast, chronic sciatic crush injury has no effect on dorsal root GABA sensitivity [24]. Two to four weeks after a unilateral neurectomy of the sciatic nerve, $GABA_B$-receptor binding in lamina II of the spinal cord is downregulated [4]. In contrast, expression of $GABA_A$ receptors may remain unchanged in laminae I and II after a spared nerve injury [34], and $GABA_A$-receptor binding is enhanced following nerve transection [4].

Furthermore, receptor functions may be modulated by neuroactive substances released in the spinal dorsal horn during inflammation. For example, prostaglandin E_2 is released in the spinal cord during peripheral inflammation. Subsequent activation of EP_2 receptors (a subtype of prostaglandin E_2 receptor), cholera-toxin-sensitive G proteins, and cyclic adenosine monophosphate (cAMP)-dependent protein kinase depresses glycine receptor subtype α_3 function [18] and reduces glycinergic currents [1]. This pathway seems to be relevant for peripheral inflammation, but not for neuropathic pain, in mice with a CCI of the sciatic nerve [20].

Altered Driving Force for Chloride Ions

Even if all of the elements of the inhibitory chain mentioned above were to remain the same, inhibition through ionotropic $GABA_A$ or glycine receptors could still be reduced, eliminated, or converted into paradoxical excitation by changes in the driving force for chloride ions.

Diminished Postsynaptic Inhibition

Activation of $GABA_A$ or glycine receptors opens Cl^--permeable ion channels. The direction of Cl^- flux is generally determined by the level of the Cl^- equilibrium potential (E_{Cl}-) with respect to the resting membrane potential (V_{Rest}) of the cell. In most neurons of mature animals, E_{Cl}- is more negative than V_{Rest}, partly because of the continuous removal of Cl^- from the cells, e.g., via the potassium-chloride cotransporter KCC2. Thus, given the relatively low Cl^- concentration in neurons, Cl^- will move into the cell when the Cl^- conductance increases upon activation of $GABA_A$ or glycine receptors, thus causing membrane hyperpolarization. This situation could, however, be quite different under conditions of a neuropathy. CCI of the sciatic nerve leads to the activation of spinal microglia and to the release of brain-derived neurotrophic factor in the spinal cord. These events depress the function of the KCC2 potassium-chloride cotransporter and thereby enhance the Cl^- concentration inside the neurons. This, in turn, leads to a reduced (or even inverted) driving force for Cl^- and thus causes reduced postsynaptic inhibition [10] (see also Chapter 8 by De Koninck, this volume).

Paradoxical Postsynaptic Excitation

In its most extreme case, the activation of postsynaptic $GABA_A$ or glycine receptors may lead to depolarization and eventually excitation. This situation may occur, for example, when the function of the potassium chloride cotransporter is severely impaired and E_{Cl}- becomes less negative than the resting membrane potential. This event reverses the direction of Cl^- flux across the membrane, leading to a Cl^- efflux and membrane depolarization rather than to an influx into the cell. During development, and also minutes to weeks after trauma of cultured hypothalamic or cortical neurons, GABA may have such a depolarizing effect [53]. Thus, it is neither the kind of neurotransmitter nor the type of neurotransmitter receptor alone that determines if neurotransmission is inhibitory or excitatory. The level of the Cl⁻ concentration gradient across the cell membrane determines whether GABA and glycine are hyper- or depolarizing [11]. In animals with a CCI of the sciatic nerve, KCC2 may be downregulated so severely that the driving force of Cl⁻ is reversed and in extreme cases may even cause action potential firing of the postsynaptic neuron (paradoxical postsynaptic excitation) [10,11].

Paradoxical Presynaptic Excitation

The anion gradient across the membrane of primary afferent nerve terminal is different as compared to most other neurons in mature animals. Here, the activity of the sodium-potassium-chloride cotransporter NKCC1 enhances the Cl⁻ concentration in the nerve terminals, so that E_{Cl}- is normally less negative than the resting membrane potential. This activity regularly results in a Cl⁻ efflux and membrane depolarization upon binding of GABA to the $GABA_A$ receptor. Thus, under normal conditions, activation of $GABA_A$ receptors will depolarize the terminals of primary afferent nerve fibers. This primary afferent depolarization is not strong enough to cause action potential firing (i.e., excitation) under normal conditions. Primary afferent depolarization inactivates voltage-gated ion channels, which are required for the release of neurotransmitter(s) from the terminals and may shunt currents of the incoming action potentials [37,54]. Thereby, moderate depolarization of the terminals may inhibit neurotransmitter release. It has been proposed that under conditions of inflammation or neuropathy, depolarization at primary afferent C fibers may become steeper and stronger, eventually reaching the thresholds for activating voltage-gated sodium channels and for triggering action potential firing. This event would cause paradoxical presynaptic excitation by GABA [7,36].

Role of Normal and Impaired Spinal Inhibition in Pain

Virtually all neurons in the spinal dorsal horn are subject to a powerful tonic and phasic inhibitory control via GABAergic, glycinergic, or other inhibitory spinal interneurons or descending inhibitory systems arising from supraspinal sites. The functional consequences of impaired or altered inhibition critically depend on the site within the neuronal network where inhibition is altered. Inhibitory spinal dorsal horn neurons serve at least four crucial functions for proper nociception (see Table I): (1) attenuating nociceptive responses, (2) muting nociceptive neurons in the absence of a noxious stimulus, (3) separating information from different sensory modalities, and (4) limiting the spread of excitation in the spinal cord to appropriate somatotopic borders.

Table I
Four crucial functions of inhibitory spinal dorsal horn neurons in nociception

Role of Inhibition	Mechanism of Action	Desired Effect	Pain Type upon Failure
Attenuation	Pre- and postsynaptic inhibition of nociceptive spinal dorsal horn neurons	Proper response level to noxious stimulation	Hyperalgesia
Muting	Inhibition of nociceptive dorsal horn neurons and the interneurons that drive them	Silencing of nociceptive neurons in the absence of noxious stimuli	Spontaneous pain
Separating	Inhibition of excitatory interneurons linking Aβ-fiber input to nociceptive-specific neurons	Inhibition of excitatory crosstalk between sensory modalities	Allodynia
Limiting	Inhibition of excitatory interneurons that cross somatotopic borders	Limiting spread of excitation to somatotopically appropriate areas	Radiating pain, referred pain, mirror-image pain

Attenuation of Nociception

Glycinergic inhibition is postsynaptic, whereas inhibition by GABA may be pre- or postsynaptic. This includes presynaptic inhibition at terminals of nociceptive nerve fibers, inhibition of spinal nociceptive projection neurons, and inhibition of any neuron that is part of the ascending nociceptive pathways. Blocking either spinal $GABA_A$ or glycine receptors greatly increases spinal dorsal horn neuronal responses to noxious stimuli in vivo [41,58] as well as responses to stimulation of dorsal root afferents at Aδ- or C-fiber intensity in slice preparations [2,23]. Thus, the magnitude of nociceptive responses and the intensity of perceived pain are not a simple monotonic or even linear function of stimulus intensity but rather result from the balance between the strength of excitatory input and attenuation by inhibitory systems. Fluctuations in the activity of endogenous antinociceptive systems contribute to variations in pain sensitivity among human subjects and account for stress-induced analgesia and diurnal variations in pain thresholds [30,42].

Muting Nociceptive Circuits

In the absence of any noxious stimulus, nociceptive-specific spinal dorsal horn neurons are largely silent and do not display any significant spontaneous activity [6,22], whereas the background activity of wide-dynamic-range neurons may be more variable under the given recording conditions [6,17]. The quiescence of these neurons requires a permanent inhibitory control. If GABA or glycine receptors are blocked in the spinal cord, virtually all neurons—including nociceptive-specific neurons—become spontaneously active, and many may also discharge rhythmically and in synchrony [38,45]; see Fig. 2. This form of spinal network activity resembles epileptiform activity in cortical neurons during epileptic seizures and also engages nociceptive-specific neurons in the superficial spinal dorsal horn with a direct projection to the brain [38]. In behaving animals, blockade of spinal $GABA_A$ receptors leads to scratching and biting behavior, which is often interpreted as an indication for spontaneous pain and/or dysesthesia [28]. If similar epileptiform activity also occurs in nociceptive spinal or trigeminal neurons of pain patients, it could underlie spontaneous paroxysmal pain attacks.

Separating Sensory Modalities

Labeled lines that exclusively subserve either nociception or touch exist at the level of the spinal cord. Nociceptive Aδ and C fibers may excite nociceptive-specific neurons in the superficial spinal dorsal horn, some of which have a direct projection to the brain. On the other hand, low-threshold Aβ fibers may excite low-threshold neurons in the deep dorsal horn that have different projection areas in the brain. In addition to these labeled lines, some neurons in spinal dorsal horn receive afferent input from Aδ and C fibers and from Aβ fibers ("wide-dynamic-range neurons"). Their function in nociception has been discussed extensively [9,12,13,35,47], but it is unlikely that these neurons discriminate between

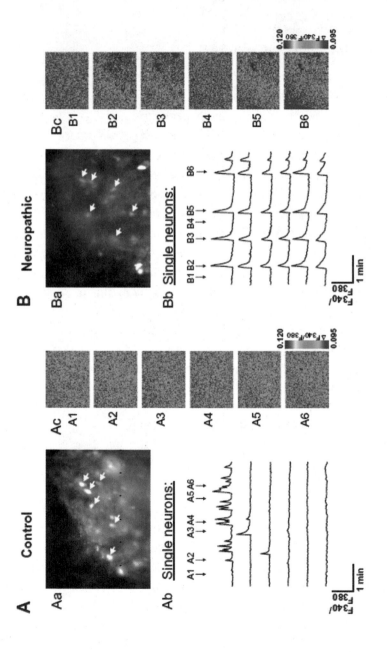

A Control

Aa

Ab Single neurons:

A1 A2   A3 A4   A5 A6

$\frac{F340}{F380}$

1 min

Ac
A1
A2
A3
A4
A5
A6

$\Delta F340/F380$

0.120

0.095

B Neuropathic

Ba

Bb Single neurons:

B1 B2   B3 B4 B5   B6

$\frac{F340}{F380}$

1 min

Bc
B1
B2
B3
B4
B5
B6

$\Delta F340/F380$

0.120

0.095

the sensory modalities of touch and pain [8,56]. In any case, to prevent touch from becoming painful, these sensory modalities must be kept separate. By definition, nociceptive-specific neurons are not excited by Aβ fibers; however, activity in Aβ fibers may activate inhibitory interneurons, which in turn depress the activity in nociceptive spinal dorsal horn neurons. Presently, three mechanisms are proposed by which impaired or altered inhibition in the spinal cord may initiate an excitatory crosstalk between low-threshold Aβ fibers and nociceptive-specific neurons in the superficial spinal dorsal horn.

1) The postsynaptic GABAergic inhibition of nociceptive-specific neurons in the superficial spinal dorsal horn may turn into excitation. Some of these GABAergic neurons may receive excitatory input from low-threshold Aβ fibers. Thus, touch stimuli may lead to activation of GABAergic neurons, which then would no longer depress, but rather excite, nociceptive-specific neurons in the spinal dorsal horn lamina I [10,11], possibly leading to touch-evoked pain. This mechanism is discussed in greater detail in Chapter 8 by De Koninck. However, spinal application of a $GABA_A$-receptor agonist attenuates, rather than evokes, pain or allodynia [15,21,25]. This finding suggests that the overall pharmacological effect of GABA is still antinociceptive. Possibly, the paradoxical excitation by GABA at specific sites along the nociceptive pathways is overruled by global depressant effects.

Fig. 2. Blockade of $GABA_A$ and glycine receptors induces synchronous network activity in laminae I/II of SNI rats. Examples are shown of the network activity in slices from the lumbar spinal cord of (A) control or (B) neuropathic animals arising after preincubation with bicuculline (10 µM) and strychnine (4 µM). (A) Panel Aa shows a 380-nm image of the region selected for recording. In slices from control animals, spinal disinhibition did not evoke simultaneous Ca^{2+}-transients. (Ab) Original traces show the time course (10–15 minutes after bicuculline/strychnine application) of the Ca^{2+} concentration of the neurons that are marked by arrows in panel Aa. Pseudocolor F340/F380 ratio images taken at the time points marked in panel Ab (arrows, A1–A6) are displayed in panel Ac. Red indicates a high intracellular Ca^{2+} concentration. While some spontaneous activity was seen, it was not synchronized between neurons. (B) In the slice from a neuropathic animal, blockade of $GABA_A$ and glycine receptors induced repetitive spontaneous Ca^{2+} transients that were synchronized in many of the recorded neurons, as illustrated in the original traces (Bb). (Bc) Pseudocolor F340/F380 ratio images of the time points marked in panel Bb (arrows, B1–B6) show that intracellular Ca^{2+} concentration was high at the time of simultaneous Ca^{2+} transients and intracellular Ca^{2+} concentration was low between two transients in spinal dorsal horn neurons. Modified from [45], with permission.

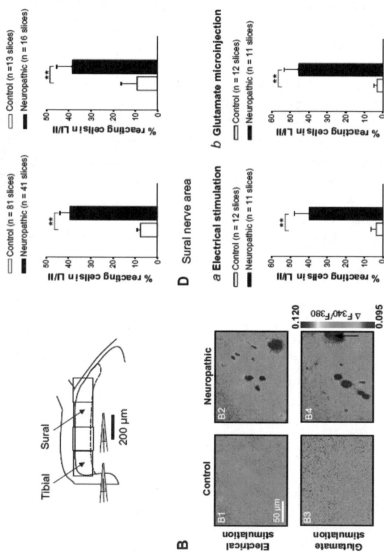

A

Tibial Sural 200 μm

B

Electrical stimulation

Glutamate stimulation

Control Neuropathic

B1 B2 B3 B4

50 μm

ΔF340/F380 0.095 0.120

C Tibial nerve area

a Electrical stimulation

□ Control (n = 81 slices) ■ Neuropathic (n = 41 slices)

% reacting cells in L/II 0 10 20 30 40 50

**

b Glutamate microinjection

□ Control (n = 13 slices) ■ Neuropathic (n = 16 slices)

% reacting cells in L/II 0 10 20 30 40 50

**

D Sural nerve area

a Electrical stimulation

□ Control (n = 12 slices) ■ Neuropathic (n = 11 slices)

% reacting cells in L/II 0 10 20 30 40 50 60

**

b Glutamate microinjection

□ Control (n =12 slices) ■ Neuropathic (n = 11 slices)

% reacting cells in L/II 0 10 20 30 40 50 60

**

2) It has further been proposed that presynaptic GABAergic inhibition at C-fiber terminals may also turn into excitation. The evidence for this proposal has been reviewed [7,36]. GABAergic neurons that contact C-fiber terminals may be activated by low-threshold Aβ fibers, normally mediating Aβ-fiber-induced inhibition of C-fiber-evoked responses in the spinal dorsal horn. If a paradoxical presynaptic excitation were to be triggered by activity in Aβ fibers, pain evoked by touch may be the consequence. In an attempt to test this hypothesis, we made intracellular recordings from DRG cells in a transverse spinal cord slice preparation with dorsal roots, DRG, and spinal nerves left intact. Preparations were from animals with a CCI of the sciatic nerve and from sham-treated animals. In slices taken from control animals, electrical thresholds for action potential discharges were low in A-type neurons attached to A fibers and high in C-type neurons attached to C fibers. If a paradoxical excitation of C-fiber terminals were to occur in neuropathic animals, action potentials would be antidromically transmitted to the site of recording in the DRG, and some C fibers should be activated at low, A-fiber intensities. Under the given experimental conditions, however, there were no differences in the stimulus-response functions of C-type

Fig. 3. Electrical stimulation and glutamate microinjection in the deep dorsal horn excite superficial dorsal horn neurons in neuropathic animals. (A) Outline of the dorsal quadrant of a transverse spinal cord slice. The dashed line indicates the approximate border between laminae II and III. The superficial dorsal horn regions in the somatotopic area of the transected tibial and the intact sural nerve selected for imaging are shown by the boxes. The sites of electrical stimulation or glutamate microinjection are indicated by the tip of the stimulation pipettes. (B) Slices were incubated with fura-2 AM. The ratio of the images captured at 340 and 380 nm illuminations was then used to detect changes in intracellular Ca^{2+} concentration. Examples of ratio images of control animals (B1, B3) and neuropathic animals (B2, B4) 500 ms after stimulation are shown in pseudocolor. Pseudocolor images show values of the difference between the F340/F380 ratio images before stimulation and at the time of the usual peak reaction to stimulation (0.5 seconds after stimulation). Red indicates areas that were excited by the stimulation, whereas blue indicates unexcited areas. Superficial dorsal horn neurons of control animals did not show Ca^{2+} transients in the frame after electrical stimulation (B1) or glutamate microinjection (B3) in the deep dorsal horn. However, in neuropathic animals, numerous superficial dorsal horn neurons were excited following electrical (stimulation B2) and glutamate microinjection (B4). (C and D) Summary of the results showing that electrical stimulation and glutamate microinjection in the deep dorsal horn in the area of the tibial (C) or the sural nerve (D) excited superficial dorsal horn neurons significantly more often in neuropathic than in control animals (**$P < 0.01$ in the Mann-Whitney rank sum test). Modified from [45], with permission.

neurons between control and neuropathic animals. Thus, we were unable to find evidence for a paradoxical excitation of C fibers [40]. Of course, this absence of evidence should not be mistaken as evidence of absence of such a mechanism.

3) There is direct evidence for an excitatory pathway from the deep to the superficial spinal dorsal horn [45]. Given that Aβ fibers terminate in the deep dorsal horn and nociceptive-specific neurons are in the superficial dorsal horn, these findings could explain the novel polysynaptic input from low-threshold Aβ fibers to nociceptive-specific neurons [52] in animals with a neuropathy [45] or a peripheral inflammation [3].

To demonstrate the existence of this excitatory pathway, we used a transverse slice preparation from the rat lumbar spinal cord with long dorsal roots attached. Calcium-imaging techniques were employed to simultaneously monitor neuronal activity in the deep dorsal horn (laminae III–IV) and in the superficial dorsal horn (laminae I and II; see Fig. 3). We microinjected glutamate through fine glass micropipettes into the deep dorsal horn in order to excite a few neurons, while leaving fibers that pass through the site of injection unaffected. In slices taken from control animals and with spinal inhibition intact, these microinjections excited no or very few neurons in the superficial dorsal horn (see Fig. 3). When GABA$_A$ and glycine receptors were blocked, however, the same microinjections of glutamate in the deep dorsal horn now excited numerous superficial dorsal horn neurons [45]. These data provide direct evidence for the existence of an excitatory pathway from the deep to the superficial dorsal horn that is tonically depressed by GABAergic and/or glycinergic interneurons.

We next used slices taken from animals with a CCI of the sciatic nerve and mechanical hyperalgesia. In these slices, glutamate microinjections into the deep dorsal horn caused excitation of numerous neurons in the superficial dorsal horn, even in the absence of GABA$_A$ or glycine receptor blockers (Fig. 3) [45]. These data suggest that the excitatory pathway from the deep to superficial dorsal horn is closed in sham-treated animals but open in neuropathic animals with mechanical hyperalgesia and allodynia.

Finally, we provided evidence that this pathway can apparently be activated not only by microinjections of glutamate at or near the

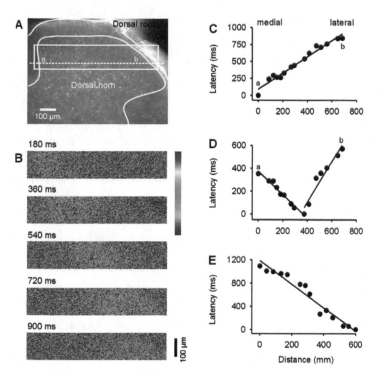

Fig. 4. Initiation and propagation of Ca²⁺ waves in the superficial dorsal horn. (A) A spinal slice section is shown at 380-nm illumination with a superimposed outline of the dorsal horn. Fura-2-loaded cells are visible as small bright spots. (B) A sequence of images taken of the region indicated by the box in (A) during a population Ca²⁺ transient is shown. To highlight the wave front moving over the spinal dorsal horn, the difference between the 380 nm image at the indicated point in time and the image obtained 180 ms previously is displayed in pseudocolor. On the color scale, red indicates large changes of fluorescence, and blue indicates little or no change. The points in time indicated above the images correspond to the time scale in (C) that illustrates the same Ca²⁺ wave as (B). (C and D) The time courses of two different Ca²⁺ waves recorded from the slice shown in (A) are illustrated. Fifteen neurons lying near the dashed line in (A) were selected, and the onset of their individual Ca²⁺ transients during a population transient were analyzed. The latency relative to the neuron with the earliest onset was then plotted against the distance from the most medial neuron, and the plots were fitted by linear regression. The mediolateral location of the neurons marked with "a" and "b" is shown in (A). (E) A lateromedially propagating wave from another slice. Examples (C–E) illustrate that Ca²⁺ waves can be initiated at various sites in the superficial dorsal horn and that these waves propagate laterally as well as medially. Modified from [39], with permission.

termination sites of primary afferent Aβ fibers in the deep dorsal horn, but also by activation of Aβ fibers. In slices from animals with a CCI but not in sham-treated animals, a substantial proportion of lamina I/II neurons were excited by stimulation of Aβ fibers [45]. Similar results were found by recording from single cells in superficial dorsal horn neurons of animals with a peripheral inflammation [3].

In behaving animals, blocking GABA or glycine receptors leads to agitation in response to light tactile stimuli [56] and to a drastic reduction of mechanical withdrawal thresholds [48]. This finding suggests that an excitatory crosstalk between Aβ-fiber afferents and nociceptive pathways has been initiated, causing Aβ-fiber-mediated mechanical allodynia. If similar mechanisms apply to human pain patients, impaired separation of sensory modalities in the spinal dorsal horn would cause touch-evoked pain.

Limiting the Spread of Excitation

The known termination patterns of primary afferents suggest that sensory information from different modalities and different regions of the body is processed in a highly organized and spatially segregated fashion [50,55]. However, when spinal $GABA_A$ and glycine receptors are blocked, excitation may spread to virtually all sites in the spinal dorsal horn, both ipsilateral and contralateral to the site of afferent stimulation [39]; see Fig. 4. Thus, somatotopic borders are not secured anatomically but need to be actively maintained by the function of inhibitory systems in the spinal dorsal horn. If similar violations of somatotopic borders were to occur in humans, then lancinating, projecting, and mirror-image pain would be the result.

Acknowledgments

Our own work described in this chapter was supported by grants from the Austria Science Fund (FWF) and the Vienna Science and Technology Fund (WWTF). I wish to thank Drs. Ruth Ruscheweyh and Doris Schoffnegger for helpful comments on an earlier version of the manuscript and Lila Czarnecki for excellent maintenance of our literature database.

References

[1]   Ahmadi S, Lippross S, Neuhuber WL, Zeilhofer HU. PGE_2 selectively blocks inhibitory glycinergic neurotransmission onto rat superficial dorsal horn neurons. Nat Neurosci 2002;5:34–40.
[2]   Ataka T, Kumamoto E, Shimoji K, Yoshimura M. Baclofen inhibits more effectively C-afferent than Aδ-afferent glutamatergic transmission in substantia gelatinosa neurons of adult rat spinal cord slices. Pain 2000;86:273–82.

[3] Baba H, Doubell TP, Woolf CJ. Peripheral inflammation facilitates Aβ-fiber-mediated synaptic input to the substantia gelatinosa of the adult rat spinal cord. J Neurosci 1999;19:859–67.

[4] Castro-Lopes JM, Malcangio M, Pan BH, Bowery NG. Complex changes of GABA$_A$ and GABA$_B$ receptor binding in the spinal cord dorsal horn following peripheral inflammation or neurectomy. Brain Res 1995;679:289–97.

[5] Castro-Lopes JM, Tavares I, Coimbra A. GABA decreases in the spinal cord dorsal horn after peripheral neurectomy. Brain Res 1993;620:287–91.

[6] Cervero F, Iggo A, Ogawa H. Nociceptor-driven dorsal horn neurones in the lumbar spinal cord of the cat. Pain 1976;2:5–24.

[7] Cervero F, Laird JM, García-Nicas E. Secondary hyperalgesia and presynaptic inhibition: an update. Eur J Pain 2003;7:345–51.

[8] Coghill RC, Mayer DJ, Price DD. The roles of spatial recruitment and discharge frequency in spinal cord coding of pain: a combined electrophysiological and imaging investigation. Pain 1993;53:295–309.

[9] Coghill RC, Mayer DJ, Price DD. Wide dynamic range but not nociceptive-specific neurons encode multidimensional features of prolonged repetitive heat pain. J Neurophysiol 1993;69:703–16.

[10] Coull JAM, Beggs S, Boudreau D, Boivin D, Tsuda M, Inoue K, Gravel C, Salter MW, De Koninck Y. BDNF from microglia causes the shift in neuronal anion gradient underlying neuropathic pain. Nature 2005;438:1017–21.

[11] Coull JAM, Boudreau D, Bachand K, Prescott SA, Nault F, Sik A, De Koninck P, De Koninck Y. Trans-synaptic shift in anion gradient in spinal lamina I neurons as a mechanism of neuropathic pain. Nature 2003;424:938–42.

[12] Craig AD. Pain mechanisms: labeled lines versus convergence in central processing. Annu Rev Neurosci 2003;26:1–30.

[13] Craig AD. Lamina I, but not lamina V, spinothalamic neurons exhibit responses that correspond with burning pain. J Neurophysiol 2004;92:2604–9.

[14] Eaton MJ, Plunkett JA, Karmally S, Martinez MA, Montanez K. Changes in GAD- and GABA-immunoreactivity in the spinal dorsal horn after peripheral nerve injury and promotion of recovery by lumbar transplant of immortalized serotonergic precursors. J Chem Neuroanat 1998;16:57–72.

[15] Eaton MJ, Plunkett JA, Martinez MA, Lopez T, Karmally S, Cejas P, Whittemore SR. Transplants of neuronal cells bioengineered to synthesize GABA alleviate chronic neuropathic pain. Cell Transplant 1999;8:87–101.

[16] Gassner M, Schoffnegger D, Sandkühler J. Properties of spinal lamina III GABAergic neurons in neuropathic mice. Abstracts of the 12th World Congress on Pain 2008;PF 346.

[17] Handwerker HO, Iggo A, Zimmermann M. Segmental and supraspinal actions on dorsal horn neurons responding to noxious and non-noxious skin stimuli. Pain 1975;1:147–65.

[18] Harvey RJ, Depner UB, Wässle H, Ahmadi S, Heindl C, Reinold H, Smart TG, Harvey K, Schütz B, Abo-Salem OM, et al. GlyRα3: an essential target for spinal PGE$_2$-mediated inflammatory pain sensitization. Science 2004;304:884–7.

[19] Heinke B, Ruscheweyh R, Forsthuber L, Wunderbaldinger G, Sandkühler J. Physiological, neurochemical and morphological properties of a subgroup of GABAergic spinal lamina II neurones identified by expression of green fluorescent protein in mice. J Physiol 2004;560:249–66.

[20] Hösl K, Reinold H, Harvey RJ, Müller U, Narumiya S, Zeilhofer HU. Spinal prostaglandin E receptors of the EP2 subtype and the glycine receptor α3 subunit, which mediate central inflammatory hyperalgesia, do not contribute to pain after peripheral nerve injury or formalin injection. Pain 2006;126:46–53.

[21] Hwang JH, Yaksh TL. The effect of spinal GABA receptor agonists on tactile allodynia in a surgically-induced neuropathic pain model in the rat. Pain 1997;70:15–22.

[22] Iggo A, Molony V, Steedman WM. Membrane properties of nociceptive neurones in lamina II of lumbar spinal cord in the cat. J Physiol 1988;400:367–80.

[23] Kangrga I, Jiang MC, Randic M. Actions of (-)-baclofen on rat dorsal horn neurons. Brain Res 1991;562:265–75.

[24] Kingery WS, Fields RD, Kocsis JD. Diminished dorsal root GABA sensitivity following chronic peripheral nerve injury. Exp Neurol 1988;100:478–90.

[25] Knabl J, Witschi R, Hösl K, Reinold H, Zeilhofer UB, Ahmadi S, Brockhaus J, Sergejeva M, Hess A, Brune K, et al. Reversal of pathological pain through specific spinal GABA$_A$ receptor subtypes. Nature 2008;451:330–4.

[26] Leitner J, Jäger T, Sandkühler J. Impaired excitatory drive to spinal GABAergic neurons as a novel potential mechanism of neuropathic pain. Abstracts of the 12th World Congress on Pain 2008;PF 356.

[27] Lever I, Cunningham J, Grist J, Yip PK, Malcangio M. Release of BDNF and GABA in the dorsal horn of neuropathic rats. Eur J Neurosci 2003;18:1169–74.

[28] Loomis CW, Khandwala H, Osmond G, Hefferan MP. Coadministration of intrathecal strychnine and bicuculline effects synergistic allodynia in the rat: an isobolographic analysis. J Pharmacol Exp Ther 2001;296:756–61.

[29] Miletic G, Draganic P, Pankratz MT, Miletic V. Muscimol prevents long-lasting potentiation of dorsal horn field potentials in rats with chronic constriction injury exhibiting decreased levels of the GABA transporter GAT-1. Pain 2003;105:347–53.

[30] Millan MJ. Descending control of pain. Prog Neurobiol 2002;66:355–474.

[31] Moore KA, Kohno T, Karchewski LA, Scholz J, Baba H, Woolf CJ. Partial peripheral nerve injury promotes a selective loss of GABAergic inhibition in the superficial dorsal horn of the spinal cord. J Neurosci 2002;22:6724–31.

[32] Obata K, Yamanaka H, Fukuoka T, Yi D, Tokunaga A, Hashimoto N, Yoshikawa H, Noguchi K. Contribution of injured and uninjured dorsal root ganglion neurons to pain behavior and the changes in gene expression following chronic constriction injury of the sciatic nerve in rats. Pain 2003;101:65–77.

[33] Polgár E, Hughes DI, Arham AZ, Todd AJ. Loss of neurons from laminas I-III of the spinal dorsal horn is not required for development of tactile allodynia in the spared nerve injury model of neuropathic pain. J Neurosci 2005;25:6658–66.

[34] Polgár E, Todd AJ. Tactile allodynia can occur in the spared nerve injury model in the rat without selective loss of GABA or GABA$_A$ receptors from synapses in laminae I-II of the ipsilateral spinal dorsal horn. Neuroscience 2008;156:193–202.

[35] Price DD, Dubner R. Neurons that subserve the sensory-discriminative aspects of pain. Pain 1977;3:307–38.

[36] Price TJ, Cervero F, De Koninck Y. Role of cation-chloride-cotransporters (CCC) in pain and hyperalgesia. Curr Top Med Chem 2005;5:547–55.

[37] Rudomin P, Schmidt RF. Presynaptic inhibition in the vertebrate spinal cord revisited. Exp Brain Res 1999;129:1–37.

[38] Ruscheweyh R, Sandkühler J. Epileptiform activity in rat spinal dorsal horn in vitro has common features with neuropathic pain. Pain 2003;105:327–38.

[39] Ruscheweyh R, Sandkühler J. Long-range oscillatory Ca^{2+} waves in rat spinal dorsal horn. Eur J Neurosci 2005;22:1967–76.

[40] Ruscheweyh R, Schoffnegger D, Sandkühler J. Does excitation of Aβ-fibres trigger action potentials in primary afferent C-fibres to cause allodynia? Abstracts of the 12th World Congress on Pain 2008;PH 361.

[41] Saadé NE, Jabbur SJ, Wall PD. Effects of 4-aminopyridine, GABA and bicuculline on cutaneous receptive fields of cat dorsal horn neurons. Brain Res 1985;344:356–9.

[42] Sandkühler J. The organization and function of endogenous antinociceptive systems. Prog Neurobiol 1996;50:49–81.

[42a] Sandkühler J. Models and mechanisms of hyperalgesia and allodynia. Physiol Rev 2009;89:in press.

[43] Satoh O, Omote K. Roles of monoaminergic, glycinergic and GABAergic inhibitory systems in the spinal cord in rats with peripheral mononeuropathy. Brain Res 1996;728:27–36.

[44] Schoffnegger D, Heinke B, Sommer C, Sandkühler J. Physiological properties of spinal lamina II GABAergic neurons in mice following peripheral nerve injury. J Physiol 2006;577:869–78.

[45] Schoffnegger D, Ruscheweyh R, Sandkühler J. Spread of excitation across modality borders in spinal dorsal horn of neuropathic rats. Pain 2008;135:300–10.

[46] Shih A, Miletic V, Miletic G, Smith LJ. Midazolam administration reverses thermal hyperalgesia and prevents γ-aminobutyric acid transporter loss in a rodent model of neuropathic pain. Anesth Analg 2008;106:1296–302.

[47] Simone DA, Sorkin LS, Oh U, Chung JM, Owens C, LaMotte RH, Willis WD. Neurogenic hyperalgesia: central neural correlates in responses of spinothalamic tract neurons. J Neurophysiol 1991;66:228–46.

[48] Sivilotti L, Woolf CJ. The contribution of GABA$_A$ and glycine receptors to central sensitization: disinhibition and touch-evoked allodynia in the spinal cord. J Neurophysiol 1994;72:169–79.

[49]   Somers DL, Clemente FR. Dorsal horn synaptosomal content of aspartate, glutamate, glycine and GABA are differentially altered following chronic constriction injury to the rat sciatic nerve. Neurosci Lett 2002;323:171–4.

[50]   Takahashi Y, Aoki Y, Doya H. Segmental somatotopic organization of cutaneous afferent fibers in the lumbar spinal cord dorsal horn in rats. Anat Sci Int 2007;82:24–30.

[51]   Todd AJ, McKenzie J. GABA-immunoreactive neurons in the dorsal horn of the rat spinal cord. Neuroscience 1989;31:799–806.

[52]   Torsney C, MacDermott AB. Disinhibition opens the gate to pathological pain signaling in superficial neurokinin 1 receptor-expressing neurons in rat spinal cord. J Neurosci 2006;26:1833–43.

[53]   van den Pol AN, Obrietan K, Chen G. Excitatory actions of GABA after neuronal trauma. J Neurosci 1996;16:4283–92.

[54]   Willis WD Jr. Dorsal root potentials and dorsal root reflexes: a double-edged sword. Exp Brain Res 1999;124:395–421.

[55]   Wilson P, Meyers DER, Snow PJ. The detailed somatotopic organization of the dorsal horn in the lumbosacral enlargement of the cat spinal cord. J Neurophysiol 1986;55:604–17.

[56]   Yaksh TL. Behavioral and autonomic correlates of the tactile evoked allodynia produced by spinal glycine inhibition: effects of modulatory receptor systems and excitatory amino acid antagonists. Pain 1989;37:111–23.

[57]   Zeilhofer HU, Studler B, Arabadzisz D, Schweizer C, Ahmadi S, Layh B, Bösl MR, Fritschy JM. Glycinergic neurons expressing enhanced green fluorescent protein in bacterial artificial chromosome transgenic mice. J Comp Neurol 2005;482:123–41.

[58]   Zieglgänsberger W, Sutor B. Responses of substantia gelatinosa neurons to putative neurotransmitters in an in vitro preparation of the adult rat spinal cord. Brain Res 1983;279:316–20.

Correspondence to: Jürgen Sandkühler, MD, PhD, Center for Brain Research, Department of Neurophysiology, A-1090 Vienna, Austria. Email: juergen.sandkuehler@meduniwien.ac.at.

Neurobiology of Itch and Pain: Scratching for Answers

5

E. Carstens

Department of Neurobiology, Physiology and Behavior, University of California, Davis, Davis, California, USA

Itch is often defined as an unpleasant sensation associated with the desire to scratch. It is commonly evoked by insect bites, allergic reactions, or contact with certain plants such as cowhage. Acute itch sensation provides a warning to the organism of surface stimuli that can be removed by scratching or rubbing. In contrast, pain sensation also provides a warning signal, which, however, is exacerbated by scratching and instead is usually coupled with protective limb withdrawal from the stimulus. Following tissue injury or other conditions, persistent pain can develop. Likewise, chronic itch frequently accompanies a wide variety of dermatological conditions such as atopic dermatitis, as well as kidney and liver diseases, HIV, and many other conditions [49]. With few exceptions, the itch is resistant to antihistamines [113]. Like chronic pain, chronic itch disrupts sleep and other aspects of life and carries a heavy economic and social burden. There is a great need to better understand mechanisms of itch and to develop more effective treatments.

Current Topics in Pain: 12th World Congress on Pain
edited by José Castro-Lopes
IASP Press, Seattle, © 2009

Incidence of Chronic Itch

Recent epidemiological studies emphasize the high incidence and economic costs of chronic itch. Large retrospective cross-sectional studies revealed that 8–12.4% of respondents had experienced chronic itch within the past 12 months [23,133]. Over 50% of Dutch patients with some form of skin disease reported itching, with half experiencing that the problem was severe [120]. Several recent epidemiological studies have quantified the incidence of itch in a variety of conditions (summarized in Table I). Incidences of chronic itch in psoriasis patients in the United States and other industrialized countries range from 64% to 84% [88,103,139]. Psoriatic itch is poorly controlled by currently available therapies [139]. Atopic dermatitis has itch as its most common symptom, affecting 87% of patients on a daily basis [140]. A recent large-scale survey of >116,000 U.S. citizens reported a 17% incidence of atopic dermatitis [40]. Another study [17] reported that 5–20% of children are affected by this skin condition worldwide. The itch associated with this condition is poorly controlled by antihistamines [58], and improved treatment of this symptom represents a major challenge.

Table I
Epidemiological studies of chronic itch incidence

Cause of Itch	Incidence	Reference
Psoriasis	64–84%	[88,103,139]
Atopic dermatitis	87%	[140]
Kidney disease	42–52%	[68,85,129]
Liver disease	37–68%	[6]
Burn injury, small	47%	[21]
Burn injury, large (>20%)	87%	[121]
Herpes zoster	17–58%	[81]
Spinal opiates	46–95%	[5,126]
Psychiatric/unknown	32%	[65]

Chronic itch is associated with a wide variety of other skin conditions and systemic diseases. Moderate to extreme itch was reported by 42–52% of hemodialysis patients [68,85,129], with variations by country

(36–50%) and medical facility (5–75%). Treatment of uremic itch remains a major challenge, with gabapentin [35] and the κ-opioid agonist nalfurafine [130] showing antipruritic potential. Itch is also a common symptom of liver disease, occurring in 37–68% of patients with primary biliary cirrhosis (reviewed in [6]). Available treatments, including antihistamines, μ-opiate antagonists, 5-HT$_3$ receptor antagonists, and gabapentin (among many others), have met with low or variable degrees of success [6]. Itch was reported to occur in 47% of patients with small burn injuries [21] and in 87% of patients with large burn injuries covering ~20% of the body surface [121]. High percentages (17–58%) of patients with acute shingles (herpes zoster) or postherpetic neuralgia report moderate to severe itch [81], which, in an extreme case, led to the patient scratching through the skull to expose the brain [82]. Itch is the main symptom of pruritic papular eruption in HIV patients [87], and it is also common in scabies [41] and onchocerciasis [71]. Spinal administration of opiates was reported to induce itch in 46% of patients during parturition (reviewed in [5]); in another study the percentage was as high as 95% [126]. Itch was reported by 32% of psychiatric inpatients for whom skin conditions and systemic itch-related diseases were excluded [65]. Itch also occurs in other disease states for which epidemiological data are not yet available. It has been estimated that annual costs associated with atopic dermatitis in the United States alone total nearly $1 billion [17]. Given the high incidence of itch under other conditions, it is easy to imagine that costs could be several-fold higher, approaching some fraction of the estimated $100 billion in annual costs associated with chronic pain in the United States [74]. Thus, like chronic pain, chronic itch is a widespread, costly, and poorly treated health issue that requires research directed toward a better mechanistic understanding for the rational development of more effective treatments.

Scratching

Our knowledge of itch mechanisms, while less extensive compared to the data available on pain, has been advanced by animal studies assessing itch-related scratching behavior. Sherrington [96] first described the "scratch reflex" in spinalized dogs. Intrathecal microinjection of many agents elicits hindlimb scratching in rats and mice [29,131], even after spinalization [12]. Intradermal pruritogens evoke scratching that occurs in bouts of back-and-forth movements of the hindpaw against the itchy skin. Within-bout scratching movements have a constant frequency (~8 Hz for rats, ~12 Hz for mice) and duration (~2 seconds), while the number of scratching bouts varies with itch intensity [76]. These observations support a model in which a suprathreshold level of pruritic input activates spinal central pattern generators to initiate scratching, which reduces pruritic input to a subthreshold level. With increased intensity of the pruritic stimulus, the threshold to trigger scratching is reached sooner, resulting in a greater number of scratching bouts per unit of time. Furthermore, while stereotyped scratching is normally coupled with itch sensation, it can occur in its absence, just as reflexive limb withdrawals can be uncoupled from pain sensation by spinalization. To be useful, the scratching should be directed toward the site of itch. Rats with transections at the pontomedullary junction still exhibit grooming behavior [11], suggesting that the medulla and spinal cord may be sufficient for directed limb movements. Spinalized frogs exhibit hindlimb wiping that is accurately directed toward a stimulus on the forelimb, indicating that propriospinal systems are sufficient to accurately direct the limb toward an irritant stimulus [31]. It is tempting to speculate that mammals also possess propriospinal pathways that support accurate directed limb scratching in the absence of conscious sensation, as occurs when patients with chronic itch scratch themselves while asleep.

Animal Models of Itch

Scratching is a spinally organized motor response; it forms part of normal grooming behavior and may also occur under conditions of pain or irritation [26]. To be a useful behavioral measure in animals, scratching should reflect the properties of itch. Scratching should be selectively induced by stimuli that induce itch, but not pain, in humans. This criterion is satisfied for hindlimb scratching directed toward a site of pruritic stimulation, usually the rostral back of mice or rats [19]. Furthermore, algogens (capsaicin, formalin) that are painful in humans do not elicit dose-related scratching in rats [53] or mice [61]. In rats, the only reliable scratch inducer is 5-HT;

other pruritic agents tested, including histamine, do not elicit scratching [53,106]. In mice, a larger array of agents that are itchy to humans elicit dose-related scratching behavior [19,61]. Table II is a partial listing of such

Table II
Agents that are pruritic in humans and elicit hindlimb scratching in mice, and possible mechanisms (with references indicated in brackets)

Agent	Human Itch	Mouse Scratching	Mechanism
Histamine	+ [98]	+/– * [34,39,50]	H1/H4 receptor; phospholipase C-β
Serotonin	+ [28,36]	+ [136]	5-HT$_2$ receptor
Substance P	+ [37]	+ [1,2]	Mast cell degranulation
Tryptase, PAR-2 agonists	+ [101]	+ [97]	PAR-2
Compound 48/80	+ [123]	+ [61]	Mast cell degranulation
Chloroquine	+ [84]	+ [34]	?
Endothelin-1	+ [127]	+ [110]	?
Platelet-activating factor	+ [28]	+ [134]	PAF receptor
Leukotriene B4	+ [16]	+ [2]	LB4 receptor

Note: + pruritic or scratch-inducing; – not pruritic. PAR-2 = protease-activated receptor 2.
* Strain-dependent.

agents and possible mechanisms of action. These data suggest that the mouse may be a useful model for human itch.

An itchy area, such as a mosquito bite, is often surrounded by a region of normal skin within which light touch elicits itch, a phenomenon called alloknesis or itchy skin [33] that appears analogous to allodynia (pain elicited by a normally innocuous touch stimulus). Alloknesis may reflect central sensitization of itch-signaling neurons, discussed below. To my knowledge, alloknesis has not been tested in animal models. Another well-known hallmark of itch is that it is often evoked or enhanced by opioids and reduced by μ-opioid antagonists [43]. The latter dose-dependently suppressed 5-HT-evoked hindlimb scratching in rats [76,80] and mice [136], while morphine did not suppress 5-HT-evoked scratching or spinal c-fos expression, although it significantly attenuated capsaicin-evoked spinal c-fos expression [80]. Finally, an animal itch model should be sensitive to other factors that modulate itch, such as noxious and innocuous counterstimuli including heating, rubbing, or irritant chemicals [125,138], cooling [13,30,70], or psychological factors such as stress. As yet, such factors have been largely unexplored in animal models.

Two additional approaches have been used to assess acute itch. One is ocular scratching in guinea pigs [134], a model used to show dose-dependent hindlimb scratching directed toward a conjunctival site of application of histamine and platelet-activating factor in a pharmacologically specific manner. Another model is biting of the hindpaw following intradermal injection of serotonin in mice [38]. Serotonin dose-dependently elicited approximately equal numbers of bites and licks, whereas formalin elicited licking with almost no biting.

Intracranial [57,60,107], intramedullary [105], and intrathecal microinjection of opioids [29,131] elicits scratching behavior, possibly by activating central itch-signaling pathways (intracranial injections) or central pattern generators (spinal injections). Intracranial injection of several neuropeptides also elicits scratching and grooming, including substance P [93,117], thyrotropin-releasing hormone, bombesin, neurotensin, and neuromedin [57,115,116,118,119]. Scratching elicited by some of these agents was antagonized by naloxone [115,116], suggesting a role for opioid receptors.

There are several animal models of chronic itch, including the spontaneously "itchy" (NC/jic) mouse [108,135]; the hairless guinea pig [134]; and neonatal capsaicin treatment in rats, which resulted in spontaneous scratching by adults that was reduced by naloxone and enhanced by morphine [104]. Dry skin itch can be produced by daily treatment of the skin with diethyl ether and acetone to result in increased spontaneous scratching [67,77]. These models have been discussed previously [19].

There are also several animal models of allergic itch and contact dermatitis. A common cause of allergic itch is a mosquito bite. When given daily injections of the salivary gland extract from female mosquitoes, mice do not initially scratch but exhibit a marked increase in scratching over time as they become sensitized to the allergen [83]. Scratching in sensitized mice was not reduced by antagonists of histamine H1 or H2 receptors or other mast cell mediators, or by leukotriene B4 antagonists, but it was reduced by the 5-lipoxygenase inhibitor zileuton, suggesting a role for some 5-lipoxygenase metabolite other than leukotriene B4 in allergic itch following a mosquito bite [62]. Another model of allergic itch involves sensitization with an allergen such as dinitrofluorobenzene, followed by challenge with that allergen. This model was used to show allergic scratching that was not affected by serotonin 5-HT$_2$ or 5-HT$_3$ receptor antagonists [78].

In a promising new model of cholestatic itch, daily injections of small doses of ethynylestradiol in rats resulted in biliary cholestasis and a doubling of spontaneous scratching that was attenuated by the κ-opioid agonist nalfurafine [51]. Although previous experiments with biliary stenosis in rats did not reveal enhanced scratching [7], the stenotic animals exhibited increased hepatic opioids and mRNA for preproenkephalin [8,10]. Interestingly, plasma extracts taken from patients suffering from cholestatic itch, when injected into the medulla of monkeys, evoked scratching behavior that was reversed by naloxone [9]. These data suggest that under conditions of chronic itch due to liver cholestasis, there is an increase in circulating opioids that induce itch in a manner that is modulated via μ- and κ-opioid receptors.

Neural Transmission of Itch versus Pain: Separate or Overlapping Pathways?

Since von Frey's seminal publication of 1922 [122], researchers have debated whether itch represents a mild form of pain signaled by a common pathway (intensity theory), or whether itch and pain are distinct qualities with separate but interacting sensory pathways (specificity theory). The weight of current evidence supports specificity theory. As noted above, itch and pain have several distinguishing features, including different motor responses (scratch vs. withdrawal) and differential effects of opioids (increased itch, reduced pain). Furthermore, localized skin or intraneural electrical stimulation can elicit itch that becomes more intense but does not transform to pain at higher frequencies [92,111], nor does pain transform to itch at low stimulus frequencies.

Major support for specificity theory derives from recent observations of human mechanically insensitive C-fiber afferents that responded to cutaneous histamine over a time course matching concomitant itch sensation [90]. Spinothalamic tract neurons with similar properties are located in lamina I [4]. The superficial dorsal horn is implicated in itch as well as in pain, based on pruritogen-evoked activation of neurons there [54,72,80]. Very recently, the gastrin-releasing peptide receptor was identified as a candidate for spinal neurotransmission of itch [102], as discussed below. Collectively, these data support the existence of an itch-selective pathway. However, it would be an oversimplification to conclude that itch and pain are conveyed separately. Recent new information on peripheral receptors and central pathways and neuroimaging findings, detailed further below, blur the picture and indicate substantial overlap in the neural processing of itch and pain.

Peripheral Receptors

Histamine elicits a nearly pure sensation of itch in humans, causing a wheal at the injection site and flare in surrounding skin [98]. A subpopulation of mechanically insensitive C fibers responds to histamine over a time course that parallels concomitant itch sensation [90]. However, most of these fibers additionally respond to capsaicin and prostaglandin E_2 [91], indicating that they are selective but not specific for itch mediators. Moreover, electrocutaneous stimulation at thresholds too low to excite histamine-responsive C fibers also elicits itch sensation, suggesting the existence of other itch-signaling primary afferents [47]. Cutaneous application of spicules from the pods of the bean plant, cowhage, elicits itch [94] in the absence of flare [56]. Cowhage-induced itch was unaffected by antihistamines and was reduced by capsaicin desensitization of the skin, which, in contrast, did not significantly attenuate histamine-evoked itch [56]. The pruritogen in cowhage, originally called mucunain [95], was recently identified to be a cysteine protease that acts at protease-activated receptor (PAR) subtypes PAR-2 and PAR-4 [86]. PAR-2 has been implicated in nonhistaminergic itch [101]. Cowhage excites mechano- and heat-sensitive polymodal C-fiber nociceptors in cats [112], monkeys [55], and humans [73]. Interestingly, histamine elicited weaker responses, or was ineffective, in cowhage-responsive nociceptors [55,73], whereas cowhage did not excite mechanically insensitive C-fibers, including those responsive to histamine [73]. These data suggest that histaminergic and nonhistaminergic types of itch may be signaled by largely separate peripheral fibers. However, it is a challenge to the specificity theory that cowhage, which is itchy, excites C-fiber polymodal nociceptors that are thought to signal burning pain sensation.

Spinal Cord

Neurons in superficial laminae of the spinal dorsal horn have been implicated in itch as well as pain. Both pruritic and algesic agents evoke Fos expression in superficial dorsal horn neurons [54,80]. Lamina I neurons project in the spinothalamic tract of monkeys [132], cats [20], and rats [15,32]. Rodent lamina I neurons also project to the parabrachial nucleus and periaqueductal gray [66,100,109]. Both itch and pain are thought to be conveyed via the spinothalamic tract, at least in higher primates, since these sensory qualities are lost below the level of spinothalamic tractotomy in humans [128].

The vast majority of wide-dynamic-range (WDR) and nociceptive-specific (NS) neurons in lamina I of rats [52,53] and monkeys, including cells identified as spinothalamic tract neurons [25,99], respond to both pruritic and algesic stimuli. In the influential study of Andrew and Craig [4], two of four histamine-responsive, mechanically insensitive feline lamina I spinothalamic tract neurons tested also responded to the algesic agent mustard oil; none were tested with capsaicin. The prolonged time course of rat lamina I neuronal responses to 5-HT paralleled that of scratching behavior [53], and monkey spinothalamic tract neuronal responses to pruritogens were inhibited by scratching [25], consistent with a role for such neurons in itch. Subpopulations of primate spinothalamic tract WDR and NS neurons responded either to histamine or cowhage, but not both, and all units additionally responded to capsaicin [25]. Intradermal injection of the PAR-2 agonist SLIGRL-NH2 resulted in Fos expression in lamina I of mice, while intradermal histamine evoked Fos in inner lamina II [72]. These data are consistent with the differential responsiveness of mechanosensitive and mechanoinsensitive C-fiber afferents (see above), and suggest that histamine- and protease-evoked itch may be signaled by different neuronal subpopulations.

We have recently identified WDR- and NS-type lamina I neurons in the mouse lumbar spinal cord that respond to intradermal microinjection of SLIGRL-NH2 over a time course matching the 20–30-minute duration of scratching elicited by this agonist (Fig. 1). A large percentage of such neurons additionally responded to 5-HT (a scratch-inducer in mice), to noxious heating, and to the algesic agents mustard oil and capsaicin. We are currently investigating whether separate neurons respond to the PAR-2 agonist versus histamine.

Gastrin-releasing peptide (GRP) receptor is normally expressed in superficial dorsal horn neurons, and mutant mice lacking this receptor exhibit reduced scratching to pruritic agents while retaining normal pain sensitivity [102]. This finding suggests a role for GRP as an itch-specific neurotransmitter in the superficial dorsal horn. Another candidate is substance P, which is released from unmyelinated primary afferents terminating in the superficial dorsal horn to act at neurokinin-1 (NK1) receptors expressed by many lamina I neurons [14]. 5-HT-evoked scratching behavior was not reduced in mice lacking substance P [22]. However, this finding might be attributed to developmental compensation, given that destruction of superficial neurons expressing NK1 receptors by application of substance P-saporin in adult rats significantly attenuated 5-HT-evoked scratching behavior [18]. This finding suggests that superficial NK1-receptor-expressing neurons may be involved in signaling itch. Conceivably, substance P may excite superficial neurons involved in signaling itch, in addition to the accepted role it plays in spinal pain neurotransmission [75]. It is also conceivable that superficial NK1-expressing neurons coexpress other receptors, such as the GRP receptor, which mediates spinal itch transmission.

Neuroimaging of Brain Activation

Recent neuroimaging studies in humans indicate substantial overlap in cortical and subcortical regions that are activated during itch versus pain sensation [24,27,42,45,64,69,70,114,124]. Brain regions exhibiting increased metabolic activity during itch include the prefrontal, anterior insular, primary and secondary somatosensory, mid-cingulate, inferior parietal, premotor, and supplementary motor cortical areas, as well as the thalamus, caudate nucleus, and cerebellum. Activation of the ipsilateral supplementary motor cortex may represent an "urge to scratch." Importantly, recent studies using functional magnetic resonance imaging to directly compare cortical activation patterns during pain and itch reported

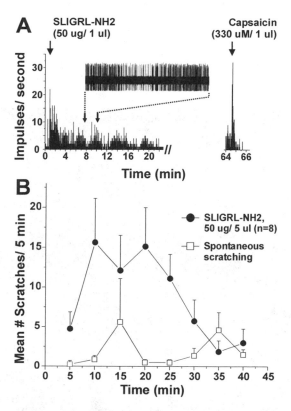

Fig. 1. Scratching and superficial dorsal horn neuronal activity elicited by intradermal microinjection of a protease-activated receptor-2 (PAR-2) agonist. (A) Peristimulus-time histogram (bins: 1 sec) of response of a mouse lumbar superficial dorsal horn neuron to intradermal microinjection of PAR-2 agonist SLIGRL-NH2 (50 µg/1 µL) into the hind-paw receptive field. Inset shows a train of action potentials taken from the time between arrows. The right-hand histogram shows the same neuron's response to intradermal microinjection of capsaicin. (B) Graph of the mean (± SEM) number of hindlimb scratching bouts at 5-minute intervals following intradermal microinjection of PAR-2 agonist SLIGRL-NH2 (50 µg/10 µL, ⊠) into the nape of neck of mice. Open squares show mean spontaneous scratching recorded separately in the same animals. Note that neuronal activity (A) increased immediately following the injection but persisted over a time course similar to that of scratching behavior (B).

substantial overlap in insular, cingulate, and prefrontal cortical areas, as well as the cerebellum [42,69] (Fig. 2). Notably, Herde et al. [42] repeatedly induced phasic itch by intracutaneous microdialysis of histamine and stopped the itch by infusion of a local anesthetic agent. In addition to the pattern of activation already described, the authors noted deactivation in the anterior cingulate cortex and amygdala, which they speculated might

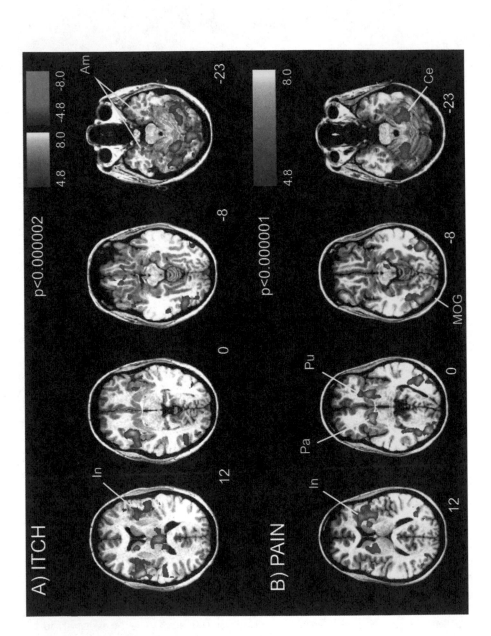

represent preparation to scratch [42]. Another recent study reported activation in similar areas (secondary somatosensory, insular, prefrontal, and inferior parietal cortex and cerebellum) as well as deactivation in the cingulate cortex, when subjects were passively scratched in the absence of itch [141].

Itch Theories

The preceding indicates that, to a large extent, itch and pain share common neural pathways. Mammalian superficial dorsal horn neurons respond to pruritic agents, but any involvement of such neurons in the central transmission of itch sensation must account for the finding that most, if not all, such neurons are also excited by noxious stimuli. One possibility is that itch and pain are signaled by a common neural population, consistent with frequency theory. Such an explanation belies the marked differences between itch and pain noted earlier. However, it should be remembered that WDR neurons can also respond at equivalent rates to noxious heat and innocuous brush stimuli [63], and it remains enigmatic how the central nervous system (CNS) distinguishes qualitatively distinct inputs from such multimodal neurons. Another possibility is that the CNS uses a population code. Activation of pruritogen-sensitive WDR and NS neurons signals itch, while increasing levels of noxious stimulation additionally recruit a larger population of pruritogen-insensitive WDR and NS neurons to signal pain and concomitantly suppress itch by occlusion or masking (Fig. 3).

← *Fig. 2.* Brain activation patterns recorded using functional magnetic resonance imaging (fMRI) under conditions of (A) histamine-induced itch or (B) noxious heat-evoked pain. (A) A mixture of histamine and codeine was delivered intracutaneously by microdialysis to elicit phasic itch, which was halted by microdialysis of a local anesthetic agent. (B) Heat pain was elicited by a Peltier thermode that increased in temperature until the subject reported moderate pain (60% on a visual analogue scale). Note overlapping regions of activation by both itch and pain in the insular and middle occipital cortical areas and cerebellum. Modified from Fig. 3 of reference [42], with permission. Abbreviations: Am = amygdala, Ce = cerebellum, In = insular cortex, MOG = middle occipital gyrus, Pa = pallidum, Pu = putamen.

E. Carstens

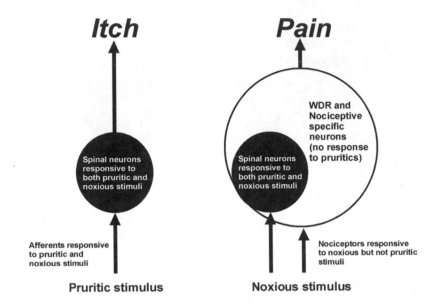

Fig. 3. Population coding of itch vs. pain. Pruritogens excite primary afferent fibers, which in turn excite wide-dynamic-range (WDR) and nociceptive-specific (NS) neurons in the superficial dorsal horn that transmit itch (left). Noxious stimulation excites nociceptors to recruit a larger population of pruritogen-insensitive spinal WDR and NS neurons that signal pain and simultaneously mask or occlude itch (right).

Sensitization of Itch

Just as pain may be exacerbated by sensitization of peripheral nociceptors and/or by central sensitization of WDR and NS neurons following injury, it is thought that itch transmission may be enhanced by analogous mechanisms under pathological conditions [137]. Central sensitization has been suggested to underlie the chronic itch of atopic dermatitis, since histamine elicits greater itch, and noxious stimuli elicit itch instead of pain in lesional skin [44,46,48], even though axon reflex flare (a measure of peripheral C-fiber activity) is reduced. Central sensitization may be triggered by spontaneous firing of pruriceptors from lesional skin [89], and the switch from pain to itch may reflect a pathological reduction in the normal inhibitory effect of pain on itch transmission. Few animal studies have thus far investigated central sensitization of itch due to limitations in our understanding of central itch transmission. We showed a significant increase in Fos expression in the superficial dorsal horn ipsilateral to dry skin treatment of one hindpaw in mice that were prevented from accessing the dry skin area by wearing an Elizabethan collar [79]. One possibility is that the dry skin itch sensation provided ongoing pruriceptive input to sensitize superficial itch-signaling neurons. Future studies of itch-signaling neurons under normal and pathological conditions will be useful in identifying mechanisms of sensitization related to chronic itch and showing how the process might be interrupted to relieve itch. Still in its infancy, research on itch mechanisms will benefit greatly from the wealth of information already available regarding chronic pain mechanisms.

Acknowledgments

The author's work was supported by grants from the National Institutes of Health.

References

[1]   Andoh T, Katsube N, Maruyama M, Kuraishi Y. Involvement of leukotriene B_4 in substance P-induced itch-associated response in mice. J Invest Dermatol 2001;117:1621–6.
[2]   Andoh T, Kuraishi Y. Intradermal leukotriene B4, but not prostaglandin E2, induces itch-associated responses in mice. Eur J Pharmacol 1998;353:93–6.
[3]   Andoh T, Nagasawa T, Satoh M, Kuraishi Y. Substance P induction of itch-associated response mediated by cutaneous NK1 tachykinin receptors in mice. J Pharmacol Exp Ther 1998;286:1140–5.
[4]   Andrew D, Craig AD. Spinothalamic lamina I neurons selectively sensitive to histamine: a central neural pathway for itch. Nat Neurosci 2001;4:72–7.
[5]   Ballantyne JC, Loach AB, Carr DB. Itching after epidural and spinal opiates. Pain 1988;33:149–60.
[6]   Bergasa NV. The pruritus of cholestasis. J Hepatol 2005;43:1078–88.
[7]   Bergasa NV, Alling DW, Vergalla J, Jones EA. Cholestasis in the male rat is associated with naloxone-reversible antinociception. J Hepatol 1994;20:85–90.
[8]   Bergasa NV, Sabol SL, Young WS, Kleiner DE, Jones EA. Cholestasis is associated with preproenkephalin mRNA expression in the adult rat liver. Am J Physiol 1995;268:G346–54.
[9]   Bergasa NV, Thomas DA, Vergalla J, Turner ML, Jones EA. Plasma from patients with the pruritus of cholestasis induces opioid receptor-mediated scratching in monkeys. Life Sci 1993;53:1253–7.
[10]   Bergasa NV, Vergalla J, Swain MG, Jones EA. Hepatic concentrations of proenkephalin-derived opioids are increased in a rat model of cholestasis. Liver 1996;16:298–302.
[11]   Berridge KC. Progressive degradation of serial grooming chains by descending decerebration. Behav Brain Res 1989;33:241–53.
[12]   Bossut D, Frenk H, Mayer DJ. Is substance P a primary afferent neurotransmitter for nociceptive input? II. Spinalization does not reduce and intrathecal morphine potentiates behavioral responses to substance P. Brain Res 1988;455:232–9.
[13]   Bromm B, Scharein E, Darsow U, Ring J. Effects of menthol and cold on histamine-induced itch and skin reactions in man. Neurosci Lett 1995;187:157–60.
[14]   Brown JL, Liu H, Maggio JE, Vigna SR, Mantyh PW, Basbaum AI. Morphological characterization of substance P receptor-immunoreactive neurons in the rat spinal cord and trigeminal nucleus caudalis. J Comp Neurol 1995;356:327–44.

[15] Burstein R, Dado RJ, Giesler GJ Jr. The cells of origin of the spinothalamic tract of the rat: a quantitative reexamination. Brain Res 1990;511:329–37.

[16] Camp RD, Coutts AA, Greaves MW, Kay AB, Walport MJ. Responses of human skin to intradermal injection of leukotrienes C4, D4 and B4. Br J Pharmacol 1983;80:497–502.

[17] Carroll CL, Balkrishnan R, Feldman SR, Fleischer AB Jr, Manuel JC. The burden of atopic dermatitis: impact on the patient, family, and society. Pediatr Dermatol 2005;22:192–9.

[18] Carstens E, Iodi-Carstens M, Simons CT. Reduced scratching in rats receiving intracisternal substance P-saporin to ablate cervical superficial dorsal horn neurons that express NK-1 receptors. Soc Neurosci Abstracts 2003;908.2.

[19] Carstens E, Kuraishi Y. Animal models of itch: scratching away at the problem. In: Yosipovitch G, Greaves MW, Fleischer AB, McGlone F, editors. Itch: basic mechanisms and therapy. Monticello, NY: Marcel Dekker; 2004. p. 35–50.

[20] Carstens E, Trevino DL. Laminar origins of spinothalamic projections in the cat as determined by the retrograde transport of horseradish peroxidase. J Comp Neurol 1978;182:161–5.

[21] Casaer M, Kums V, Wouters PJ, Van den Kerckhove E, Van den Berghe G. Pruritus in patients with small burn injuries. Burns 2008;34:185–91.

[22] Cuellar JM, Jinks SL, Simons CT, Carstens E. Deletion of the preprotachykinin A gene in mice does not reduce scratching behavior elicited by intradermal serotonin. Neurosci Lett 2003;339:72–6.

[23] Dalgard F, Dawn AG, Yosipovitch G. Are itch and chronic pain associated in adults? Results of a large population survey in Norway. Dermatology 2007;214:305–9.

[24] Darsow U, Drzezga A, Frisch M, Munz F, Weilke F, Bartenstein P, Schwaiger M, Ring J. Processing of histamine-induced itch in the human cerebral cortex: a correlation analysis with dermal reactions. J Invest Dermatol 2000;115:1029–33.

[25] Davidson S, Zhang X, Yoon CH, Khasabov SG, Simone DA, Giesler GJ Jr. The itch-producing agents histamine and cowhage activate separate populations of primate spinothalamic tract neurons. J Neurosci 2007;27:10007–14.

[26] De Castro-Costa M, Gybels J, Kupers R, Van Hees J. Scratching behaviour in arthritic rats: a sign of chronic pain or itch? Pain 1987;29:123–31.

[27] Drzezga A, Darsow U, Treede RD, Siebner H, Frisch M, Munz F, Weilke F, Ring J, Schwaiger M, Bartenstein P. Central activation by histamine-induced itch: analogies to pain processing: a correlational analysis of O-15 H_2O positron emission tomography studies. Pain 2001;92:295–305.

[28] Fjellner B, Hägermark O. Pruritus in polycythemia vera: treatment with aspirin and possibility of platelet involvement. Acta Derm Venereol 1979;59:505–12.

[29] Frenk H, Bossut D, Urca G, Mayer DJ. Is substance P a primary afferent neurotransmitter for nociceptive input? I. Analysis of pain-related behaviors resulting from intrathecal administration of substance P and 6 excitatory compounds. Brain Res 1988;455:223–31.

[30] Fruhstorfer H, Hermanns M, Latzke L. The effects of thermal stimulation on clinical and experimental itch. Pain 1986;24:259–69.

[31] Fukson OI, Berkinblit MB, Feldman AG. The spinal frog takes into account the scheme of its body during the wiping reflex. Science 1980;209:1261–3.

[32] Giesler GJ Jr, Ménétrey D, Basbaum AI. Differential origins of spinothalamic tract projections to medial and lateral thalamus in the rat. J Comp Neurol 1979;184:107–26.

[33] Graham DT, Goddell H, Woolf HG. Neural mechanisms involved in itch, itchy skin, and tickle sensations. J Clin Invest 1951;30:37–49.

[34] Green AD, Young KK, Lehto SG, Smith SB, Mogil JS. Influence of genotype, dose and sex on pruritogen-induced scratching behavior in the mouse. Pain 2006;124:50–8.

[35] Gunal AI, Ozalp G, Yoldas TK, Gunal SY, Kirciman E, Celiker H. Gabapentin therapy for pruritus in haemodialysis patients: a randomized, placebo-controlled, double-blind trial. Nephrol Dial Transplant 2004;19:3137–9.

[36] Hägermark O. Peripheral and central mediators of itch. Skin Pharmacol 1992;5:1–8.

[37] Hägermark O, Hökfelt T, Pernow B. Flare and itch induced by substance P in human skin. J Invest Dermatol 1978;71:233–5.

[38] Hagiwara K, Nojima H, Kuraishi Y. Serotonin-induced biting of the hind paw is itch-related response in mice. Pain Res 1999;14:53–9.

[39] Han SK, Mancino V, Simon MI. Phospholipase C beta 3 mediates the scratching response activated by the histamine H1 receptor on C-fiber nociceptive neurons. Neuron 2006;52:691–703.

[40] Hanifin JM, Reed ML; Eczema Prevalence and Impact Working Group. A population-based survey of eczema prevalence in the United States. Dermatitis 2007;18:82–91.

[41] Hengge UR, Currie BJ, Jäger G, Lupi O, Schwartz RA. Scabies: a ubiquitous neglected skin disease. Lancet Infect Dis 2006;6:769–79.

[42] Herde L, Forster C, Strupf M, Handwerker HO. Itch induced by a novel method leads to limbic deactivations a functional MRI study. J Neurophysiol 2007;98:2347–56.

[43] Heyer G, Dotzer M, Diepgen TL, Handwerker HO. Opiate and H1 antagonist effects on histamine induced pruritus and alloknesis. Pain 1997;73:239–43.

[44] Hosogi M, Schmelz M, Miyachi Y, Ikoma A. Bradykinin is a potent pruritogen in atopic dermatitis: a switch from pain to itch. Pain 2006;126:16–23.

[45] Hsieh JC, Hägermark O, Ståhle-Bäckdahl M, Ericson K, Eriksson L, Stone-Elander S, Ingvar M. Urge to scratch represented in the human cerebral cortex during itch. J Neurophysiol 1994;72:3004–8.

[46] Ikoma A, Fartasch M, Heyer G, Miyachi Y, Handwerker H, Schmelz M. Painful stimuli evoke itch in patients with chronic pruritus: central sensitization for itch. Neurology 2004;62:212–7.

[47] Ikoma A, Handwerker H, Miyachi Y, Schmelz M. Electrically evoked itch in humans. Pain 2005;113:148–54.

[48] Ikoma A, Rukwied R, Ständer S, Steinhoff M, Miyachi Y, Schmelz M. Neuronal sensitization for histamine-induced itch in lesional skin of patients with atopic dermatitis. Arch Dermatol 2003;139:1455–8.

[49] Ikoma A, Steinhoff M, Ständer S, Yosipovitch G, Schmelz M. The neurobiology of itch. Nat Rev Neurosci 2006;7:535–47.

[50] Inagaki N, Nagao M, Igeta K, Kawasaki H, Kim JF, Nagai H. Scratching behavior in various strains of mice. Skin Pharmacol Appl Skin Physiol 2001;14:87–96.

[51] Inan S, Cowan A. Nalfurafine, a kappa opioid receptor agonist, inhibits scratching behavior secondary to cholestasis induced by chronic ethynylestradiol injections in rats. Pharmacol Biochem Behav 2006;85:39–43.

[52] Jinks SL, Carstens E. Superficial dorsal horn neurons identified by intracutaneous histamine: chemonociceptive responses and modulation by morphine. J Neurophysiol 2000;84:616–27.

[53] Jinks SL, Carstens E. Responses of superficial dorsal horn neurons to intradermal serotonin and other irritants: comparison with scratching behavior. J Neurophysiol 2002;87:1280–9.

[54] Jinks SL, Simons CT, Dessirier JM, Carstens MI, Antognini JF, Carstens E. C-fos induction in rat superficial dorsal horn following cutaneous application of noxious chemical or mechanical stimuli. Exp Brain Res 2002;145:261–9.

[55] Johanek LM, Meyer RA, Friedman RM, Greenquist KW, Shim B, Borzan J, Hartke T, LaMotte RH, Ringkamp M. A role for polymodal C-fiber afferents in non-histaminergic itch. J Neurosci 2008;28:7659–69.

[56] Johanek LM, Meyer RA, Hartke T, Hobelmann JG, Maine DN, LaMotte RH, Ringkamp M. Psychophysical and physiological evidence for parallel afferent pathways mediating the sensation of itch. J Neurosci 2007;27:7490–7.

[57] Johnson MD, Ko M, Choo KS, Traynor JR, Mosberg HI, Naughton NN, Woods JH. The effects of the phyllolitorin analogue [desTrp(3), Leu(8)] phyllolitorin on scratching induced by bombesin and related peptides in rats. Brain Res 1999;839:194–8.

[58] Klein PA, Clark RA. An evidence-based review of the efficacy of antihistamines in relieving pruritus in atopic dermatitis. Arch Dermatol 1999;135:1522–5.

[59] Ko MC, Naughton NN. An experimental itch model in monkeys: characterization of intrathecal morphine-induced scratching and antinociception. Anesthesiology 2000;92:795–805.

[60] Königstein H. Experimental study of itch stimuli in animals. Arch Dermatol Syphilol 1948;57:829–49.

[61] Kuraishi Y, Nagasawa T, Hayashi K, Satoh M. Scratching behavior induced by pruritogenic but not algesiogenic agents in mice. Eur J Pharmacol 1995;275:229–33.

[62] Kuraishi Y, Ohtsuka E, Nakano T, Kawai S, Andoh T, Nojima H, Kamimura K. Possible involvement of 5-lipoxygenase metabolite in itch-associated response of mosquito allergy in mice. J Pharmacol Sci 2007;105:41–7.

[63] LeBars D, Chitour D. Do convergent neurones in the spinal dorsal horn discriminate nociceptive from non-nociceptive information? Pain 1983;17:1–19.

[64] Leknes SG, Bantick S, Willis CM, Wilkinson JD, Wise RG, Tracey I. Itch and motivation to scratch: an investigation of the central and peripheral correlates of allergen- and histamine-induced itch in humans. J Neurophysiol 2007;97:415–22.

[65] Mazeh D, Melamed Y, Cholostoy A, Aharonovitzch V, Weizman A, Yosipovitch G. Itching in the psychiatric ward. Acta Derm Venereol 2008;88:128–31.

[66] Menétrey D, De Pommery J. Origins of spinal ascending pathways that reach central areas involved in visceroception and visceronociception in the rat. Eur J Neurosci 1991;3:249–59.

[67] Miyamoto T, Nojima H, Shinkado T, Nakahashi T, Kuraishi Y. Itch-associated response induced by experimental dry skin in mice. Jpn J Pharmacol 2002;88:285–92.

[68] Mistik S, Utas S, Ferahbas A, Tokgoz B, Unsal G, Sahan H, Ozturk A, Utas C. An epidemiology study of patients with uremic pruritus. J Eur Acad Dermatol Venereol 2006;20:672–8.

[69] Mochizuki H, Sadato N, Saito DN, Toyoda H, Tashiro M, Okamura N, Yanai K. Neural correlates of perceptual difference between itching and pain: a human fMRI study. Neuroimage 2007;36:706–17.

[70] Mochizuki H, Tashiro M, Kano M, Sakurada Y, Itoh M, Yanai K. Imaging of central itch modulation in the human brain using positron emission tomography. Pain 2003;105:339–46.

[71] Murdoch ME, Asuzu MC, Hagan M, Makunde WH, Ngoumou P, Ogbuagu KF, Okello D, Ozoh G, Remme J. Onchocerciasis: the clinical and epidemiological burden of skin disease in Africa. Ann Trop Med Parasitol 2002;96:283–96.

[72] Nakano T, Andoh T, Lee JB, Kuraishi Y. Different dorsal horn neurons responding to histamine and allergic itch stimuli. Neuroreport 2008;19:723–6.

[73] Namer B, Carr R, Johanek LM, Schmelz M, Handwerker HO, Ringkamp M. Separate peripheral pathways for pruritus in man. J Neurophysiol 2008;100:2062–9.

[74] National Institutes of Health. NIH guide: new directions in pain research I. Bethesda, MD: National Institutes of Health; September 4, 1998.

[75] Nichols ML, Allen BJ, Rogers SD, Ghilardi JR, Honore P, Luger NM, Finke MP, Li J, Lappi DA, Simone DA, Mantyh PW. Transmission of chronic nociception by spinal neurons expressing the substance P receptor. Science 1999;286:1558–61.

[76] Nojima H, Carstens E. Quantitative assessment of directed hind limb scratching behavior as a rodent itch model. J Neurosci Methods 2003;126:137–43.

[77] Nojima H, Carstens MI, Carstens E. c-fos expression in superficial dorsal horn of cervical spinal cord associated with spontaneous scratching in rats with dry skin. Neurosci Lett 2003;347:62–4.

[78] Nojima H, Carstens E. 5-Hydroxytryptamine (5-HT)2 receptor involvement in acute 5-HT-evoked scratching but not in allergic pruritus induced by dinitrofluorobenzene in rats. J Pharmacol Exp Ther 2003;306:245–52.

[79] Nojima H, Cuellar JM, Simons CT, Carstens MI, Carstens E. Spinal c-fos expression associated with spontaneous biting in a mouse model of dry skin pruritus. Neurosci Lett 2004;361:79–82.

[80] Nojima H, Simons CT, Cuellar JM, Carstens MI, Moore JA, Carstens E. Opioid modulation of scratching and spinal c-fos expression evoked by intradermal serotonin. J Neurosci 2003;23:10784–90.

[81] Oaklander AL, Bowsher D, Galer B, Haanpää M, Jensen MP. Herpes zoster itch: preliminary epidemiologic data. J Pain 2003;4:338–43.

[82] Oaklander AL, Cohen SP, Raju SV. Intractable postherpetic itch and cutaneous deafferentation after facial shingles. Pain 2002;96:9–12.

[83] Ohtsuka E, Kawai S, Ichikawa T, Nojima H, Kitagawa K, Shirai Y, Kamimura K, Kuraishi Y. Roles of mast cells and histamine in mosquito bite-induced allergic itch-associated responses in mice. Jpn J Pharmacol 2001;86:97–105.

[84] Okor RS. Onset of pruritogenicity of chloroquine and the implication for the timing of suppressive therapy. J Clin Pharm Ther 1991;16:463–5.

[85] Pisoni RL, Wikström B, Elder SJ, Akizawa T, Asano Y, Keen ML, Saran R, Mendelssohn DC, Young EW, Port FK. Pruritus in haemodialysis patients: international results from the Dialysis Outcomes and Practice Patterns Study (DOPPS). Nephrol Dial Transplant 2006;21:3495–505.

[86] Reddy VB, Iuga AO, Shimada SG, LaMotte RH, Lerner EA. Cowhage-evoked itch is mediated by a novel cysteine protease: a ligand of protease-activated receptors. J Neurosci 2008;28:4331–5.

[87] Resneck JS Jr, Van Beek M, Furmanski L, Oyugi J, LeBoit PE, Katabira E, Kambugu F, Maurer T, Berger T, Pletcher MJ, Machtinger EL. Etiology of pruritic papular eruption with HIV infection in Uganda. JAMA 2004;292:2614–21.

[88] Sampogna F, Gisondi P, Melchi CF, Amerio P, Girolomoni G, Abeni D; IDI Multipurpose Psoriasis Research on Vital Experiences Investigators. Prevalence of symptoms experienced by patients with different clinical types of psoriasis. Br J Dermatol 2004;151:594–9.

[89] Schmelz M, Hilliges M, Schmidt R, Ørstavik K, Vahlquist C, Weidner C, Handwerker HO, Torebjörk HE. Active "itch fibers" in chronic pruritus. Neurology 2003;61:564–6.

[90] Schmelz M, Schmidt R, Bickel A, Handwerker HO, Torebjörk HE. Specific C-receptors for itch in human skin. J Neurosci 1997;17:8003–8.

[91] Schmelz M, Schmidt R, Weidner C, Hilliges M, Torebjork HE, Handwerker HO. Chemical response pattern of different classes of C-nociceptors to pruritogens and algogens. J Neurophysiol 2003;89:2441–8.

[92] Schmidt R, Torebjork E, Jorum E. Pain and itch from intraneural microstimulation. In: Abstracts of the 7th World Congress on Pain. Seattle: IASP; 1993. p. 143.

[93] Share NN, Rackham A. Intracerebral substance P in mice: behavioral effects and narcotic agents. Brain Res 1981;211:379–86.

[94] Shelley WB, Arthur RP. Studies on cowhage (Mucuna pruriens) and its pruritogenic proteinase, mucunain. AMA Arch Derm 1955;72:399–406.

[95] Shelley WE, Arthur RP. Mucunain, the active pruritogenic proteinase of cowhage. Science 1955;122:469–70.

[96] Sherrington CS. Observations on the scratch-reflex in the spinal dog. J Physiol 1906;34:1–50.

[97] Shimada SG, Shimada KA, Collins JG. Scratching behavior in mice induced by the proteinase-activated receptor-2 agonist, SLIGRL-NH2. Eur J Pharmacol 2006;530:281–3.

[98] Simone DA, Ngeow JY, Whitehouse J, Becerra-Cabal L, Putterman GJ, LaMotte RH. The magnitude and duration of itch produced by intracutaneous injections of histamine. Somatosens Res 1987;5:81–92.

[99] Simone DA, Zhang X, Li J, Zhang JM, Honda CN, LaMotte RH, Giesler GJ Jr. Comparison of responses of primate spinothalamic tract neurons to pruritic and algogenic stimuli. J Neurophysiol 2004;91:213–22.

[100] Spike RC, Puskár Z, Andrew D, Todd AJ. A quantitative and morphological study of projection neurons in lamina I of the rat lumbar spinal cord. Eur J Neurosci 2003;18:2433–48.

[101] Steinhoff M, Neisius U, Ikoma A, Fartasch M, Heyer G, Skov PS, Luger TA, Schmelz M. Proteinase-activated receptor-2 mediates itch: a novel pathway for pruritus in human skin. J Neurosci 2003;23:6176–80.

[102] Sun YG, Chen ZF. A gastrin-releasing peptide receptor mediates the itch sensation in the spinal cord. Nature 2007;448:700–3.

[103] Szepietowski JC, Reich A, Wiśnicka B. Itching in patients suffering from psoriasis. Acta Dermatovenerol Croat 2002;10:221–6.

[104] Thomas DA, Dubner R, Ruda MA. Neonatal capsaicin treatment in rats results in scratching behavior with skin damage: potential model of non-painful dysesthesia. Neurosci Lett 1994;171:101–4.

[105] Thomas DA, Hammond DL. Microinjection of morphine into the rat medullary dorsal horn produces a dose-dependent increase in facial scratching. Brain Res 1995;695:267–70.

[106] Thomsen JS, Petersen MB, Benfeldt E, Jensen SB, Serup J. Scratch induction in the rat by intradermal serotonin: a model for pruritus. Acta Derm Venereol 2001;81:250–4.

[107] Tohda C, Yamaguchi T, Kuraishi Y. Intracisternal injection of opioids induces itch-associated response through mu-opioid receptors in mice. Jpn J Pharmacol 1997;74:77–82.

[108] Tohda C, Yamaguchi T, Kuraishi Y. Increased expression of mRNA for myocyte-specific enhancer binding factor (MEF) 2C in the cerebral cortex of the itching mouse. Neurosci Res 1997;29:209–15.

[109] Todd AJ, Spike RC, Young S, Puskár Z. Fos induction in lamina I projection neurons in response to noxious thermal stimuli. Neuroscience 2005;131:209–17.

[110] Trentin PG, Fernandes MB, D'Orléans-Juste P, Rae GA. Endothelin-1 causes pruritus in mice. Exp Biol Med (Maywood) 2006;231:1146–51.

[111] Tuckett RP. Itch evoked by electrical stimulation of the skin. J Invest Dermatol 1982;79:368–73.

[112] Tuckett RP, Wei JY. Response to an itch-producing substance in cat. II. Cutaneous receptor populations with unmyelinated axons. Brain Res 1987;413:95–103.

[113] Twycross R, Greaves MW, Handwerker H, Jones EA, Libretto SE, Szepietowski JC, Zylicz Z. Itch: scratching more than the surface. QJM 2003;96:7–26.

[114] Valet M, Pfab F, Sprenger T, Wöller A, Zimmer C, Behrendt H, Ring J, Darsow U, Tölle TR. Cerebral processing of histamine-induced itch using short-term alternating temperature modulation: an FMRI study. J Invest Dermatol 2008;128:426–33.

[115] Van Wimersma Greidanus TB. Effects of naloxone and neurotensin on excessive grooming behavior of rats induced by bombesin, beta-endorphin and ACTH. NIDA Res Monogr 1986;75:477–80.

[116] Van Wimersma Greidanus TB, Maigret C. Neuromedin-induced excessive grooming/scratching behavior is suppressed by naloxone, neurotensin and a dopamine D1 receptor antagonist. Eur J Pharmacol 1991;209:57–61.

[117] Van Wimersma Greidanus TB, Maigret C. Grooming behavior induced by substance P. Eur J Pharmacol 1988;154:217–20.

[118] Van Wimersma Greidanus TB, Maigret C, Krechting B. Excessive grooming induced by somatostatin or its analog SMS 201-995. Eur J Pharmacol 1987;144:277–85.

[119] Van Wimersma Greidanus TB, Maigret C, Rinkel GJ, Metzger P, Panis M, Van Zinnicq Bergmann FE, Poelman PJ, Colbern DL. Some characteristics of TRH-induced grooming behavior in rats. Peptides 1988;9:283–8.

[120] Verhoeven EW, Kraaimaat FW, van de Kerkhof PC, van Weel C, Duller P, van der Valk PG, van den Hoogen HJ, Bor JH, Schers HJ, Evers AW. Prevalence of physical symptoms of itch, pain and fatigue in patients with skin diseases in general practice. Br J Dermatol 2007;156:1346–9.

[121] Vitale M, Fields-Blache C, Luterman A. Severe itching in the patient with burns. J Burn Care Rehabil 1991;12:330–3.

[122] von Frey M. Zur Physiologie der Juckempfindung. Arch Neerland Physiol 1922;7:142–5.

[123] Wahlgren CF, Hägermark O, Bergström R. Patients' perception of itch induced by histamine, compound 48/80 and wool fibres in atopic dermatitis. Acta Derm Venereol 1991;71:488–94.

[124] Walter B, Sadlo MN, Kupfer J, Niemeier V, Brosig B, Stark R, Vaitl D, Gieler U. Brain activation by histamine prick test-induced itch. J Invest Dermatol 2005;125:380–2.

[125] Ward L, Wright E, McMahon SB. A comparison of the effects of noxious and innocuous counterstimuli on experimentally induced itch and pain. Pain 1996;64:129–38.

[126] Wells J, Paech MJ, Evans SF. Intrathecal fentanyl-induced pruritus during labour: the effect of prophylactic ondansetron. Int J Obstet Anesth 2004;13:35–9.

[127] Wenzel RR, Zbinden S, Noll G, Méier B, Lüscher T. Endothelin-1 induces vasodilation in human skin by nociceptor fibres and release of nitric oxide. Br J Clin Pharmacol 1998;45:441–6.

[128] White JC, Sweet WH. Pain and the neurosurgeon: a forty year experience. New York: Thomas; 1969.

[129] Wikstrom B. Itchy skin—a clinical problem for haemodialysis patients. Nephrol Dial Transplant 2007;22(Suppl 5):v3–v7.

[130] Wikström B, Gellert R, Ladefoged SD, Danda Y, Akai M, Ide K, Ogasawara M, Kawashima Y, Ueno K, Mori A, Ueno Y. Kappa-opioid system in uremic pruritus: multicenter, randomized, double-blind, placebo-controlled clinical studies. J Am Soc Nephrol 2005;16:3742–7.

[131] Wilcox GL. Pharmacological studies of grooming and scratching behavior elicited by spinal substance P and excitatory amino acids. Ann N Y Acad Sci 1988;525:228–36.

[132] Willis WD, Kenshalo DR Jr, Leonard RB. The cells of origin of the primate spinothalamic tract. J Comp Neurol 1979;188:543–73.

[133] Wolkenstein P, Grob JJ, Bastuji-Garin S, Ruszczynski S, Roujeau JC, Revuz J; Société Française de Dermotologie. French people and skin diseases: results of a survey using a representative sample. Arch Dermatol. 2003;139:1614–9.

[134] Woodward DF, Nieves AL, Spada CS, Williams LS, Tuckett RP. Characterization of a behavioral model for peripherally evoked itch suggests platelet-activating factor as a potent pruritogen. J Pharmacol Exp Ther 1995;272:758–65.

[135] Yamaguchi T, Maekawa T, Nishikawa Y, Nojima H, Kaneko M, Kawakita T, Miyamoto T, Kuraishi Y. Characterization of itch-associated responses of NC mice with mite-induced chronic dermatitis. J Dermatol Sci 2001;25:20–8.

[136] Yamaguchi T, Nagasawa T, Satoh M, Kuraishi Y. Itch-associated response induced by intradermal serotonin through 5-HT2 receptors in mice. Neurosci Res 1999;35:77–83.

[137] Yosipovitch G, Carstens E, McGlone F. Chronic itch and chronic pain: analogous mechanisms. Pain 2007;131:4–7.

[138] Yosipovitch G, Duque MI, Fast K, Dawn AG, Coghill RC. Scratching and noxious heat stimuli inhibit itch in humans: a psychophysical study. Br J Dermatol 2007;156:629–34.

[139] Yosipovitch G, Goon A, Wee J, Chan YH, Goh CL. The prevalence and clinical characteristics of pruritus among patients with extensive psoriasis. Br J Dermatol 2000;143:969–73.

[140] Yosipovitch G, Goon AT, Wee J, Chan YH, Zucker I, Goh CL. Itch characteristics in Chinese patients with atopic dermatitis using a new questionnaire for the assessment of pruritus. Int J Dermatol 2002;41:212–6.

[141] Yosipovitch G, Ishiuji Y, Patel TS, Hicks MI, Oshiro Y, Kraft RA, Winnicki E, Coghill RC. The brain processing of scratching. J Invest Dermatol 2008;128:1806–11.

Correspondence to: E. Carstens, PhD, Department of Neurobiology, Physiology and Behavior, University of California, Davis, 1 Shields Avenue, Davis, CA 95616, USA. Email: eecarstens@ucdavis.edu.

The Role of Cytokines in Pain

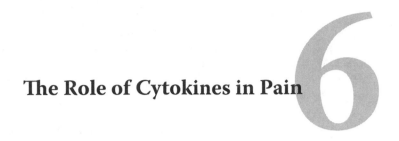

Claudia Sommer

Department of Neurology, University of Würzburg, Würzburg, Germany

Proinflammatory cytokines induce or enhance pain, whereas anti-inflammatory cytokines can have analgesic effects. For some cytokines, the mechanisms leading to pain have recently been clarified at the molecular level. Knowledge about the role of cytokines in pain, derived mainly from animal experiments, is increasingly being corroborated by clinical data. Gene therapy has been used to exploit the analgesic role of anti-inflammatory cytokines experimentally, and drugs modulating the cytokine system have started to find their way into clinical trials. This chapter will give a short overview of research on cytokines and pain during the last few decades and then focus on the latest data from cytokine research from bench to bedside, with a summary of current knowledge about clinical implications.

Proinflammatory Cytokines and Pain: Early Findings and Clues about Mechanisms

Pioneering work in this field was performed by the group of Sergio Ferreira, who first identified interleukin (IL)-1β as a mediator of inflammatory hyperalgesia [20] and recognized tumor necrosis factor (TNF) as a pivotal molecule in pain induced by carrageenin [13] in the periphery. Linda Watkins' and Joyce DeLeo's groups focused on the role of cytokines in the central nervous system, mostly in the spinal cord, and identified glial cells as the most important players in central hyperalgesia [16]. Interestingly, one of the very early studies on cytokines and pain found an analgesic action of high doses of centrally applied IL-1 [54]. A later study found an algesic action of low doses and an analgesic action of higher doses, which also depended on the precise site of injection [31].

Further interest in the modulation of pain by cytokines arose through observations on the "sickness response," the response of organisms to infection, associated with fever, fatigue, loss of appetite, and hyperalgesia [110]. In this context, hyperalgesia is regarded as one of the cytokine-mediated adaptive changes occurring during illness or injury, which are proposed to promote recuperation by decreasing energy use. Another factor that stimulated research on the role of cytokines in pain was research on chronic inflammatory diseases such as rheumatoid arthritis, where TNF and IL-1β are important pathogenic molecules, and where specific inhibitors can reduce both disease progression and pain [4].

In the early studies, cytokines were mostly regarded as molecules that induce algesic substances including prostaglandins or bradykinin, the known inducers of pain [60,77]. While this may be true in models of inflammatory pain, cyclooxygenase inhibition could only marginally reduce pain behavior after nerve injury or intraneural injection of TNF, indicating additional mechanisms [71]. Other factors induced by cytokines are the neuropeptides substance P and calcitonin gene-related peptide (CGRP), bradykinin, and nerve growth factor (NGF).

Later on, more and more direct actions of cytokines on nociceptors were identified (Fig. 1). TNF applied to peripheral nerve fibers lowers mechanical activation thresholds in C nociceptors, rapidly evokes ongoing activity in C fibers, increases plasma permeability and extravasation, and elicits mechanical allodynia [38,91]. Injection of IL-1β induces transient spontaneous discharges and hyperalgesia within 1 minute [21]. In a skin-nerve in vitro preparation, brief exposure of the skin to IL-1β facilitates heat-evoked CGRP release [58] from peptidergic neurons, which is a direct effect independent of changes in gene expression or receptor upregulation.

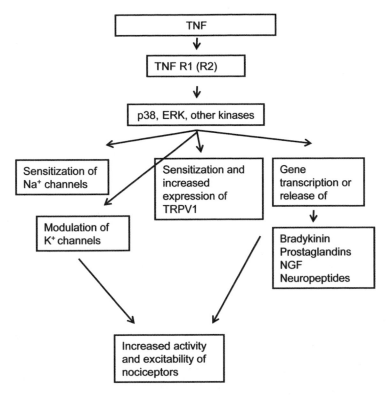

Fig. 1. Diagram with examples of peripheral mechanisms of how tumor necrosis factor (TNF), as a prototypic proinflammatory cytokine, might increase neuronal excitability in primary afferents. ERK = extracellular regulated kinase, NGF = nerve growth factor, TRPV1 = transient receptor potential vanilloid 1.

In vitro perfusion of dorsal root ganglia (DRG) with TNF elicits neuronal discharges in both A and C fibers and induces allodynia (for review see [72]). Application of nucleus pulposus to the DRG also induces spontaneous firing in dorsal horn wide-dynamic-range neurons; this activation is blocked by TNF antagonists, implying that the activity is cytokine mediated [12]. After nerve injury, subthreshold quantities of TNF injected into the DRG result in faster onset of allodynia and increased spontaneous pain behavior, suggesting increased sensitivity of nerve-injured DRG to TNF [70]. Furthermore, in the spinal nerve ligation (SNL) model with lesion of L5 and L6, the neighboring uninjured L4 DRG was sensitized to TNF just as much as the injured L5 ganglion. The reason for this finding has not been fully explained. Fibers from L4 and L5 intermingle in the sciatic nerve, such that uninjured L4 fibers are also in contact with the inflammatory mediators released because of the L5 lesion. Furthermore, a phenotype shift has been shown in uninjured neurons adjacent to injured ones, such that their expression of neurotransmitters, sodium channels, α-adrenergic receptors, and growth factors may change. For instance, in naive DRG, TNF was expressed only in small neurons, but after chronic constriction injury (CCI) it was also expressed in small and medium-sized neurons of injured nerves [69]. Using retrograde labeling with fluorophores, we could show that this phenotype shift was most prominent in neurons from the neighboring uninjured fibers. The pathophysiological role of this phenotype shift is as yet unknown, but it may well be related to the hypersensitivity of neighboring intact neurons observed in the electrophysiological experiments.

In a model of low back pain, TNF administered to a compressed DRG also enhanced ongoing allodynia [30], and after mechanical compression of the DRG, TNF-induced neuronal firing was enhanced [47]. IL-1β applied to dorsal roots increased the mechanosensitivity of the peripheral receptive fields [59]. While most investigators have used peripheral nerve or DRG preparations to show possible effects of cytokines on excitability, a recent study showed that lamina II neurons increase their activity after application of TNF, IL-1β, or IL-6 in spinal cord slices from rats [41]. Interestingly, TNF and IL-1β enhanced currents induced by amino-3-hydroxy-5-methyl-4-isoxazolepropionate (AMPA) or N-methyl-D-aspartate (NMDA), and IL-1β and IL-6 suppressed γ-aminobutyric acid (GABA)- and glycine-induced currents. Accordingly, in hippocampal neurons, TNF increases cell surface expression of the AMPA-receptor subunit GluR1 [6]. The increase in AMPA-receptor surface expression is triggered by the TNF receptor TNFR1 and requires phosphatidylinositol-3 kinase (PI3K) activity [92]. Thus, these cytokines were able to increase excitatory synaptic transmission and to decrease inhibitory synaptic transmission (Fig. 2). This finding may be important in the context of understanding the possible pathogenic role of proinflammatory cytokine profiles in patients with chronic pain, discussed below.

One pathway of cytokine-induced neuronal sensitization may involve the heat and proton sensor transient receptor potential vanilloid 1 (TRPV1). Brief applications of IL-1β to DRG potentiated heat-activated

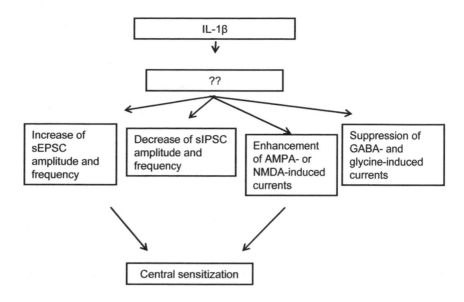

Fig. 2. Diagram with examples of central mechanisms of how interleukin (IL)-1β, as a prototypic proinflammatory cytokine, might increase neuronal excitability in spinal cord lamina II neurons. AMPA = α-amino-3-hydroxy-5-methyl-4-isoxazol-propionate, GABA = γ-aminobutyric acid, NMDA = *N*-methyl-D-aspartate, sEPSC = spontaneous excitatory postsynaptic current, sIPSC = spontaneous inhibitory postsynaptic current.

inward currents and shifted of activation thresholds toward lower temperatures without altering intracellular calcium levels. This IL-1β-induced heat sensitization was dependent on protein kinase C. IL-1 receptor I was found to be present on DRG neurons, such that IL-1β would be able to act on sensory neurons directly to increase their susceptibility to noxious heat [56]. TNF enhances TRPV1-mediated currents in DRG neurons [55], as was also found for brief applications of IL-1β [57]. Further, TNF increases the proportion of DRG neurons expressing TRPV1 via TNFR1 and increases the activation of extracellular regulated kinase (ERK) [29]. Topical application of TNF to nerve roots of rats increases phosphorylation of ERK with an onset time of several hours [95], whereas acute application of TNF to cultured DRG neurons induces phosphorylation of c-Jun terminal kinase (JNK) and protein kinase p38 (p38), but not ERK [61]. These findings suggest different roles for all three families of mitogen-activated protein kinases (MAPK).

Cytokines may also have direct effects on voltage-dependent ion channels. Recently, TNF was shown to rapidly enhance Na^+ currents [15].

The underlying mechanism may be that TNF induces tetrodotoxin-resistant (TTX-R) Na^+ currents in DRG neurons via activation of TNFR1 and p38 MAPK [36]. Indeed, phosphorylation of the sodium channel subtype $Na_V1.8$ by p38 MAPK occurred at the second transmembrane loop, which increased $Na_V1.8$ current density [33]. In addition, cytokine modulation of K^+ channels might contribute to regulation of action potentials [17,32]. Cytokine-induced modulation of voltage-gated Ca^{2+} currents has also been the subject of investigation. L-type Ca^{2+}-currents were increased by extended, but not acute, incubation of hippocampal neuronal cell cultures with TNF [22]. In DRG neurons, voltage-dependent Ca^{2+} channel (VDCC) currents were decreased voltage-dependently by TNF [15].

Phosphorylation of p38-MAPK, as needed for sensitization of $Na_V1.8$, also occurs in the spinal cord following nerve injury; the vast majority of phosphorylated p38 (phospho-p38) is found in the activated microglia [35,97], with only a small fraction being found in neurons. We observed the onset of spinal phospho-p38 at 5 hours after nerve injury, with levels reaching their peak at day 1 [75]. There were similar differences between pretreatment and post-treatment pain behavior in rats with spinal administration of the TNF antagonist etanercept or the p38 inhibitor SB203580 [75], again implying a triggering function for phospho-p38. Intrathecal administration of etanercept, starting pre-injury, blocked phosphorylation of p38 in the spinal cord [93]. These data imply that TNF acts both up- and downstream of p38 in the spinal cord.

In summary, the major net effect of proinflammatory cytokines, at least of those that have been studied in this regard, seems to be to enhance neuronal activity by a variety of nonexclusive mechanisms.

Cytokines in Neuropathic Pain: Experimental Studies

As a neurologist, I am exposed to the clinical problem of neuropathic pain, so my own work has focused on the role of cytokines in experimental neuropathic pain. The first impulse in this direction came from Bob Myers in San Diego, who hypothesized that TNF might be the major player in hyperalgesia induced in the then-novel animal model of neuropathic pain, CCI of the rat sciatic nerve [7]. In this model, we observed morphological changes that could very well be related to known actions of TNF, such as angiogenesis, endothelial hypertrophy, and narrowing of the vessel lumina [85]. Whether there was indeed a causal connection between TNF and these findings was not certain at the time, but our findings led to the first experiments trying to block TNF in this model. Using thalidomide, a readily available and relatively specific inhibitor of TNF, we were able reduce hyperalgesia and TNF levels in this model [26,84]. Later on, we confirmed this reduction of pain behavior by treating CCI mice with more specific TNF inhibitors such as the metalloprotease inhibitor TAPI, which blocks cleavage of cell-surface TNF and thus reduces levels of the mature 17-kDa TNF polypeptide [90], with antibodies to TNF and to its receptors [46,83,89], and with etanercept [88]. An antihyperalgesic action of the TNF inhibitors thalidomide, pentoxifylline, and others was then confirmed by several investigators [18,48,62,78,112]. Likewise, blocking IL-1 and IL-6 in neuropathic pain models reduced hyperalgesia in our studies and those of other groups [67,76,82,86]. The findings with inhibitors were corroborated by work in knockout mice [52,105,106,113,115] and in mice with delayed Wallerian degeneration and concomitantly delayed cytokine upregulation [53,87]. Blockade of an individual cytokine was never sufficient to entirely block pain behavior in our studies, so we tested local combinations of neutralizing antibodies, which had an additive affect [67], as shown even more impressively by DeLeo's group with intrathecal application [94].

Given that cytokine blockade was quite successful in reducing neuropathic pain behavior, the question arose as to where the cytokines in nerves came from. IL-1 was the first cytokine to be shown to be produced in Schwann cell cultures [8]. Wagner and Myers first showed by in situ hybridization that Schwann cells produce cytokines in intact nerves, and that cytokine production increases after nerve injury [108]. We measured cytokine contents at the protein level in injured nerves and found a rapid and sustained increase of TNF in sciatic nerves with CCI, and to a lesser extent in other nerve injury models [27]. When reverse transcription PCR became more widely available, several groups set out to measure cytokine gene expression in injured nerves, showing rapid, sustained, and sometimes biphasic increases in TNF, IL-1β, IL-6, and other cytokines (for review see [100]). Remarkably, after unilateral CCI, IL-1β also increases in the contralateral homologue nerve, sparing the neighboring femoral nerve [42]. This selective contralateral cytokine induction is mediated by NMDA receptors and indicates a spinal mechanism.

Having seen a peak of TNF induction at 1 day after CCI, we investigated TNF regulation at very early time points and found an increase of TNF and IL-1β gene expression as early as 1 hour after CCI. Unlike the peak at 24 hours, this early increase could not be blocked by the NMDA antagonist MK 801, but was abolished by the calpain inhibitor MDL-28170 [101]. We knew that the cytokines would not be able to act without their cognate receptors, so we and others investigated the temporal course of expression of TNF receptors R1 and R2 after nerve injury, finding a fast increase in TNFR1, but a delayed and sustained increase in TNFR2 in the injured nerve itself [24] and a biphasic increase of the receptors in injured and neighboring uninjured DRG neurons [73].

Studies on the mechanism of cytokine-induced hyperalgesia had led to the speculation that a portion of the large amount of cytokines produced in an injured nerve might be transported retrogradely to the DRG and there induce changes in gene transcription and thus in the properties of the DRG neurons [111]. We therefore investigated transport of endogenous and exogenously applied TNF in the sciatic nerve of rats. Transport of endogenous TNF was studied using the double ligature model [96]. Rat recombinant 125I-TNF was used to study transport of exogenously applied TNF. CGRP served as a positive control for anterograde transport, and NGF for retrograde transport. We were able to show with both methods that TNF was anterogradely transported in the peripheral nerve after intraneural injection and that it accumulated in the muscle [68]. Thus, muscular pain may contribute to neuropathic pain, given that muscle afferents produce ectopic activity after nerve injury [49]. Retrograde transport of TNF to the dorsal root ganglion (DRG) did not occur in our model, in contrast to retrograde transport of 125I-NGF. However, retrograde transport of TNF in the rat sciatic nerve could be demonstrated using biotinylated TNF [79]. Properties that have been elegantly demonstrated for the chemokine CCL2 (packing into synaptic vesicles, transport, and the ability to act as a neurotransmitter) [37] have not yet been shown for any of the cytokines.

The finding that TNF is transported from nerves to muscles prompted us to investigate what would happen if a muscle is injected with TNF directly. Using concentrations in the nanogram range, we found dose-dependent hyperalgesia in the animals with only minimal histological changes in the muscle. However, the muscle content of CGRP, NGF, and prostaglandin E_2 markedly increased [74], in accordance with a proalgesic effect. This TNF-induced experimental muscle pain could be blocked by drugs used to treat neuropathic pain [9]. One might speculate that cytokines produced intraneurally in nerve lesions and neuropathies in humans might also be transported into muscles and might partly explain why some neuropathic pains tend to change their character over time and resemble myofascial pain. Direct injection of proinflammatory cytokines into naive nerves also led to pain behavior [114]. In contrast to previous investigators, we used very low concentrations, similar to those detectable in injured tissue. We found a bell-shaped dose-response curve for both IL-1β and TNF, very similar to that seen in electrophysiological studies [38,70]. As already mentioned above, this peculiar dose-response curve may explain some of the apparent discrepancies in the literature, showing algesic or analgesic effects for the same cytokine.

Most studies on neuropathic pain have investigated cytokines related to the innate immune system. However, there is no reason why cytokines of the adaptive immune system should not be involved. Moalem and Tracey identified T-lymphocyte infiltration as a critical factor in CCI, and could furthermore show that pain was dependent on T-helper-1 (Th1) cells, the subtype producing proinflammatory cytokines [50]. We found a monophasic expression of IL-17A in degenerating nerves at day 7 after CCI, while transcripts for the IL-17A regulatory cytokines IL-23 and IL-15 peaked earlier. Accordingly, IL-17A-positive T cells were detectable within the endoneurium of the injured nerves by immunocytochemistry. RAG-1 knockout mice lacking functional T lymphocytes did not express IL-17A mRNA and had less thermal hyperalgesia and reduced mRNA levels for the macrophage marker molecule F4/80 and the chemokine CCL-2 after CCI, supporting the notion that T cells and T-cell-derived cytokines contribute to the inflammatory response after peripheral nerve injury [43].

Looking at the expression of the anti-inflammatory cytokine IL-10 after nerve injury, we found a rapid increase at the mRNA level, but a long-lasting depletion at the protein level, indicating loss of IL-10 as a possible cofactor in the maintenance of neuropathic pain [25]. Treatment with

thalidomide not only attenuated the increase in TNF and hyperalgesia after experimental nerve injury, but also helped to restore the decreased levels of IL-10 more rapidly [26]. This result is in accordance with the finding
of several groups that anti-inflammatory cytokines can attenuate hyperalgesia in pain models. A single 250-ng dose of IL-10 at the site and time of
a CCI had a long-lasting effect attenuating hyperalgesia [107]. In studies
with plantar inflammation in rats, IL-4 reduced hyperalgesia by inhibiting
the production of TNF, IL-1β, and IL-8 [14]. IL-4, IL-10, and IL-13 also
displayed analgesic activity in the writing test and in zymosan-induced
arthritis in mice [103].

Cytokines in Human Pain States

Rheumatoid Arthritis

The best-known human disease demonstrating an important role of proinflammatory cytokines in pain is rheumatoid arthritis, a chronic inflammatory disorder, in which the role of cytokines in disease progression
and pain generation has been recognized for many years [63]. Pain was
markedly reduced in patients receiving TNF antagonists during controlled
trials, a result that was later confirmed in clinical practice. The TNF antagonists etanercept and infliximab are now widely used in patients with
rheumatoid arthritis refractory to other treatments, as well as in other
chronic inflammatory diseases. The IL-1 antagonist anakinra is also effective in combination with methotrexate in patients with rheumatoid arthritis [11].

Back Pain

Following up on the experimental data indicating that cytokines mediate
pain in disk herniation, researchers measured cytokine levels in the vicin-
ity of herniated disks, in the cerebrospinal fluid, and in serum in humans.
Cytokine production was found in human disk material [10], and higher
levels of IL-8 correlated with pain [1]. Patients with persisting pain after
diskectomy had higher serum IL-6 levels than those without pain [23]. A
functional IL-1α polymorphism that increases IL-1α synthesis was found
to be associated with low back pain [81].

In a randomized controlled trial using etanercept in ankylosing spondylitis, etanercept was more efficient than placebo in reducing back pain [28]. The first preliminary studies using TNF inhibition in patients with chronic back pain of other etiologies have been reported. Case reports have shown perispinal etanercept to be efficacious in patients with chronic diskogenic pain, and an open-label study [40] and further case reports found an improvement in patients with low back pain with intravenous infliximab. Randomized controlled long-term trials will be necessary to show whether this treatment is really effective.

Temporomandibular Joint Dysfunction

Pain associated with dysfunction of the temporomandibular joint is another condition in which cytokines have been studied for several years (for review see [44]). IL-1β, IL-6, and TNF were found in joint fluid and were associated with worse outcome, with an emphasis on IL-6. In synovial cell fibroblasts, IL-1β induced expression of IL-8 and CCL-5. A deficiency in the anti-inflammatory mediators IL-1Ra, IL-10, and transforming growth factor (TGF)-β was also found in patients with temporomandibular dysfunction. Arthrocentesis with a perfusate volume of 300 to 400 mL can reduce inflammatory mediators and IL-6 in the temporomandibular joint fluid as a therapeutic measure [39].

Neuropathic Pain

Peripheral neuropathies may be painful or painless. One factor determining the painfulness of a neuropathy may be the individual tendency to react with high or low production of proinflammatory cytokines upon nerve injury [64]. The classical example of a correlation between cytokine levels and neuropathic pain is leprosy, in which a subgroup of patients have elevated serum levels of TNF and IL-1β and suffer from excruciating pain [66]. Treatment with thalidomide reduces TNF secretion in peripheral blood mononuclear cells by more than 90% and significantly reduces pain in these patients [5]. In two series of sural nerve biopsies, cytokine levels were increased more often in patients with painful neuropathies [19,45]. In a recent study we investigated the systemic mRNA and protein expression profile of patients with painful and painless neuropathies.

Independent of the underlying etiology, patients with painful neuropathy had higher blood mRNA and protein levels of TNF and IL-2. Patients with painless neuropathies had higher levels of the anti-inflammatory and analgesic cytokines IL-4 and IL-10 [99].

Small-fiber neuropathy describes a subgroup of sensory neuropathies with spontaneous burning pain or painful dysesthesias in the distal extremities as the main clinical symptoms. It is characterized by the functional and morphological involvement of the intraepidermal Aδ or C fibers. It can be associated with diabetes mellitus, Sjögren's syndrome, or Fabry's disease. In the majority of cases, however, no underlying reason can be found, and the cases remain idiopathic. Given that small-fiber neuropathy is characterized by localized pain, we assumed that there were alterations in cytokine expression in the affected skin. In a prospective study, we investigated the systemic (blood) and local (skin) cytokine profiles of 27 consecutive patients with small-fiber neuropathy and compared the results with healthy controls. In a subgroup of patients, cytokine expression in the painful skin was greatly increased compared to unaffected skin, whereas we found no changes in systemic cytokine profiles.

Fibromyalgia Syndrome and Chronic Widespread Pain

Chronic widespread pain (CWP) and fibromyalgia (FM) are disorders of largely unknown pathophysiology. Wallace and colleagues were the first to assume a connection between the pathogenesis of FM and cytokines. They observed that patients with malignancies, when treated with interleukin 2 (IL-2), developed FM-like symptoms, consisting of fatigue, poor sleep, and pain [109]. The results of further studies analyzing local or systemic cytokine expression in CWP and FM are divergent, mostly due to varying methodologies and the heterogeneity of the patient groups investigated. We examined a group of 55 patients and age- and gender-matched healthy controls with regard to their blood mRNA and serum protein levels of selected pro- and anti-inflammatory cytokines. Gene expression of the proinflammatory cytokines IL-2, IL-8, and TNF did not differ between patients and healthy controls, but expression of the anti-inflammatory cytokines IL-4 and IL-10 was significantly lower in patients compared with controls [102]. Serum protein levels of IL-4 and IL-10 were also significantly lower in the patient group compared to controls. The reason for the observed reduction of IL-4 and IL-10 expression at both the mRNA and protein level in the patients with CWP is unknown. No correlation was found between individual cytokine expression profile and the assessment of items including mood, sleep quality, fatigue, cognitive function, and pain. It is conceivable that restoring cytokine balance may be therapeutically useful in CWP and FM.

Complex Regional Pain Syndrome

Complex regional pain syndrome (CRPS) is another condition in which the cytokine system has been implicated. No differences in blood cytokine levels were found in a study comparing 26 patients with CRPS to controls [104]. However, in a study and comparing cytokine levels in blister fluid from the affected and the unaffected side, a local increase in IL-1β and TNF was found [34]. Recently, we found an increase in TNF and IL-2 mRNA and protein levels in the blood of patients with CRPS, along with a reduction in the anti-inflammatory cytokines IL-4, IL-10, and TGF-β [98]. In the cerebrospinal fluid, a proinflammatory profile was found by some researchers [3], but not by others [51].

Other Diseases

An extensive literature describes the role of cytokines in the pathogenesis of the disease and the related pain in endometriosis (for review see [80]), cystitis and other types of pelvic pain, angina [2], pancreatitis [65], myeloma, AIDS, and sepsis. Discussion of these disorders is beyond the scope of this chapter, but looking at parallels between these disorders and other chronic pain conditions may lead to a better understanding of their pathophysiology.

Open Questions

In contrast to the in vitro and in vivo animal studies, it is difficult to judge cause-and-effect relationships in most of the human studies. Obviously, most of these studies show associations between a painful disorder and a certain cytokine profile, but whether the cytokines involved are causally related to the pain remains unclear in most cases. Furthermore, most studies are cross-sectional, and few longitudinal data are available. However, sometimes a successful treatment with a cytokine inhibitor does point to a causal relationship between a cytokine and pain. More work will have to be done in this area. Furthermore, although a number of known mechanisms can explain how cytokines might directly or indirectly excite or sensitize nociceptors, the relative importance of these different mechanisms remains to be explored. Signal transduction pathways are being investigated, and it remains to be determined whether drugs interacting with these pathways might lead to useful analgesics. Also, we would like to know more about cytokine and chemokine interactions, and whether these mediators act in a cascade or in a network. The latter question is of importance in devising treatment directed at pathologically increased cytokines or altered cytokine profiles in patients with chronic pain.

Conclusions

A large amount of preclinical data has emerged over the last few years to elucidate the role of cytokines in different pain models and the molecular mechanisms by which cytokines may alter the function of nociceptive neurons. Clinical data on the function of cytokines in human pain states are also accumulating, supporting the relevance of these molecules for pain in clinical practice. Further work is needed to elucidate possible causal relationships and their impact on the treatment of pain.

Acknowledgments

The authors' work was supported by the German Bundesministerium für Bildung und Forschung (BMBF), Deutscher Forschungsverbund Neuropathischer Schmerz (DFNS), by Deutsche Forschungsgemeinschaft SFB 581, and by intramural funds from the University of Würzburg.

References

[1] Ahn SH, Cho YW, Ahn MW, Jang SH, Sohn YK, Kim HS. mRNA expression of cytokines and chemokines in herniated lumbar intervertebral discs. Spine 2002;27:911–7.
[2] Alam SE, Nasser SS, Fernainy KE, Habib AA, Badr KF. Cytokine imbalance in acute coronary syndrome. Curr Opin Pharmacol 2004;4:166–70.

[3] Alexander GM, Perreault MJ, Reichenberger ER, Schwartzman RJ. Changes in immune and glial markers in the CSF of patients with Complex Regional Pain Syndrome. Brain Behav Immun 2007;21:668–76.

[4] Arend WP, Dayer JM. Cytokines and cytokine inhibitors or antagonists in rheumatoid arthritis. Arthritis Rheum 1990;33:305–15.

[5] Barnes PF, Chatterjee D, Brennan PJ, Rea TH, Modlin RL. Tumor necrosis factor production in patients with leprosy. Infection and immunity 1992;60:1441–6.

[6] Beattie EC, Stellwagen D, Morishita W, Bresnahan JC, Ha BK, Von Zastrow M, Beattie MS, Malenka RC. Control of synaptic strength by glial TNFalpha. Science 2002;295:2282–5.

[7] Bennett GJ, Xie YK. A peripheral mononeuropathy in rat that produces disorders of pain sensation like those seen in man. Pain 1988;33:87–107.

[8] Bergsteinsdottir K, Kingston A, Mirsky R, Jessen KR. Rat Schwann cells produce interleukin-1. J Neuroimmunol 1991;34:15–23.

[9] Beyreuther BK, Geis C, Stöhr T, Sommer C. Antihyperalgesic efficacy of lacosamide in a rat model for muscle pain induced by TNF. Neuropharmacology 2007;52:1312–7.

[10] Burke JG, RW GW, Conhyea D, McCormack D, Dowling FE, Walsh MG, Fitzpatrick JM. Human nucleus pulposus can respond to a pro-inflammatory stimulus. Spine 2003;28:2685–93.

[11] Cohen SB, Moreland LW, Cush JJ, Greenwald MW, Block S, Shergy WJ, Hanrahan PS, Kraishi MM, Patel A, Sun G, Bear MB. A multicentre, double blind, randomised, placebo controlled trial of anakinra (Kineret), a recombinant interleukin 1 receptor antagonist, in patients with rheumatoid arthritis treated with background methotrexate. Ann Rheum Dis 2004;63:1062–8.

[12] Cuellar JM, Montesano PX, Carstens E. Role of TNF-alpha in sensitization of nociceptive dorsal horn neurons induced by application of nucleus pulposus to L5 dorsal root ganglion in rats. Pain 2004;110:578–87.

[13] Cunha FQ, Poole S, Lorenzetti BB, Ferreira SH. The pivotal role of tumour necrosis factor alpha in the development of inflammatory hyperalgesia. Br J Pharmacol 1992;107:660–4.

[14] Cunha FQ, Poole S, Lorenzetti BB, Veiga FH, Ferreira SH. Cytokine-mediated inflammatory hyperalgesia limited by interleukin-4. Br J Pharmacol 1999;126:45–50.

[15] Czeschik JC, Hagenacker T, Schafers M, Busselberg D. TNF-alpha differentially modulates ion channels of nociceptive neurons. Neurosci Lett 2008;434:293–8.

[16] DeLeo JA, Tanga FY, Tawfik VL. Neuroimmune activation and neuroinflammation in chronic pain and opioid tolerance/hyperalgesia. Neuroscientist 2004;10:40–52.

[17] Diem R, Meyer R, Weishaupt JH, Bahr M. Reduction of potassium currents and phosphatidylinositol 3-kinase-dependent AKT phosphorylation by tumor necrosis factor-alpha rescues axotomized retinal ganglion cells from retrograde cell death in vivo. J Neurosci 2001;21:2058–66.

[18] Dorazil-Dudzik M, Mika J, Schafer MK, Li Y, Obara I, Wordliczek J, Przewlocka B. The effects of local pentoxifylline and propentofylline treatment on formalin-induced pain and tumor necrosis factor-alpha messenger RNA levels in the inflamed tissue of the rat paw. Anesth Analg 2004;98:1566–73.

[19] Empl M, Renaud S, Erne B, Fuhr P, Straube A, Schaeren-Wiemers N, Steck AJ. TNF-alpha expression in painful and nonpainful neuropathies. Neurology 2001;56:1371–7.

[20] Ferreira SH, Lorenzetti BB, Bristow AF, Poole S. Interleukin-1 beta as a potent hyperalgesic agent antagonized by a tripeptide analogue. Nature 1988;334:698–700.

[21] Fukuoka H, Kawatani M, Hisamitsu T, Takeshige C. Cutaneous hyperalgesia induced by peripheral injection of interleukin-1 beta in the rat. Brain Res 1994;657:133–40.

[22] Furukawa K, Mattson MP. The transcription factor NF-kappaB mediates increases in calcium currents and decreases in NMDA- and AMPA/kainate-induced currents induced by tumor necrosis factor-alpha in hippocampal neurons. J Neurochem 1998;70:1876–86.

[23] Geiss A, Rohleder N, Kirschbaum C, Steinbach K, Bauer HW, Anton F. Predicting the failure of disc surgery by a hypofunctional HPA axis: evidence from a prospective study on patients undergoing disc surgery. Pain 2005;114:104–17.

[24] George A, Buehl A, Sommer C. Tumor necrosis factor receptor 1 and 2 proteins are differentially regulated during Wallerian degeneration of mouse sciatic nerve. Exp Neurol 2005;192:163–6.

[25] George A, Kleinschnitz C, Zelenka M, Brinkhoff J, Stoll G, Sommer C. Wallerian degeneration after crush or chronic constriction injury of rodent sciatic nerve is associated with a depletion of endoneurial interleukin-10 protein. Exp Neurol 2004;188:187–91.

[26] George A, Marziniak M, Schafers M, Toyka KV, Sommer C. Thalidomide treatment in chronic constrictive neuropathy decreases endoneurial tumor necrosis factor-alpha, increases interleukin-10 and has long-term effects on spinal cord dorsal horn met-enkephalin. Pain 2000;88:267–75.

[27] George A, Schmidt C, Weishaupt A, Toyka KV, Sommer C. Serial determination of tumor necrosis factor-alpha content in rat sciatic nerve after chronic constriction injury. Exp Neurol 1999;160:124–32.

[28] Gorman JD, Sack KE, Davis JC, Jr. Treatment of ankylosing spondylitis by inhibition of tumor necrosis factor alpha. N Engl J Med 2002;346:1349–56.

[29] Hensellek S, Brell P, Schaible HG, Brauer R, Segond von Banchet G. The cytokine TNFalpha increases the proportion of DRG neurones expressing the TRPV1 receptor via the TNFR1 receptor and ERK activation. Mol Cell Neurosci 2007;36:381–91.

[30] Homma Y, Brull SJ, Zhang JM. A comparison of chronic pain behavior following local application of tumor necrosis factor alpha to the normal and mechanically compressed lumbar ganglia in the rat. Pain 2002;95:239–46.

[31] Hori T, Oka T, Hosoi M, Aou S. Pain modulatory actions of cytokines and prostaglandin E2 in the brain. Ann NY Acad Sci 1998;840:269–81.

[32] Houzen H, Kikuchi S, Kanno M, Shinpo K, Tashiro K. Tumor necrosis factor enhancement of transient outward potassium currents in cultured rat cortical neurons. J Neurosci Res 1997;50:990–9.

[33] Hudmon A, Choi JS, Tyrrell L, Black JA, Rush AM, Waxman SG, Dib-Hajj SD. Phosphorylation of sodium channel Na(v)1.8 by p38 mitogen-activated protein kinase increases current density in dorsal root ganglion neurons. J Neurosci 2008;28:3190–201.

[34] Huygen FJ, De Bruijn AG, De Bruin MT, Groeneweg JG, Klein J, Zijlstra FJ. Evidence for local inflammation in complex regional pain syndrome type 1. Mediators Inflamm 2002;11:47–51.

[35] Jin SX, Zhuang ZY, Woolf CJ, Ji RR. p38 mitogen-activated protein kinase is activated after a spinal nerve ligation in spinal cord microglia and dorsal root ganglion neurons and contributes to the generation of neuropathic pain. J Neurosci 2003;23:4017–22.

[36] Jin X, Gereau RWt. Acute p38-mediated modulation of tetrodotoxin-resistant sodium channels in mouse sensory neurons by tumor necrosis factor-alpha. J Neurosci 2006;26:246–55.

[37] Jung H, Toth PT, White FA, Miller RJ. Monocyte chemoattractant protein-1 functions as a neuromodulator in dorsal root ganglia neurons. J Neurochem 2008;104:254–63.

[38] Junger H, Sorkin LS. Nociceptive and inflammatory effects of subcutaneous TNFalpha. Pain 2000;85:145–51.

[39] Kaneyama K, Segami N, Nishimura M, Sato J, Fujimura K, Yoshimura H. The ideal lavage volume for removing bradykinin, interleukin-6, and protein from the temporomandibular joint by arthrocentesis. J Oral Maxillofac Surg 2004;62:657–61.

[40] Karppinen J, Korhonen T, Malmivaara A, Paimela L, Kyllonen E, Lindgren KA, Rantanen P, Tervonen O, Niinimaki J, Seitsalo S, Hurri H. Tumor necrosis factor-alpha monoclonal antibody, infliximab, used to manage severe sciatica. Spine 2003;28:750–753.

[41] Kawasaki Y, Zhang L, Cheng JK, Ji RR. Cytokine mechanisms of central sensitization: distinct and overlapping role of interleukin-1beta, interleukin-6, and tumor necrosis factor-alpha in regulating synaptic and neuronal activity in the superficial spinal cord. J Neurosci 2008;28:5189–94.

[42] Kleinschnitz C, Brinkhoff J, Sommer C, Stoll G. Contralateral cytokine gene induction after peripheral nerve lesions: dependence on the mode of injury and NMDA receptor signaling. Brain Res Mol Brain Res 2005;136:23–8.

[43] Kleinschnitz C, Hofstetter HH, Meuth SG, Braeuninger S, Sommer C, Stoll G. T cell infiltration after chronic constriction injury of mouse sciatic nerve is associated with interleukin-17 expression. Exp Neurol 2006;200:480–5.

[44] Kopp S, Sommer C. Inflammatory mediators in temporomandibular joint pain. In: Türp J, Sommer C, Hugger A, editors. The puzzle of orofacial pain: integrating research into clinical management. Basel: Karger; 2007.

[45] Lindenlaub T, Sommer C. Cytokines in sural nerve biopsies from inflammatory and non-inflammatory neuropathies. Acta Neuropathol 2003;105:593–602.

[46] Lindenlaub T, Teuteberg P, Hartung T, Sommer C. Effects of neutralizing antibodies to TNF-alpha on pain-related behavior and nerve regeneration in mice with chronic constriction injury. Brain Res 2000;866:15–22.

[47] Liu B, Li H, Brull SJ, Zhang JM. Increased sensitivity of sensory neurons to tumor necrosis factor alpha in rats with chronic compression of the lumbar ganglia. J Neurophysiol 2002;88:1393–9.

[48] Liu J, Feng X, Yu M, Xie W, Zhao X, Li W, Guan R, Xu J. Pentoxifylline attenuates the development of hyperalgesia in a rat model of neuropathic pain. Neurosci Lett 2007;412:268–72.

[49] Michaelis M, Liu X, Janig W. Axotomized and intact muscle afferents but no skin afferents develop ongoing discharges of dorsal root ganglion origin after peripheral nerve lesion. J Neurosci 2000;20:2742–8.

[50] Moalem G, Xu K, Yu L. T lymphocytes play a role in neuropathic pain following peripheral nerve injury in rats. Neuroscience 2004;129:767–77.

[51] Munts AG, Zijlstra FJ, Nibbering PH, Daha MR, Marinus J, Dahan A, van Hilten JJ. Analysis of cerebrospinal fluid inflammatory mediators in chronic complex regional pain syndrome related dystonia. Clin J Pain 2008;24:30–4.

[52] Murphy PG, Ramer MS, Borthwick L, Gauldie J, Richardson PM, Bisby MA. Endogenous interleukin-6 contributes to hypersensitivity to cutaneous stimuli and changes in neuropeptides associated with chronic nerve constriction in mice. Eur J Neurosci 1999;11:2243–53.

[53] Myers RR, Heckman HM, Rodriguez M. Reduced hyperalgesia in nerve-injured WLD mice: relationship to nerve fiber phagocytosis, axonal degeneration, and regeneration in normal mice. Exp Neurol 1996;141:94–101.

[54] Nakamura H, Nakanishi K, Kita A, Kadokawa T. Interleukin-1 induces analgesia in mice by a central action. Eur J Pharmacol 1988;149:49–54.

[55] Nicol GD, Lopshire JC, Pafford CM. Tumor necrosis factor enhances the capsaicin sensitivity of rat sensory neurons. J Neurosci 1997;17:975–82.

[56] Obreja O, Rathee PK, Lips KS, Distler C, Kress M. IL-1 beta potentiates heat-activated currents in rat sensory neurons: involvement of IL-1RI, tyrosine kinase, and protein kinase C. FASEB J 2002;16:1497–503.

[57] Obreja O, Schmelz M, Poole S, Kress M. Interleukin-6 in combination with its soluble IL-6 receptor sensitises rat skin nociceptors to heat, in vivo. Pain 2002;96:57–62.

[58] Opree A, Kress M. Involvement of the proinflammatory cytokines tumor necrosis factor-alpha, IL-1 beta, and IL-6 but not IL-8 in the development of heat hyperalgesia: effects on heat-evoked calcitonin gene-related peptide release from rat skin. J Neurosci 2000;20:6289–93.

[59] Özaktay AC, Kallakuri S, Takebayashi T, Cavanaugh JM, Asik I, DeLeo JA, Weinstein JN. Effects of interleukin-1 beta, interleukin-6, and tumor necrosis factor on sensitivity of dorsal root ganglion and peripheral receptive fields in rats. Eur Spine J 2006;15:1529–37.

[60] Perkins MN, Kelly D. Interleukin-1 beta induced-desArg9bradykinin-mediated thermal hyperalgesia in the rat. Neuropharmacology 1994;33:657–60.

[61] Pollock J, McFarlane SM, Connell MC, Zehavi U, Vandenabeele P, MacEwan DJ, Scott RH. TNF-alpha receptors simultaneously activate Ca^{2+} mobilisation and stress kinases in cultured sensory neurones. Neuropharmacology 2002;42:93–106.

[62] Raghavendra V, Tanga F, Rutkowski MD, DeLeo JA. Anti-hyperalgesic and morphine-sparing actions of propentofylline following peripheral nerve injury in rats: mechanistic implications of spinal glia and proinflammatory cytokines. Pain 2003;104:655–64.

[63] Ridderstad A, Abedi-Valugerdi M, Moller E. Cytokines in rheumatoid arthritis. Ann Med 1991;23:219–23.

[64] Rutkowski JL, Tuite GF, Lincoln PM, Boyer PJ, Tennekoon GI, Kunkel SL. Signals for proinflammatory cytokine secretion by human Schwann cells. J Neuroimmunol 1999;101:47–60.

[65] Saluja A, Dudeja V, Phillips P. Inflammation and pain in pancreatic disorders: summary of the symposium sponsored by the American Pancreatic Association and the National Pancreas Foundation (Chicago, November 4–5, 2005). Pancreas 2006;33:184–191.

[66] Sarno EN, Grau GE, Vieira LM, Nery JA. Serum levels of tumour necrosis factor-alpha and interleukin-1 beta during leprosy reactional states. Clin Exp Immunol 1991;84:103–8.

[67] Schäfers M, Brinkhoff J, Neukirchen S, Marziniak M, Sommer C. Combined epineurial therapy with neutralizing antibodies to tumor necrosis factor-alpha and interleukin-1 receptor has an additive effect in reducing neuropathic pain in mice. Neurosci Lett 2001;310:113–6.

[68] Schäfers M, Geis C, Brors D, Yaksh TL, Sommer C. Anterograde transport of tumor necrosis factor-alpha in the intact and injured rat sciatic nerve. J Neurosci 2002;22:536–45.

[69] Schäfers M, Geis C, Svensson CI, Luo ZD, Sommer C. Selective increase of tumour necrosis factor-alpha in injured and spared myelinated primary afferents after chronic constrictive injury of rat sciatic nerve. Eur J Neurosci 2003;17:791–804.

[70] Schäfers M, Lee DH, Brors D, Yaksh TL, Sorkin LS. Increased sensitivity of injured and adjacent uninjured rat primary sensory neurons to exogenous tumor necrosis factor-alpha after spinal nerve ligation. J Neurosci 2003;23:3028–38.

[71] Schäfers M, Marziniak M, Sorkin LS, Yaksh TL, Sommer C. Cyclooxygenase inhibition in nerve-injury- and TNF-induced hyperalgesia in the rat. Exp Neurol 2004;185:160–8.

[72] Schäfers M, Sorkin L. Effect of cytokines on neuronal excitability. Neurosci Lett 2008;437:188–93.

[73] Schäfers M, Sorkin LS, Geis C, Shubayev VI. Spinal nerve ligation induces transient upregulation of tumor necrosis factor receptors 1 and 2 in injured and adjacent uninjured dorsal root ganglia in the rat. Neurosci Lett 2003;347:179–82.

[74] Schäfers M, Sorkin LS, Sommer C. Intramuscular injection of tumor necrosis factor-alpha induces muscle hyperalgesia in rats. Pain 2003;104:579–88.

[75] Schäfers M, Svensson CI, Sommer C, Sorkin LS. Tumor necrosis factor-alpha induces mechanical allodynia after spinal nerve ligation by activation of p38 MAPK in primary sensory neurons. J Neurosci 2003;23:2517–21.

[76] Schoeniger-Skinner DK, Ledeboer A, Frank MG, Milligan ED, Poole S, Martin D, Maier SF, Watkins LR. Interleukin-6 mediates low-threshold mechanical allodynia induced by intrathecal HIV-1 envelope glycoprotein gp120. Brain Behav Immun 2007;21:660–7.

[77] Schweizer A, Feige U, Fontana A, Muller K, Dinarello CA. Interleukin-1 enhances pain reflexes. Mediation through increased prostaglandin E$_2$ levels. Agents Actions 1988;25:246–51.

[78] Sharma S, Kulkarni SK, Agrewala JN, Chopra K. Curcumin attenuates thermal hyperalgesia in a diabetic mouse model of neuropathic pain. Eur J Pharmacol 2006;536:256–61.

[79] Shubayev VI, Myers RR. Anterograde TNF alpha transport from rat dorsal root ganglion to spinal cord and injured sciatic nerve. Neurosci Lett 2002;320:99–101.

[80] Siristatidis C, Nissotakis C, Chrelias C, Iacovidou H, Salamalekis E. Immunological factors and their role in the genesis and development of endometriosis. J Obstet Gynaecol Res 2006;32:162–70.

[81] Solovieva S, Leino-Arjas P, Saarela J, Luoma K, Raininko R, Riihimaki H. Possible association of interleukin 1 gene locus polymorphisms with low back pain. Pain 2004;109:8–19.

[82] Sommer C. Tierexperimentelle Untersuchungen bei neuropathischem Schmerz: die pathogene und therapeutische Bedeutung von Zytokinen und Zytokinrezeptoren. Schmerz 1999;13:315–23.

[83] Sommer C, Lindenlaub T, Teuteberg P, Schafers M, Hartung T, Toyka KV. Anti-TNF-neutralizing antibodies reduce pain-related behavior in two different mouse models of painful mononeuropathy. Brain Res 2001;913:86–9.

[84] Sommer C, Marziniak M, Myers RR. The effect of thalidomide treatment on vascular pathology and hyperalgesia caused by chronic constriction injury of rat nerve. Pain 1998;74:83–91.

[85] Sommer C, Myers RR. Vascular pathology in CCI neuropathy: a quantitative temporal study. Exp Neurol 1996;141:113–9.

[86] Sommer C, Petrausch S, Lindenlaub T, Toyka KV. Neutralizing antibodies to interleukin 1-receptor reduce pain associated behavior in mice with experimental neuropathy. Neurosci Lett 1999;270:25–8.

[87] Sommer C, Schäfers M. Painful mononeuropathy in C57BL/Wld mice with delayed wallerian degeneration: differential effects of cytokine production and nerve regeneration on thermal and mechanical hypersensitivity. Brain Res 1998;784:154–62.

[88] Sommer C, Schäfers M, Marziniak M, Toyka KV. Etanercept reduces hyperalgesia in experimental painful neuropathy. J Peripher Nerv Syst 2001;6:67–72.

[89] Sommer C, Schmidt C, George A. Hyperalgesia in experimental neuropathy is dependent on the TNF receptor 1. Exp Neurol 1998;151:138–42.

[90] Sommer C, Schmidt C, George A, Toyka KV. A metalloprotease-inhibitor reduces pain associated behavior in mice with experimental neuropathy. Neurosci Lett 1997;237:45–8.

[91] Sorkin LS, Xiao WH, Wagner R, Myers RR. Tumour necrosis factor-alpha induces ectopic activity in nociceptive primary afferent fibres. Neuroscience 1997;81:255–62.

[92] Stellwagen D, Beattie EC, Seo JY, Malenka RC. Differential regulation of AMPA receptor and GABA receptor trafficking by tumor necrosis factor-alpha. J Neurosci 2005;25:3219–28.

[93] Svensson CI, Schäfers M, Jones TL, Powell H, Sorkin LS. Spinal blockade of TNF blocks spinal nerve ligation-induced increases in spinal P-p38. Neurosci Lett 2005;379:209–13.

[94] Sweitzer S, Martin D, DeLeo JA. Intrathecal interleukin-1 receptor antagonist in combination with soluble tumor necrosis factor receptor exhibits an anti-allodynic action in a rat model of neuropathic pain. Neuroscience 2001;103:529–39.

[95] Takahashi N, Kikuchi S, Shubayev VI, Campana WM, Myers RR. TNF-alpha and phosphorylation of ERK in DRG and spinal cord: insights into mechanisms of sciatica. Spine 2006;31:523–9.
[96] Tonra JR, Curtis R, Wong V, Cliffer KD, Park JS, Timmes A, Nguyen T, Lindsay RM, Acheson A, DiStefano PS. Axotomy upregulates the anterograde transport and expression of brain-derived neurotrophic factor by sensory neurons. J Neurosci 1998;18:4374–83.
[97] Tsuda M, Mizokoshi A, Shigemoto-Mogami Y, Koizumi S, Inoue K. Activation of p38 mitogen-activated protein kinase in spinal hyperactive microglia contributes to pain hypersensitivity following peripheral nerve injury. Glia 2004;45:89–95.
[98] Üçeyler N, Eberle T, Rolke R, Birklein F, Sommer C. Differential expression patterns of cytokines in complex regional pain syndrome. Pain 2007;132:195–205.
[99] Üçeyler N, Rogausch JP, Toyka KV, Sommer C. Differential expression of cytokines in painful and painless neuropathies. Neurology 2007;69:42–9.
[100] Üçeyler N, Sommer C. Cytokine regulation in animal models of neuropathic pain and in human diseases. Neurosci Lett 2008;437:194–8.
[101] Üçeyler N, Tscharke A, Sommer C. Early cytokine expression in mouse sciatic nerve after chronic constriction nerve injury depends on calpain. Brain Behav Immun 2007;21:553–60.
[102] Üçeyler N, Valenza R, Stock M, Schedel R, Sprotte G, Sommer C. Reduced levels of antiinflammatory cytokines in patients with chronic widespread pain. Arthritis Rheum 2006;54:2656–64.
[103] Vale ML, Marques JB, Moreira CA, Rocha FA, Ferreira SH, Poole S, Cunha FQ, Ribeiro RA. Antinociceptive effects of interleukin-4, -10, and -13 on the writhing response in mice and zymosan-induced knee joint incapacitation in rats. J Pharmacol Exp Ther 2003;304:102–8.
[104] van de Beek WJ, Remarque EJ, Westendorp RG, van Hilten JJ. Innate cytokine profile in patients with complex regional pain syndrome is normal. Pain 2001;91:259–61.
[105] Vogel C, Lindenlaub T, Tiegs G, Toyka KV, Sommer C. Pain-related behavior in TNF-receptor deficient mice. In: Devor M, Rowbotham MC, Wiesenfeld-Hallin Z, editors. Proceedings of the 9th World Congress on Pain. Progress in Pain Research and Management, Vol. 16. Seattle: IASP Press; 2003. p. 249–57.
[106] Vogel C, Stallforth S, Sommer C. Altered pain behavior and regeneration after nerve injury in TNF receptor deficient mice. J Peripher Nerv Syst 2006;11:294–303.
[107] Wagner R, Janjigian M, Myers RR. Anti-inflammatory interleukin-10 therapy in CCI neuropathy decreases thermal hyperalgesia, macrophage recruitment, and endoneurial TNF-alpha expression. Pain 1998;74:35–42.
[108] Wagner R, Myers RR. Schwann cells produce tumor necrosis factor alpha: expression in injured and non-injured nerves. Neuroscience 1996;73:625–9.
[109] Wallace DJ, Margolin K, Waller P. Fibromyalgia and interleukin-2 therapy for malignancy. Ann Intern Med 1988;108:909.
[110] Watkins LR, Maier SF. Immune regulation of central nervous system functions: from sickness responses to pathological pain. J Intern Med 2005;257:139–55.
[111] Watkins LR, Maier SF, Goehler LE. Immune activation: the role of pro-inflammatory cytokines in inflammation, illness responses and pathological pain states. Pain 1995;63:289–302.
[112] Xu JT, Xin WJ, Zang Y, Wu CY, Liu XG. The role of tumor necrosis factor-alpha in the neuropathic pain induced by Lumbar 5 ventral root transection in rat. Pain 2006;123:306–21.
[113] Xu XJ, Hao JX, Andell-Jonsson S, Poli V, Bartfai T, Wiesenfeld-Hallin Z. Nociceptive responses in interleukin-6-deficient mice to peripheral inflammation and peripheral nerve section. Cytokine 1997;9:1028–33.
[114] Zelenka M, Schäfers M, Sommer C. Intraneural injection of interleukin-1beta and tumor necrosis factor-alpha into rat sciatic nerve at physiological doses induces signs of neuropathic pain. Pain 2005;116:257–63.
[115] Zhong J, Dietzel ID, Wahle P, Kopf M, Heumann R. Sensory impairments and delayed regeneration of sensory axons in interleukin-6-deficient mice. J Neurosci 1999;19:4305–13.

Correspondence to: Prof. Dr. Claudia Sommer, Department of Neurology, University of Würzburg, Josef-Schneider-Str. 11, D-97080 Wuerzburg, Germany. Tel: +49-931-201-23763; fax: +49-931-201-23697; email: sommer@uni-wuerzburg.de.

Neuronal Mechanisms of Joint Pain

Hans-Georg Schaible

Department of Neurophysiology, Institute of Physiology, Jena University Clinic, Jena, Germany

Joint pain is a frequent and debilitating problem. In a recent survey, Breivik et al. [8] reported on the prevalence of chronic pain in Europe, its impact on daily life, and the success of treatment. Of the 46,394 people interviewed from 15 European countries, 19% complained about chronic pain. Chronic pain had to fulfil the following criteria: pain lasting at least 6 months, pain occurring in the last month at least twice per week, and pain intensity of at least 5 on a scale from 0 to 10. Eight percent of the respondents complained about pain in the hip, 9% about pain in the shoulder, 10% about pain in the joints (unspecified), and 16% about pain in the knee. Major causes of joint pain were rheumatoid arthritis (8% of respondents); arthritis/osteoarthritis (34% of respondents); cartilage damage (4% of respondents); and traumatic injury, which often affects joints (12% of respondents) [8]. These data clearly show that deep tissue, including the joints, is a major site of clinically relevant pain and that major causes of such pain are inflammation, trauma, and degeneration.

Current Topics in Pain: 12th World Congress on Pain
edited by José Castro-Lopes
IASP Press, Seattle, © 2009

The Nociceptive System of the Joint

Selective mechanical stimulation of structures in the joint can evoke sensations. Dye et al. [19] performed neurosensory mapping of the internal structures of the human knee without intraarticular anesthesia (the skin was anesthetized). In all structures of the joint—including the ligaments, fibrous capsule, adipose tissue, meniscus, periosteum, and synovial layer—it was possible to evoke conscious sensations. Only stimulation of the cartilage did not elicit sensations. Evoked conscious sensations ranged from nonpainful awareness to slight or moderate discomfort to severe pain. The findings of Dye et al. [19] confirmed a previous study of Kellgren and Samuel [44], who were able to evoke nonpainful pressure sensations with innocuous mechanical stimulation and pain with noxious mechanical and chemical stimulation of the internal structures of the joint in conscious human subjects.

Pain in a normal, healthy joint is elicited only by movements that exceed the working range of motion of the joint (for example, twisting the joint against the resistance of the joint structures) or by strong pressure on the joint. Movements in the working range of a normal joint are not usually painful, and palpation of a normal joint does not hurt. By contrast, when the joint is inflamed, movements within the working range of motion are often painful, and pain may be elicited by palpation of the joint, indicating mechanical hyperalgesia. Pain in the joints and other deep tissues is often dull and aching, and it is poorly localized, in contrast to cutaneous pain [49]. The different character of cutaneous and deep somatic tissue pain led to the proposal that the neuronal organization of cutaneous and deep-tissue nociceptive transmission is different [49]. In addition to the unpleasant sensation, patients often report that joint pain leads to a loss of strength.

Types of Joint Afferents That Encode Noxious Mechanical Stimuli Applied to the Joint

In order to identify nociceptive joint afferents, various researchers on joint afferents have made recordings from the nerves of large joints such as the knee, ankle, or elbow. The joint nerves contain Aβ, Aδ, and C fibers. Thick myelinated Aβ fibers are proprioceptors because most of them respond to innocuous mechanical stimuli such as light pressure onto the joint structures and movements within the working range of the joint. The majority of these fibers do not encode noxious stimuli, although they are coactivated by noxious stimulation. Most of the nociceptive fibers are unmyelinated C fibers, but some belong to a subgroup of thin myelinated Aδ fibers. They either show a weak response to innocuous mechanical stimuli (such as a rotation of the joint to the limit of its normal working range) and a pronounced response to noxious stimuli (such as rotation against the resistance of the tissue), or they respond only to noxious but not to innocuous stimuli. A further group of fibers do not respond to any innocuous and noxious mechanical stimulus as long as the joint is unaffected. Many of these fibers are "silent nociceptors," which are initially mechanoinsensitive but become mechanosensitive when inflammation develops in the joint [68,70].

Fig. 1 shows the typical setup for recordings from afferent fibers of the medial articular nerve of the knee joint of the rat (Fig. 1a), typical receptive fields of C fibers in the joint (Fig. 1b), and the response pattern of a C fiber that responds weakly to innocuous stimuli (outward or inward rotation) but shows a pronounced response to noxious outward rotation of the joint (Fig. 1c). Most Aδ and C fibers are not only mechanosensitive but also chemosensitive. This property is important for activation and sensitization during inflammation.

Spinal Neurons with Nociceptive Joint Input

Afferent fibers of large joints project to several segments of the spinal cord. Studies using horseradish peroxidase labeling have identified projection fields of joint afferents of the knee joint in both the superficial and deep dorsal horn [14]. In general, the localization of fibers in these laminae matches the localization of spinal cord cells expressing c-Fos protein, such as during urate arthritis in the rat ankle joint [52]. Thus, information from the knee joint is processed in the superficial as well as the deep dorsal horn of the spinal cord.

Electrophysiological recordings from the spinal cord of anesthetized cats and rats have revealed two main types of spinal cord neurons with input from the joints. Most neurons show convergent inputs from the skin and from deep tissues such as the joints and the adjacent muscles.

Often the receptive field in the skin is located more distally than the receptive fields in the deep tissue, thus enabling distinct stimulation of receptive fields in the deep tissue versus the skin. The other type of neurons have convergent inputs from deep tissue such as the joints and other deep structures, but not from the skin. Most of the neurons with convergent inputs from skin and deep tissue are wide-dynamic-range neurons that show small responses to innocuous stimuli (for example,

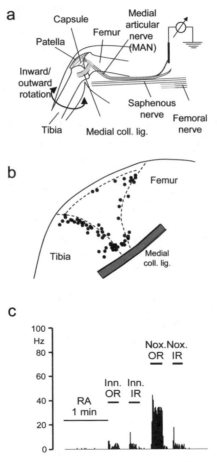

Fig. 1. (a) Experimental set-up for recording from single fibers of the medial articular nerve (MAN) of the exposed rat knee joint. (b) Centers of mechanical receptive fields of C fibers (dots) in the joint capsule. (c) Peristimulus time histogram showing responses of a C fiber to movements of the knee joint. RA = resting activity, Inn. OR = innocuous outward rotation, Inn. IR = innocuous inward rotation, Nox. OR = noxious outward rotation, Nox. IR = noxious inward rotation. Reproduced from Brenn et al. [9].

light to moderate pressure) and strong responses to noxious stimuli applied to the joint (such as noxious pressure or twisting movements). The remaining neurons and most of the neurons with deep input are nociceptive-specific neurons, which respond only to noxious stimuli applied to the joint and other tissues. Neurons with deep-tissue input are either ascending tract neurons or local interneurons [68,70].

Supraspinal Neurons with Nociceptive Joint Input

Nociceptive neurons with input from the joints (and other deep tissues) have also been identified in the thalamus, cortex, and amygdala. In the cat, nociceptive neurons with input from muscles and tendons have been identified in the ventral and dorsolateral periphery of the ventroposterolateral nucleus (VPL) and in the transitional zone between the VPL and the ventrolateral nucleus. While most of these neurons had convergent inputs from the skin and deep tissue, a small proportion of neurons responded only to noxious stimulation of the muscle and tendon [45]. In the cat, electrical stimulation of Aδ fibers in the medial articular nerve of the knee joint [38] and injection of algesic substances into the knee joint artery [39] activated thalamic wide-dynamic-range neurons with convergent cutaneous and deep inputs in this region. By contrast, in the rat, nociceptive neurons with input from the skin and joints have been found intermingled with tactile neurons throughout the ventrobasal complex [33]. In the cat, nociceptive neurons with very large and often bilateral receptive fields with convergent inputs from the skin and deep tissue have been identified in the posterior complex [18,38] and in the medial nucleus of the thalamus [18].

In the rat, the somatosensory cortex contains a large proportion of neurons that respond to noxious stimulation, and a small proportion of these neurons are driven by deep input [46]. Electrical stimulation of Aβ and Aδ fibers in the posterior articular nerve of the rat knee evoked field potentials in the primary and secondary somatosensory cortices [36]. More recently, neurons were identified in the amygdala that are also driven by joint stimulation [34,41,50].

Thus, nociceptive input from the joint is processed in neurons of the central nervous system that show convergent inputs from the skin and deep tissue, as well as in neurons that show only deep input. The relative contribution of these types of neurons to joint pain is unknown. However, both types of neurons show similar changes in their discharge properties during inflammation, suggesting that both types are important in inflammation-evoked pain.

Models of Joint Inflammation

Experimental models are being used to investigate neuronal mechanisms of clinically relevant inflammatory joint pain. Acute inflammation that develops within 2 to 4 hours can be induced by injection of kaolin and carrageenan or of carrageenan alone into the joint [72]. Within 4 hours the joint becomes significantly swollen, and infiltration of inflammatory cells can be observed. Awake animals develop significant limping to protect the injected joint. The mechanical threshold for withdrawal responses at the injected knee is significantly lowered within the first 4 hours and remains stable between 6 and 12 hours, when inflammation is fully established. The advantages of acute inflammatory models are that identified neurons can be recorded throughout the development of inflammation and that the generation of hyperexcitability can be monitored directly [73,74]. In fact, most neurophysiological studies on joint pain have used the kaolin/carrageenan model. Although these models are mainly used as acute models of inflammation, they can also be adapted as chronic models.

Because human joint inflammation is often chronic (such as in rheumatoid arthritis), chronic models are necessary to study the full range of neurobiological reactions to inflammation. Chronic models of inflammation can be unilateral or may present as polyarthritis. Chronic unilateral forms of inflammation are arthritis induced by complete Freund's adjuvant (CFA) or antigen-induced arthritis (AIA), an immune-mediated inflammation that is dependent on T cells. To produce CFA-induced arthritis, CFA is injected into the joint cavity or around the joint [30]. In order to induce AIA, rats or mice are immunized against the antigen methylated bovine serum albumin (m-BSA). Two weeks later, m-BSA is injected into the knee joint. Unilateral AIA shows an acute phase and spontaneously progresses into a chronic inflammation [27,64,77]. Examples of chronic forms of polyarthritis are CFA polyarthritis [13] or collagen-induced arthritis (CIA). The latter is induced by immunization with type II collagen in CFA that causes an autoimmune disease directed against the cartilage in the joint [40,85]. In particular, CIA and AIA are used in rheumatological research because they are immunologically induced and show many similarities to human rheumatoid arthritis. A repeated injection of m-BSA into the knee joint induces a pronounced flare-up of inflammation in the AIA model [11].

More recently, CIA and AIA have been used in pain research. The course of mechanical hyperalgesia at the knee joint in the AIA model is shown in Fig. 2a, and the swelling is displayed in Fig. 2b. Mechanical hyperalgesia is most pronounced on days 1–7 of AIA (the acute phase, characterized by fibrin exudation and invasion of granulocytes), but it is still present up to day 21 after knee injection (the chronic phase, characterized by infiltration of mononuclear cells, synovial hyperplasia, fibrosis in the periarticular structures, and some cartilage and bone destruction). Rats also show significant changes in their locomotor behavior. The guarding score in locomotor behavior (for details see [7,77]) is highest on days 1–3 of AIA, but some guarding persists up to day 21. In addition, the rats show thermal hyperalgesia in the paw, which is interpreted as secondary hyperalgesia [7].

Peripheral Sensitization
(Sensitization of Joint Afferents)

An important mechanism of inflammation-induced mechanical hyperalgesia is the sensitization of joint afferents to mechanical stimuli applied to the inflamed joint. Mechanical sensitization of joint nociceptors can be shown easily and reliably. It is induced within the first few hours after onset of inflammation [72,73], and it can persist over weeks in chronic models of inflammation [32]. Low-threshold $A\delta$ fibers show increased responses to innocuous and noxious mechanical stimulation of the joint. High-threshold $A\delta$ and C fibers show a reduced mechanical threshold and enhanced responses to noxious stimuli. Finally, numerous silent nociceptors develop sensitivity to mechanical stimulation of the inflamed joint. This recruitment of fibers significantly increases the input into the spinal cord [28,72,73].

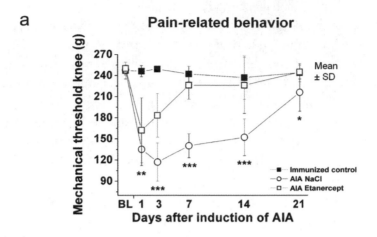

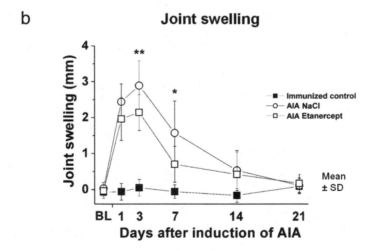

Fig. 2. Outcome of treatment of rats with antigen-induced arthritis (AIA) with systemic etanercept (open squares) or saline (NaCl, circles) for 21 days. Immunized rats without inflammation and treatment are also displayed (filled squares). The first intraperitoneal (i.p.) injection of etanercept or saline was given 6 hours after antigen injection into the knee, and the i.p. injections were repeated every third day. All animals were tested twice during the immunization procedure and at 1, 3, 7, 14, and 21 days of AIA. (a) Mechanical threshold at the inflamed knee for withdrawal response. (b) Knee joint swelling as an indicator of inflammation. BL = baseline. * $P < 0.05$, ** $P < 0.01$, *** $P < 0.001$; asterisks show the significance of the differences between saline- and etanercept-treated rats. Reproduced from Boettger et al. [7].

It is thought that sensitization of primary afferent fibers for mechanical stimuli is produced by the action of inflammatory mediators on the sensory endings of nerve fibers in the joint. Changes in the intrinsic properties of the neurons may also play a role, because neurons from inflamed tissue maintain enhanced excitability even when the neurons are removed and acutely dissociated several days after inflammation of the joint [25].

A number of mediators have been shown to sensitize joint nociceptors for mechanical stimuli. These include bradykinin, prostaglandin E_2 (PGE_2), prostaglandin I_2 (PGI_2), serotonin, substance P, and vasoactive intestinal polypeptide (for a comprehensive review see [68,71]). These mediators affect subpopulations of $A\delta$ and/or C fibers with low and high mechanical thresholds but do not affect $A\beta$ fibers. In addition, they alter some initially mechanoinsensitive afferent fibers such that they become mechanosensitive. The increase in mechanosensitivity is observed soon after close intraarterial injection of these mediators, and it usually lasts several minutes. In addition, PGE_2 and PGI_2 sensitize joint afferents to the effects of bradykinin; a combination of bradykinin and PGE_2 can cause a stronger sensitization to mechanical stimulation than either substance alone. Conversely, nonsteroidal anti-inflammatory drugs such as aspirin and indomethacin, which block prostaglandin synthesis, reduce spontaneous discharges from acutely and chronically inflamed joints and attenuate the responses to mechanical stimulation. A number of other mediators, including adenosine triphosphate, adenosine, capsaicin, and anandamide, briefly excite proportions of joint afferents, but their effect on mechanosensitivity is unclear. Notably, somatostatin and endomorphin and other opioids reduce mechanosensitivity in numerous afferents, suggesting that mechanosensitivity can be up- and downregulated by mediators. The peptides galanin, neuropeptide Y, and nociceptin sensitize some neurons and reduce responses in other neurons [cf. 68].

More recent studies have focused on the role of the cytokines tumor necrosis factor-α (TNF-α) and interleukin-6 (IL-6) in the development and maintenance of mechanical sensitization of joint afferents. These cytokines play an important role in the pathology of rheumatoid arthritis. In particular, neutralization of TNF-α with etanercept or infliximab has significantly improved rheumatoid arthritis in many patients [23,51,56,63,79]. It is of great interest, therefore, to determine whether and how these mediators are involved in nociception.

Etanercept-treated rats showed significantly less mechanical hyperalgesia than saline-treated rats at the injected knee joint in both the acute and chronic phase of AIA (Fig. 2a), and locomotor behavior was significantly improved. The inflammation per se was only weakly attenuated (see reduction of swelling in Fig. 2b), and no significant differences were found between saline- and etanercept-treated groups regarding histopathological scoring on days 3 and 21 [7]. Thus, the antinociceptive effect of etanercept (and infliximab) in that study was probably mainly due to a direct action at a neuronal target and less to an attenuation of the inflammation. In fact, the injection of etanercept into the knee joint of rats at day 3 of AIA significantly reduced the responses of C fibers to innocuous and noxious outward rotation of the inflamed knee within 1 hour. The injection of etanercept into the normal knee joint did not influence the responses of C fibers to innocuous and noxious outward rotation. Thus, the effect of etanercept was specific to the inflammatory situation [7]. A neuronal effect of TNF-α is plausible because TNF receptors were identified on primary afferent neurons [35,62,67,68] and because TNF-α can evoke direct effects at nerve cell membranes [43,61]. Over the long term, the reduction of the disease process itself may be more important for the reduction of pain.

The proinflammatory cytokine IL-6 plays an important role in the pathogenesis of rheumatoid arthritis. Its concentration is elevated in the serum and synovial fluid of arthritic patients [3,16]. Neuronal effects of IL-6 are likely because most DRG neurons express the transmembrane signal-transducing subunit gp130, to which the complex of IL-6 and its (soluble or membrane-bound) receptor IL6-R bind [60,76]. The concentration of soluble IL-6R is also elevated in synovial tissue in rheumatoid arthritis and correlates with the degree of leukocyte infiltration [15,59]. Injection of IL-6 at 20 ng into the normal knee joint caused a slow increase of the responses of C fibers (but not of Aδ fibers) to noxious outward rotation; the increase became significant after about 100 minutes (Fig. 3a). Injection of 100 ng IL-6 caused a stronger effect. A more rapid sensitization (significantly higher responses to noxious pressure after about 45 minutes) and a significant increase in responses to innocuous outward rotation were observed after coadministration of IL-6 and its soluble receptor (Fig. 3b). The IL-6 neutralizing compound sgp130 prevented the IL-6-induced sensitization of joint afferents (Fig. 3c), showing that the effects of IL-6 were specific [9]. Interestingly, however, IL-6-induced mechanical sensitization was not reversed when sgp130 was administered about 1 hour after IL-6, showing that the IL-6-induced sensitization was persistent. A similar finding was recently reported by Dina et al. [17], who investigated the role of IL-6 in chronic muscle hyperalgesia. They found that PGE_2 has a stronger effect on the nociceptive threshold 24 hours after IL-6 treatment than under control conditions, which suggests that IL-6 has a role in "priming" of muscle afferents.

In addition to their effect on mechanical thresholds of afferent fibers, cytokines have other actions on primary afferent neurons. Some forms of inflammation lead to an increase in the proportion of DRG neurons that express TRPV1 receptors [2,10,42], and inflammation-evoked thermal hyperalgesia is thought to be dependent on TRPV1 receptors [12]. In cultured DRG neurons from adult rats, the expression of the TRPV1 receptor was upregulated after long-term incubation (at least 24 hours) with TNF-α (Fig. 4a) [35]. No such upregulation occurred in DRG neurons from *tnfr1/2$^{-/-}$* and *tnfr1$^{-/-}$* mice, showing that TNFR1 receptors in particular are responsible for this effect (Fig. 4b). After long-term treatment with TNF-α, significantly more DRG neurons responded to capsaicin with an increase of intracellular Ca^{2+} concentration, indicating that the newly expressed TRPV1 receptors were functional. The upregulation was dependent on extracellular signal-regulated kinase but not on p38 kinase or cyclooxygenases [35]. Thus, TNF-α may have an important role in the generation of thermal hyperalgesia via an upregulation of the TRPV1 receptor.

At present, our understanding of the molecular process of peripheral sensitization is still incomplete. It is unclear whether some of the mediators are key mediators that govern the process of sensitization. The remarkably long-lasting effects of TNF-α and of IL-6 on mechanosensitivity suggest that cytokines may be key molecules of inflammation-evoked mechanical sensitization. However, they probably act in concert with other mediators.

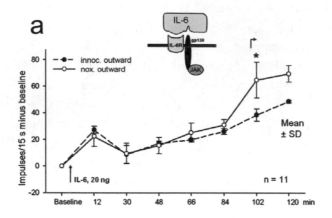

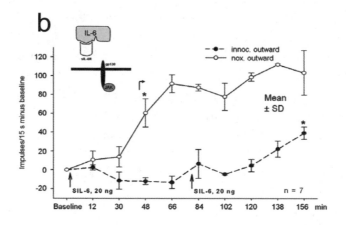

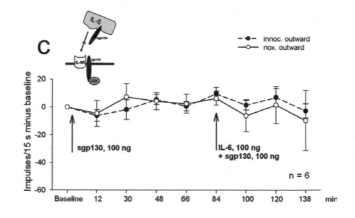

◄— **Fig. 3.** Effects of interleukin-6 (IL-6) and SuperIL-6 (SIL-6: IL-6 plus soluble IL-6R) on responses of C fibers to mechanical stimulation of the normal joint. Curves show the change in responses of groups of fibers to innocuous (dashed lines, filled circles) or noxious outward rotation (solid lines, hollow circles) of the knee from baseline (mean ± SD, n = number of fibers). The baseline was set at zero; arrows indicate the injections of the compounds. (a) Effect of intraarticular injection of 20 ng IL-6. (b) Effect of 20 ng Super-IL-6 (SIL-6; 20 ng IL-6 + 20 ng sIL-6R). (c) No effect of soluble glycoprotein 130 (sgp130) alone and of the subsequent coadministration of sgp130 and IL-6. Asterisks show first statistically significant differences to baseline (Wilcoxon matched-pairs signed-rank test, $P < 0.05$). Reproduced from Brenn et al. [9].

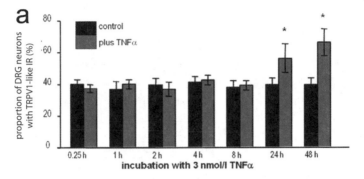

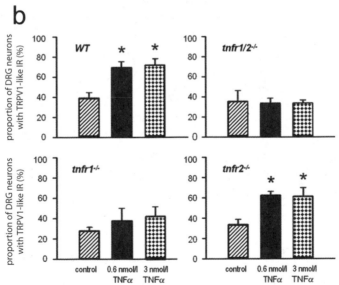

Fig. 4. Influence of tumor necrosis factor-α (TNF-α) on the expression of TRPV1-receptor-like immunoreactivity (IR) in cultured dorsal root ganglion (DRG) neurons. (a) Proportion of DRG neurons from adult rats with TRPV1-receptor-like IR in control cultures and in cultures exposed to TNF-α (doses 3 nmol/L) for 0.25 to 48 hours. (b) Proportion of neurons with TRPV1 receptor-like IR in control cultures and in cultures exposed to TNF-α (doses 0.6 nmol/L or 3 nmol/L) for 48 hours from adult wild-type (WT), *tnfr1/2-/-*, *tnfr1-/-*, and *tnfr2-/-* mice. Bars indicate standard deviation. * $P < 0.05$. Reproduced from Hensellek et al. [35].

Central Sensitization

A second important process involved in inflammatory pain is the development of hyperexcitability of spinal cord neurons with input from joints. In animal studies, Woolf and Wall [86] and Sluka [78] showed that, compared to cutaneous afferents, afferent fibers from deep tissue are particularly capable of inducing central sensitization. In fact, pronounced inflammation-evoked spinal hyperexcitability for mechanical stimulation of the knee joint is generated within 2 to 4 hours after intraarticular injection of kaolin/carrageenan into the knee joint. Wide-dynamic-range neurons with input from joints show a significant increase in their responses to innocuous and noxious pressure applied to the knee. Nociceptive-specific neurons with input from joints show enhanced responses to noxious pressure, and their threshold is lowered such that the neurons become substantially activated by innocuous pressure applied to the joint. In addition, neurons with knee input show increased responses to stimulation of adjacent, healthy tissues such as the ankle joint, and the receptive field may even expand to the paw [57]. The change in responses is even more pronounced in spinalized animals, suggesting that descending pathways dampen the generation of hyperexcitability [58]. In fact, during development of inflammation, tonic descending inhibition of neurons with input from inflamed tissue is increased [83]. Recordings from spinal cord neurons of rats with acute and chronic arthritis at the ankle joint revealed expanded receptive fields and lowered thresholds throughout several weeks, indicating that the state of central sensitization is long-lasting [30].

It is unknown whether similar changes occur in the spinal cord of humans, but testing of hyperalgesia in awake human subjects suggests that this might be the case. Local injection of hypertonic saline (6%) into the tibial anterior muscle just below the knee joint produces a zone of hyperalgesia in the entire lower limb. When the same injection is given to subjects with painful osteoarthritis, the zone of hyperalgesia expands to include the foot [6]. Such an expansion of hyperalgesic zones is likely to be caused by the process of central sensitization.

Inflammation-evoked changes were also studied in supraspinal neurons with input from joints. In polyarthritic rats, a large proportion of neurons in the ventrobasal complex respond to movements and gentle pressure applied to inflamed joints, and often long-lasting afterdischarges were noted, whereas only a few neurons respond to these stimuli in normal rats. Some neurons also displayed paroxysmal discharges. Furthermore, neurons in the centrolateral nucleus of the thalamus acquire input from the inflamed joint that is not present in normal animals [26]. Similarly, neurons in superficial cortical layers that do not respond to joint stimulation in normal rats start to respond to joint stimulation in polyarthritic rats [47,48]. These findings indicate substantial neuroplasticity at the thalamocortical level that may contribute to inflammatory deep tissue pain. It is unknown whether these alterations mirror the altered spinal processing or whether additional elements of neuroplasticity are generated in the thalamus and cortex.

The mechanisms of inflammation-evoked spinal sensitization are being continuously explored. Important elements are the enhanced intraspinal release of transmitters from sensitized joint afferents as well as an increase in the excitability of postsynaptic neurons [69,71]. Recently long-term potentiation was demonstrated in the superficial dorsal horn, suggesting that "learning-like" mechanisms may also be at work [65]. Whether long-term potentiation can be induced by joint inflammation has not yet been directly explored.

Irrespective of the precise mechanisms, we addressed the transmitters and receptors that are involved in the induction and maintenance of central sensitization. The substances involved in the kaolin/carrageenan model include excitatory amino acids; the neuropeptides substance P, neurokinin A, and calcitonin gene-related peptide (CGRP); and spinal prostaglandins. Once inflammation develops in the joint, the intraspinal release of glutamate (the main transmitter of nociceptive afferents) and neuropeptides (cotransmitters in joint afferents) is enhanced. Only noxious compression of the normal joint enhances the intraspinal release of substance P, neurokinin A, and CGRP above baseline, yet these excitatory peptides are intraspinally released even by innocuous compression when the joint is inflamed [cf. 68,71]. An experiment using antibody-coated microprobes showed that the intraspinal release of these neuropeptides peaked in the superficial dorsal horn, but enhanced release extended into the deep dorsal horn, thus matching the termination fields of joint afferents in the dorsal horn.

In addition, the intraspinal milieu is altered by the enhanced release of spinal prostaglandins. Both cyclooxygenase-1 and cyclooxygenase-2 (COX-2) are expressed in the spinal cord [80,82], and during development of joint inflammation, PGE_2 is tonically released above baseline within the dorsal and ventral horn [21]. This increase is likely to result from an upregulation of spinal COX-2 that begins 3 hours after induction of knee joint inflammation [21]. Thus, as a presynaptic mechanism, a "cocktail" of transmitters and modulators is released in the spinal cord under inflammatory conditions that is likely to influence synaptic processing.

Ionophoretic application of antagonists at the AMPA receptor, the N-methyl-D-aspartate (NMDA) receptor, and metabotropic glutamate receptors close to neurons with joint input during the development of kaolin/carrageenan-induced inflammation prevents the generation of spinal hyperexcitability. Antagonists at these receptors also markedly reduce responses of the neurons to mechanical stimulation of the joint after inflammation and spinal hyperexcitability are established, even during chronic inflammation. The release of glutamate and activation of glutamate receptors are thus key mechanisms of inflammation-evoked spinal hyperexcitability, and antagonists at these receptors are even able to reverse spinal sensitization [68,69,71].

Ionophoretic application of substance P, neurokinin A, and CGRP to spinal cord neurons with joint input increase the responses of these neurons to mechanical stimulation of the knee. Antagonists at the neurokinin-1 receptor, the neurokinin-2 receptor, and the CGRP receptor significantly attenuate, but do not prevent, the development of spinal hyperexcitability. When inflammation and spinal hyperexcitability are established, the application of these antagonists significantly reduces enhanced responses; however, unlike the antagonists at glutamate receptors, these antagonists do not completely reverse spinal hyperexcitability [68,69,71]. Thus, these neuropeptides and their receptors contribute to spinal hyperexcitability, but their role is modulatory. Ionophoretic application of CGRP to the spinal cord enhances the responses of spinal cord neurons with joint input to ionophoretic application of AMPA and NMDA, showing that CGRP increases the effects of excitatory amino acids [20].

Spinal PGE_2 is also involved in spinal hyperexcitability, but its pattern of effects is different from that of excitatory amino acids and excitatory neuropeptides. Application of PGE_2 to the spinal cord surface facilitates the responses of spinal cord neurons to mechanical stimulation of the joint, similar to joint inflammation (see Fig. 5b, top panel). Also, spinal application of the nonselective COX inhibitor indomethacin attenuates the increase of responses to mechanical stimulation of the knee joint during development of inflammation. These findings suggest that endogenous spinal prostaglandins contribute to central sensitization [84]. However, spinally applied indomethacin did not reduce the responses to stimulation of the inflamed knee after spinal hyperexcitability was established [84], although it significantly reduced spinal PGE_2 release (unpublished observations). We believe, therefore, that PGE_2 is involved in the generation of spinal hyperexcitability and that the continuous presence of spinal PGE_2 is not required for the maintenance of spinal hyperexcitability [84].

Spinal application of agonists at either the EP1, EP2, or EP4 receptor dose-dependently increased the responses of spinal cord neurons to mechanical stimulation of the normal knee joint. However, once inflammation and spinal hyperexcitability were established, only a EP1-receptor agonist further increased responses of neurons to knee stimulation, whereas agonists at the EP2 and the EP4 receptors had no further effect [5]. None of the compounds increased the responses to mechanical stimulation of the chronically inflamed knee joint (at 21 days post-induction of AIA) (unpublished observations). In our opinion, these findings also support the conclusion that the continuous presence of spinal PGE_2 does not increase spinal hyperexcitability that has already been established.

The effect of spinal prostaglandins appears more complex when another prostaglandin, PGD_2, is considered. PGD_2 is produced and released in significant amounts in the central nervous system, including the spinal cord. In rats with normal knee joints, topical application of PGD_2 to the spinal cord did not influence responses to innocuous and noxious pressure applied to the normal knee joint, except at a very high dose [81]. In slice preparations of the spinal cord from normal animals, the application of PGD_2 did not evoke effects on the membrane or the synaptic transmission, in contrast to the pronounced excitatory and facilitatory effects of PGE_2 given at the same concentration [1,4]. By contrast, spinal application of PGD_2 and of the specific DP1-receptor agonist BW245C (Fig. 5a, top) in rats with established acute kaolin/carrageenan-induced inflammation in the knee joint reduced the responses of ipsilateral spinal cord neurons to innocuous and noxious pressure on the inflamed knee [81]. Spinal application of the DP1-receptor antagonist BWA868C during knee inflammation increased responses to stimulation of the inflamed knee, suggesting that the neurons were under the inhibitory influence of endogenous PGD$_2$ (Fig. 5a, bottom). These data suggest that under inflammatory conditions, PGD$_2$ counteracts the pronociceptive effects of PGE$_2$. In fact, the spinal application of PGD$_2$ can partially reduce the increased responses of spinal cord neurons following spinal application of PGE$_2$ (Fig. 5b) [81]. In behavioral experiments in mice, Minami et al. showed that

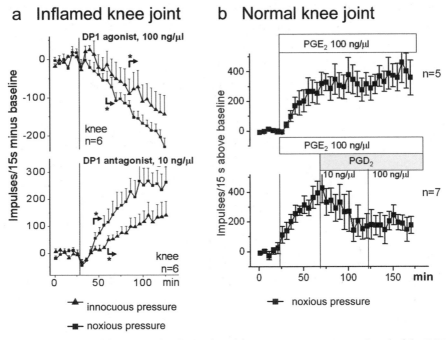

Fig. 5. (a) Effects of the prostaglandin D$_1$ (DP1) receptor agonist BW245C and of the DP1 receptor antagonist BWA868C on the responses of spinal cord neurons in rats with acute knee joint inflammation. Graphs show changes in response to innocuous and noxious pressure applied to the inflamed knee. The predrug baseline was set at 0; vertical lines show the time of drug application. Asterisks indicate the first interval of 15 minutes after drug application in which the values were significantly different from baseline ($P < 0.05$, Wilcoxon matched-pairs signed-rank test). (b) Effects of the coadministration of PGE$_2$ and PGD$_2$ on responses to mechanical stimulation of the normal knee joint. Increase in responses to noxious stimulation of the knee by PGE$_2$ alone (top) and reduction of increased responses by coapplication of PGD$_2$ at two doses (bottom). The baseline was set at 0. Reproduced from Telleria-Diaz et al. [81].

low doses of intrathecal PGD_2 reduced PGE_2-induced [53] and nociceptin-induced allodynia [54], although PGD_2 alone may cause allodynia [22,55].

The inhibitory effect of PGD_2 through DP1 receptors under inflammatory conditions could result from an activation of inhibitory GABAergic interneurons [22,54]. Such an effect would occur in particular under conditions in which neurons are hyperexcitable, such as during inflammation-evoked sensitization. The antinociceptive effect of PGD_2 under inflammatory conditions may be a form of neuroprotection (see [29]), counteracting spinal hyperexcitability during inflammation and thus protecting the spinal cord. It should be investigated whether the application of cyclooxygenase inhibitors might interfere with a neuroprotective effect of PGD_2.

Conclusions

Several mechanisms of pain in conditions of acute joint inflammation have been elucidated, but the neuronal mechanisms of chronic joint pain are poorly understood. Chronic inflammatory models may help to elucidate these mechanisms. Analytical methods must be employed that allow investigators to monitor subtle but persistent nociceptive processes.

So far the main focus of neurophysiological research on joint pain has been inflammatory pain. This research has primarily addressed pain mechanisms during inflammatory diseases, but it may also be relevant for pain arising from osteoarthritis. The correlation between radiological signs of osteoarthritis (a narrow joint space and osteophytes) and pain is poor [75], but some recent studies have shown that painful osteoarthritic knee joints exhibit more magnetic resonance abnormalities than do nonpainful osteoarthritis joints that have synovial hypertrophy and subchondral bone marrow edema lesions (which may increase intraosseous pressure) [24]. These data suggest that pain often results from inflammatory episodes in the course of osteoarthritis.

References

[1] Ahmadi S, Lippross S, Neuhuber WL, Zeilhofer HU. PGE_2 selectively blocks inhibitory glycinergic neurotransmission onto rat superficial dorsal horn neurons. Nat Neurosci 2002;5:34–40.
[2] Amaya F, Oh-Hashi K, Naruse Y, Iijima N, Ueda M, Shimosato G, Tominaga Y, Tanaka Y, Tanaka M. Local inflammation increases vanilloid receptor 1 expression within distinct subgroups of DRG neurons. Brain Res 2003;963:190–6.

[3]   Arvidson NG, Gudbjornsson B, Elfman L, Ryden AC, Tötterman TH, Hällgren R. Circadian rhythms of serum interleukin-6 in rheumatoid arthritis. Rheum Dis 1994;53:521–4.

[4]   Baba H, Kohno T, Moore KA, Woolf CJ. Direct activation of rat spinal dorsal horn neurons by prostaglandin E_2. J Neurosci 2001;21:1750–6.

[5]   Bär K-J, Natura G, Telleria-Diaz A, Teschner P, Vogel R, Vasquez E, Schaible H-G, Ebersberger A. Changes in the effect of spinal prostaglandin E_2 during inflammation: prostaglandin E (EP1–EP4) receptors in spinal nociceptive processing of input from the normal or inflamed knee joint. J Neurosci 2004;24:642–51.

[6]   Bajaj P, Bajaj P, Graven-Nielsen T, Arendt-Nielsen L. Osteoarthritis and its association with muscle hyperalgesia: an experimental controlled study. Pain 2001;93:107–14.

[7]   Boettger MK, Hensellek S, Richter F, Gajda M, Stoeckigt R, Segond von Banchet G, Braeuer R, Schaible H-G. Antinociceptive effects of TNF-α neutralization in a rat model of antigen-induced arthritis. Arthritis Rheum 2008;58:2368–78.

[8]   Breivik H, Beverly C, Ventafridda V, Cohen R, Gallacher D. Survey of chronic pain in Europe: prevalence, impact on daily life, and treatment. Eur J Pain 2006;10:287–333.

[9]   Brenn D, Richter F, Schaible H-G. Sensitization of unmyelinated sensory fibres of the joint nerve to mechanical stimuli by interleukin-6 in the rat. An inflammatory mechanism of joint pain. Arthritis Rheum 2007;56:351–9.

[10]   Bron R, Klesse LJ, Shah K, Parada L-F, Winter J. Activation of ras is necessary and sufficient for upregulation of vanilloid receptor type 1 in sensory neurons by neurotrophic factors. Mol Cell Neurosci 2003;22:118–32.

[11]   Buchner E, Braeuer R, Emmrich F, Kinne RW. Induction of flare-up reactions in rat antigen-induced arthritis. J Autoimmun 1995;8:61–74.

[12]   Caterina MJ, Schumacher MA, Tominaga M, Rosen TA, Levine JD, Julius D. The capsaicin receptor: a heat-activated ion channel in the pain pathway. Nature 1997;389:816–24.

[13]   Colpaert FC. Evidence that adjuvant arthritis in the rat is associated with chronic pain. Pain 1987;28:210–222.

[14]   Craig AD, Heppelmann B, Schaible H-G. The projection of the medial and posterior articular nerves of cat's knee to the spinal cord. J Comp Neurol 1988;276:279–88.

[15]   De Benedetti F, Massa M, Pignatti P, Albani S, Novick D, Martini A. Serum soluble interleukin-6 (IL-6) receptor and IL-6/soluble IL-6 receptor complex in systemic juvenile rheumatoid arthritis. J Clin Invest 1994;93:2114–9.

[16]   Desgeorges A, Gabay C, Silacci P, Novick D, Roux-Lombard P, Grau G, Dayer JM, Vischer T, Guerne PA. Concentrations and origins of soluble interleukin 6 receptor in serum and synovial fluid. J Rheumatol 1997;24:1510–6.

[17]   Dina OA, Green PG, Levin JD. Role of interleukin-6 in chronic muscle hyperalgesic priming. Neuroscience 2008;152:521–5.

[18]   Dong WK, Ryu H, Wagman IH. Nociceptive responses of neurons in medial thalamus and their relationship to spinothalamic pathways. J Neurophysiol 1978;41:1592–613.

[19]   Dye SF, Vaupel GL, Dye CC. Conscious neurosensory mapping of the internal structures of the human knee without intraarticular anesthesia. Am J Sports Med 1998;26:773–7.

[20]   Ebersberger A, Charbel Issa P, Vanegas H, Schaible H-G. Differential effects of CGRP and CGRP8-37 upon responses to NMDA and AMPA in spinal nociceptive neurons with knee input in the rat. Neuroscience 2000;99:171–8.

[21]   Ebersberger A, Grubb BD, Willingale HL, Gardiner NJ, Nebe J, Schaible H-G. The intraspinal release of prostaglandin E_2 in a model of acute arthritis is accompanied by an upregulation of cyclooxygenase-2 in the rat spinal cord. Neuroscience 1999;93:775–81.

[22]   Eguchi N, Minami T, Shirafuji N, Kanaoka Y, Tanaka T, Nagata A, Yoshida N, Urade Y, Ito S, Hayaishi O. Lack of tactile pain (allodynia) in lipocalin-type prostaglandin D synthase-deficient mice. Proc Natl Acad Sci USA 1999;96:726–30.

[23]   Feldmann M, Maini RN. Anti-TNF alpha therapy of rheumatoid arthritis: what have we learned? Ann Rev Immunol 2001;19:163–96.

[24]   Felson DT. The sources of pain in knee osteoarthritis. Curr Opin Rheumatol 2005;17:624–28.

[25]   Flake NM, Gold MS. Inflammation alters sodium currents and excitability of temporomandibular joint afferents. Neurosci Lett 2005;384:294–9.

[26]   Gautron M, Guilbaud G. Somatic responses of ventrobasal thalamic neurones in polyarthritic rats. Brain Res 1982;237:459–71.

[27] Griffiths RJ. Characterisation and pharmacological sensitivity of antigen arthritis induced by methylated bovine serum albumin in the rat. Agents Actions 1992;35:88–95.

[28] Grigg P, Schaible H-G, Schmidt RF. Mechanical sensitivity of group III and IV afferents from posterior articular nerve in normal and inflamed cat knee. J Neurophysiol 1986;55:635–43.

[29] Grill M, Heinemann A, Hoefler G, Peskar BA, Schuligoi R. Effect of endotoxin treatment on the expression and localization of spinal cyclooxygenase, prostaglandin synthases, and PGD_2 receptors. J Neurochem 2008:104:1345–57.

[30] Grubb BD, Stiller RU, Schaible H-G. Dynamic changes in the receptive field properties of spinal cord neurons with ankle input in rats with unilateral adjuvant-induced inflammation in the ankle region. Exp Brain Res 1993;92:441–52.

[31] Guilbaud G, Caille D, Besson J-M, Benelli G. Single unit activities in ventral posterior and posterior group thalamic nuclei during nociceptive and non nociceptive stimulations in the cat. Arch Ital Biol 1977;115:38–56.

[32] Guilbaud G, Iggo A, Tegner R. Sensory receptors in ankle joint capsules of normal and arthritic rats. Exp Brain Res 1985;58:29–40.

[33] Guilbaud G, Peschanski M, Gautron M, Binder D. Neurones responding to noxious stimulation in VB complex and caudal adjacent regions in the thalamus of the rat. Pain 1980;8:303–18.

[34] Han JS, Li W, Neugebauer V. Critical role of calcitonin gene-related peptide 1 receptors in the amygdala in synaptic plasticity and pain behaviour. J Neurosci 2005;25:10717–28.

[35] Hensellek S, Brell P, Schaible H-G, Bräuer R, Segond von Banchet G. The cytokine TNFα increases the proportion of DRG neurones expressing the TRPV1 receptor via the TNFR1 receptor and ERK activation. Mol Cell Neurosci 2007;36:381–91.

[36] Heppelmann B, Pawlak M, Just S, Schmidt RF. Cortical projection of the rat knee joint innervation and its processing in the somatosensory areas SI and SII. Exp Brain Res 2001;141:501–6.

[37] Hodge DR, Hurt EM, Farrar WL. The role of IL-6 and STAT3 in inflammation and cancer. Eur J Cancer 2005;41:2502–12.

[38] Hutchison WD, Lühn MA, Schmidt RF. Knee joint input into the peripheral region of the ventral posterior lateral nucleus of cat thalamus. J Neurophysiol 1992;67:1092–104.

[39] Hutchison WD, Lühn MAB, Schmidt RF. Responses of lateral thalamic neurons to algesic stimulation of the cat knee joint. Exp Brain Res 1994;101:452–4.

[40] Inglis JJ, Notley CA, Essex D, Wilson AW, Feldmann M, Anand P, Williams R. Collagen-induced arthritis as a model of hyperalgesia. Functional and cellular analysis of the analgesic actions of tumor necrosis factor blockade. Arthritis Rheumat 2007;56:4015–23.

[41] Ji G, Neugebauer V. Differential effects of CRF1 and CRF2 receptor antagonists on pain-related sensitization of neurons in the central nucleus of the amygdala. J Neurophysiol 2007;97:3893–904.

[42] Ji RR, Samad TA, Jin SX, Schmoll R, Woolf CJ. p38 MAPK activation by NGF in primary sensory neurons after inflammation increases TRPV1 levels and maintains heat hyperalgesia. Neuron 2002;36:57–68.

[43] Jin X, Gereau IV R. Acute p38-mediated modulation of tetrodotoxin-resistant sodium channels in mouse sensory neurons by tumor necrosis factor-α. J Neurosci 2006;26:246–55.

[44] Kellgren JH, Samuel EP. The sensitivity and innervation of the articular capsule. J Bone Joint Surg 1950;4:193–205.

[45] Kniffki K-D, Mizumura K. Responses of neurons in VPL and VPL-VL region of the cat to algesic stimulation of muscle and tendon. J Neurophysiol 1983;49:649–61.

[46] Lamour Y, Willer JC, Guilbaud G. Rat somatosensory (Sm I) cortex. I. Characteristics of neuronal responses to noxious simulation and comparison with responses to non-noxious stimulation. Exp Brain Res 1983;49:35–45.

[47] Lamour Y, Willer JC, Guilbaud G. Rat somatosensory (Sm I) cortex. II. Laminar and columnar organization of noxious and non-noxious inputs. Exp Brain Res 1983;49:46–54.

[48] Lamour Y, Willer JC, Guilbaud G. Altered properties and laminar distribution of neuronal responses to peripheral stimulation in the Sm I cortex of the arthritic rat. Brain Res 1983;273:183–87.

[49] Lewis T. Suggestions relating to the study of somatic pain. BMJ 1938;1:321–5.

[50] Li W, Neugebauer V. Block of NMDA and non-NMDA receptor activation results in reduced background and evoked activity of central amygdala neurons in a model of arthritic pain. Pain 2004;110:112–22.

[51] Lorenz H-M, Kalden JR. Perspectives for TNF-α-targeting therapies. Arthritis Res 2002;4(Suppl 3):S17–S24.

[52] Menetréy D, Gannon JD, Levine JD, Basbaum AI. Expression of c-fos protein in interneurons and projection neurons of the rat spinal cord in response to noxious somatic, articular, and visceral stimulation. J Comp Neurol 1989;285:177–95.

[53] Minami T, Okuda-Ashitaka E, Mori H, Ito S, Hayaishi O. Prostaglandin D_2 inhibits prostaglandin E_2-induced allodynia in conscious mice. J Pharmacol Exp Ther 1996;278:1146–52.

[54] Minami T, Okuda-Ashitaka E, Nishizawa M, Mori H, Ito S. Inhibition of nociceptin-induced allodynia in conscious mice by prostaglandin D_2. Br J Pharmacol 1997;122:605–10.

[55] Minami T, Uda R, Horiguchi S, Ito S, Hyodo M, Hayaishi O. Allodynia evoked by intrathecal administration of prostaglandin E_2 to conscious mice. Pain 1994;57:217–23.

[56] Möller B, Villiger PM. Inhibition of IL-1, IL-6, and TNFα in immune-mediated inflammatory diseases. Springer Semin Immun 2006;27:391–408.

[57] Neugebauer V, Luecke T, Schaible H-G. N-methyl-D-aspartate (NMDA) and non-NMDA receptor antagonists block the hyperexcitability of dorsal horn neurons during development of acute arthritis in rat's knee joint. J Neurophysiol 1993;70:1365–77.

[58] Neugebauer V, Schaible H-G. Evidence for a central component in the sensitization of spinal neurons with joint input during development of acute arthritis in cat's knee. J Neurophysiol 1990;64:299–311.

[59] Novick D, Engelmann H, Wallach D, Rubinstein M. Soluble cytokine receptors are present in normal human urine. J Exp Med 1989;170:1409–14.

[60] Obreja O, Biasio W, Andratsch M, Lips KS, Rathee PK, Ludwig A, Rose-John S, Kress M. Fast modulation of heat-activated ionic current by proinflammatory interleukin 6 in rat sensory neurons. Brain 2005;128:1634–41.

[61] Opree A, Kress M. Involvement of the proinflammatory cytokines tumor necrosis factor-alpha, IL-1 beta, and IL-6 but not IL-8 in the development of heat hyperalgesia: effects on heat-evoked calcitonin gene-related peptide release from rat skin. J Neurosci 2000;20:6289–93.

[62] Pollock J, McFarlane SM, Connell MC, Zehavi U, Vandenabeele P, MacEwan DJ, Scott RH. TNF-alpha receptors simultaneously activate Ca^{2+} mobilisation and stress kinases in cultured sensory neurones. Neuropharmacology 2002;42:93–106.

[63] Redlich K, Schett G, Steiner G, Hayer S, Wagner EF, Smolen JS. Rheumatoid arthritis therapy after tumor necrosis factor and interleukin-1 blockade. Arthritis Rheum 2003;48:3308–19.

[64] Roth A, Mollenhauer J, Wagner A, Fuhrmann R, Straub A, Venbrocks RA, Petrow P, Braeuer R, Schubert H, Ozegowski J, et al. Intra-articular injections of high-molecular-weight hyaluronic acid have biphasic effects on joint inflammation and destruction in rat antigen-induced arthritis. Arthritis Res Ther 2005;7:R677–86.

[65] Sandkuehler J. Learning and memory in pain pathways. Pain 2000;88:113–8.

[66] Schaefers M, Geis C, Brors D, Yaksh TL, Sommer C. Anterograde transport of tumor necrosis factor-alpha in the intact and injured rat sciatic nerve. J Neurosci 2002;22: 536–45.

[67] Schaefers M, Lee DH, Brors D, Yaksh TL, Sorkin LS. Increased sensitivity of injured and adjacent uninjured rat primary sensory neurons to exogenous tumour necrosis factor-alpha after spinal nerve ligation. J Neurosci 2003;23:3028–38.

[68] Schaible H-G. Basic mechanisms of deep somatic pain. In: McMahon SB, Koltzenburg M, editors. Wall and Melzack's textbook of pain, 5th ed. Elsevier Churchill Livingston; 2006. p. 621–33.

[69] Schaible H-G. Peripheral and central mechanisms of pain generation. In: Stein C, editor. Handbook of experimental pharmacology, Vol. 177. Berlin: Springer-Verlag; 2006. p. 4–28.

[70] Schaible H-G, Grubb BD. Afferent and spinal mechanisms of joint pain. Pain 1993;55:5–54.

[71] Schaible H-G, Schmelz M, Tegeder I. Pathophysiology and treatment of pain in joint disease. Adv Drug Deliv Rev 2006;58:323–42.

[72] Schaible H-G, Schmidt RF. Effects of an experimental arthritis on the sensory properties of fine articular afferent units. J Neurophysiol 1985;54:1109–22.

[73] Schaible H-G, Schmidt RF. Time course of mechanosensitivity changes in articular afferents during a developing experimental arthritis. J Neurophysiol 1988;60:2180–95.

[74] Schaible H-G, Schmidt RF, Willis WD. Enhancement of the responses of ascending tract cells in the cat spinal cord by acute inflammation of the knee joint. Exp Brain Res 1987;66:489–9.

[75] Scott DL. Osteoarthritis and rheumatoid arthritis. In: McMahon SB, Koltzenburg M, editors. Wall and Melzack's textbook of pain, 5th ed. Elsevier Churchill Livingstone; 2006. p. 653–67.

[76] Segond von Banchet G, Kiehl M, Schaible H-G. Acute and long-term effects of interleukin-6 on cultured dorsal root ganglion neurones from adult rat. J Neurochem 2005;94:238–8.

[77] Segond von Banchet G, Petrow PK, Braeuer R, Schaible H-G. Monoarticular antigen-induced arthritis leads to pronounced bilateral upregulation of the expression of neurokinin 1 and bradykinin 2 receptors in dorsal root ganglion neurones of rats. Arthritis Res 2000;2:424–7.

[78] Sluka KA. Stimulation of deep somatic tissue with capsaicin produces long-lasting mechanical allodynia and heat hypoalgesia that depends on early activation of the cAMP pathway. J Neurosci 2002;22:5687–93.

[79] Smolen JS, Steiner G. Therapeutic strategies for rheumatoid arthritis. Nature Rev Drug Discov 2003;2:473–88.

[80] Svensson CI, Yaksh TL. The spinal phospholipase-prostanoid cascade in nociceptive processing. Annu Rev Toxicol 2002;42:553–83.

[81] Telleria-Diaz A, Ebersberger A, Vasquez E, Schache F, Kahlenbach J, Schaible H-G. Different effects of spinally applied prostaglandin D_2 (PGD_2) on responses of dorsal horn neurons with knee input in normal rats and in rats with acute knee inflammation. Neuroscience 2008;156:184–92.

[82] Vanegas H, Schaible H-G. Prostaglandins and cyclooxygenases in the spinal cord. Prog Neurobiol 2001;64:327–63.

[83] Vanegas H, Schaible H-G. Descending control of persistent pain: inhibitory or facilitatory? Brain Res Rev 2004;46:295–309.

[84] Vasquez E, Bär K-J, Ebersberger A, Klein B, Vanegas H, Schaible H-G. Spinal prostaglandins are involved in the development but not the maintenance of inflammation-induced spinal hyperexcitability. J Neurosci 2001;21:9001–8.

[85] Williams RO. Models of rheumatoid arthritis. Ernst Schering Res Found Workshop 2005;50:89–117.

[86] Woolf CJ, Wall PD. Relative effectiveness of C primary afferent fibres of different origins in evoking a prolonged facilitation of the flexor reflex in the rat. J Neurosci 1986;6:1433–42.

Correspondence to: Prof. Dr. med. Hans-Georg Schaible, Institute of Physiology 1/Neurophysiology, Universitätsklinikum Jena, Teichgraben 8, D-07740 Jena, Germany. Email: hans-georg.schaible@mti.uni-jena.de.

Signaling Events and Ionic Mechanisms Disrupting Spinal Inhibition in Neuropathic Pain

Yves De Koninck

Department of Psychiatry and Division of Cellular Neurobiology, Robert Giffard Research Center, Laval University, Quebec, Canada

A large body of evidence indicates that injury to either the peripheral or central nervous system (CNS) causes a number of changes in the CNS, which lead to abnormal information processing and hyperexcitability. A decrease in synaptic inhibition, or "disinhibition," appears to be an important substrate of several pathophysiological conditions of the CNS, such as traumatic injuries, epilepsy, and chronic pain [49,69,76]. This disinhibition results in a general increase in the excitability of individual neurons and networks of neurons; it also has the potential to allow inputs to be relayed through pathways that are normally kept silent by inhibition, thus destabilizing neuronal circuits.

The important question that arises for therapeutic development is to determine what mechanisms underlie altered inhibition in the CNS under pathological conditions such as neuropathic pain. This chapter reviews recent work introducing novel perspectives on this question. First, I discuss the concept that the strength of inhibition mediated by γ-aminobutyric acid A ($GABA_A$) and glycine receptors can be modulated via alterations in the mechanisms that regulate the transmembrane gradient for chloride ions. Second, I review the concept that chloride homeostasis is dynamically modulated in adult tissue under pathological conditions by a cascade of intercellular signaling events.

In relation to these novel perspectives, the chapter also highlights another advance in our understanding of adult CNS pathophysiology: the realization that CNS immune cells play an active role in regulating neuronal excitability. Interactions between the immune and nervous systems occur at multiple levels, where different types of immune and glial cells and immune-derived substances are implicated at different stages of the pathogenesis of a wide array of syndromes, including spinal cord injury, multiple sclerosis, neuropathic pain, epilepsy, and brain ischemia, as well as neurodegenerative diseases such as Alzheimer's and Parkinson's disease and amyotrophic lateral sclerosis [22,36,43,54,55]. Importantly, many of these neuroimmune interactions occur within the CNS parenchyma. On the other hand, not only central, but also peripheral nerve injuries trigger central neuroinflammatory responses [36,43,54,55]. Yet, while immune cells of the CNS—notably microglia—are recognized as active participants in the control of neuronal function, the mechanisms by which microglia signal to neurons to alter their excitability have remained elusive until recently.

The search for mechanisms underlying impaired spinal inhibition following peripheral nerve injury has unraveled an intricate neuroimmune interplay. Following peripheral nerve injury in adults, nerve cells release mediators that cause activation, proliferation, and migration of CNS microglia toward the site of central projection of the terminals of the damaged nerves. These microglia express de novo $P2X_4$ receptors, and upon stimulation by adenosine triphosphate (ATP), they release brain-derived neurotrophic factor (BNDF). In turn, BDNF acts on neuronal tyrosine kinase B (TrkB) receptors to downregulate the potassium-chloride cotransporter KCC2, which is normally responsible for chloride extrusion from the cells. The resulting reduction in chloride extrusion capacity impairs $GABA_A$- and glycine-receptor-mediated inhibition, significantly raising neuronal excitability and allowing crosstalk between sensory modalities in spinal ascending pathways.

While continuous ATP signaling to $P2X_4$ receptors on spinal microglia appears to maintain reduced segmental inhibition, this signaling mechanism is not responsible for the initial activation of spinal microglia by peripheral nerve injury. Release of monocyte chemoattractant protein-1 (MCP-1, also known as CCL2) from sensory terminals appears to cause activation and chemotaxis of microglia and even of bone-marrow-derived monocytes via activation of the CCR2 receptor. Remarkably, the processes of activation and chemotaxis are restricted to the area of the spinal cord innervated by the damaged afferents.

The identification of the multitude of signaling events and altered ionic mechanisms involved in neuron-glia-neuron interactions after nerve injury offers a wide range of novel avenues for mechanism-based diagnosis and treatment of neuropathic pain.

Altered Chloride Homeostasis in the Spinal Dorsal Horn as a Substrate of Neuropathic Pain

Blocking Spinal Inhibition Causes Pain Hypersensitivity

Ample evidence indicates that decreasing spinal inhibition (disinhibition) causes pain hypersensitivity. Blocking inhibition mediated by GABA and glycine replicates symptoms of neuropathic and inflammatory pain [57–59,62,77]. The network of local inhibitory neurons within the dorsal horn represses a large number of established excitatory connections, and suppression of this inhibitory control unmasks a profound network of polysynaptic excitatory inputs to relay neurons. This event results in a general increase in the excitability of the network and has the potential for allowing inputs to be relayed through pathways that do not convey these inputs in normal conditions (e.g., normally nociceptive-specific pathways). For example, after blockade of $GABA_A$ and glycine receptors, spinal lamina I and II neurons with normally little or no low-threshold input can be seen to receive considerable inputs from low-threshold afferents (comparable in magnitude to inputs from high-threshold afferents) via unmasked polysynaptic links [4,68]. Nociceptive-specific lamina I neurons show responses to innocuous touch after blockade of intrinsic $GABA_A$/glycine inhibition [30]. Moreover, nociceptive-specific thalamic neurons display responses to innocuous input following blockade of glycine receptors at the lumbar

spinal level, indicating subliminal low-threshold input to normally nociceptive-specific spinal output pathways [58]. Because there are normally
no monosynaptic inputs to lamina I from low-threshold afferents, these
findings indicate that the network is organized in such a way that $GABA_A$/
glycine inhibitory neurons repress existing excitatory connections, allowing crosstalk between low- and high-threshold pathways. However, the
fact that blocking inhibition causes pain hypersensitivity does not necessarily imply that disinhibition occurs in pathological conditions. Hence,
several recent studies have been aimed at identifying substrates of impaired inhibition in experimental models of chronic pain.

Conventional Substrates of Dorsal Horn Disinhibition

Several studies have shown that peripheral nerve injury causes loss of inhibition impinging on spinal dorsal horn neurons. A potential underlying mechanism is the degeneration of inhibitory interneurons [26,40,56].
However, it has been argued that pain hypersensitivity after nerve injury
may occur without any apparent loss of interneurons [45,46]. Altered
expression of GABA (or its synthesizing enzyme, glutamate decarboxyl-
ase) or of $GABA_A$ receptors is another potential mechanism, but findings
appear to differ depending on chronic pain models and animal strains
[8–10,40,60].

Impaired Chloride Extrusion as a Novel Mechanism
of Dorsal Horn Disinhibition

In parallel with these studies, we identified another mechanism to account
for dorsal horn disinhibition in neuropathic pain conditions. It involves
a decrease in the expression of the K^+-Cl^- cotransporter KCC2 in spinal dorsal horn neurons following peripheral nerve injury [16]. Because
primary afferents do not express KCC2 in normal conditions, the loss of
KCC2 points to a mechanism specifically affecting postsynaptic inhibition
of dorsal horn neurons (not presynaptic inhibition of sensory afferent
terminals) [16]. In functional terms, this mechanism results in a shift
in the reversal potential for GABA currents (E_{GABA}) to more depolarized values, effectively eliminating the hyperpolarizing action of GABA
and glycine (Fig. 1). In most cases, the shift in E_{GABA} was sufficient to

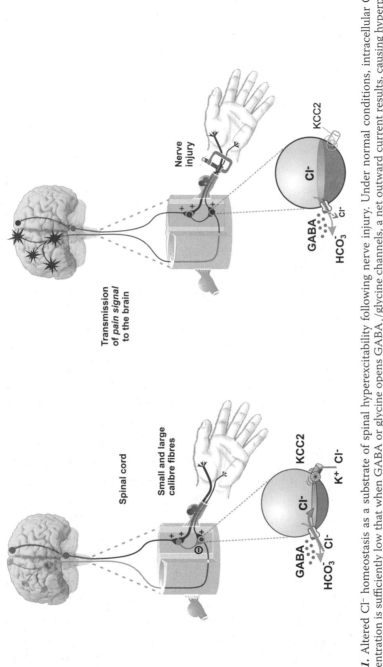

Fig. 1. Altered Cl- homeostasis as a substrate of spinal hyperexcitability following nerve injury. Under normal conditions, intracellular Cl-concentration is sufficiently low that when GABA or glycine opens GABA$_A$/glycine channels, a net outward current results, causing hyperpolarizing inhibition. Loss of KCC2 activity in spinal dorsal horn neurons following peripheral nerve injury causes an accumulation of resting intracellular Cl- and a decrease in Cl- extrusion capacity in these cells, which effectively impairs the efficacy of GABA$_A$- and glycine-receptor-mediated hyperpolarization [16]. This impairment leads to a loss of spinal inhibition and an increase in excitability of dorsal horn neurons, allowing crosstalk between non-nociceptive and nociceptive sensory channels and the aberrant relay of innocuous input via normally nociceptive-specific relay pathways to the brain, setting the stage for allodynia [30].

invert GABA/glycine-mediated hyperpolarization to depolarization, and in a subset of cells, it effectively converted inhibition into net excitation [16]. Local blockade or knockdown of spinal KCC2 in intact rats markedly reduced nociceptive threshold, confirming that disruption of chloride homeostasis in superficial dorsal horn neurons was sufficient to replicate the symptoms of neuropathic pain [16].

The net effect of a change in E_{GABA} is not necessarily obvious, however, because in addition to having a hyperpolarizing effect, activation of $GABA_A$ or glycine receptor channels produces inhibition via a significant shunt of the membrane, which can effectively attenuate concurrent excitatory input. Nevertheless, even if shunting inhibition remains unchanged after nerve injury, a loss of hyperpolarization by $GABA_A$ of glycine receptors will, by itself, produce a net deficit in inhibition (disinhibition) with respect to normal conditions.

To investigate the degree of change in neuronal excitability at the single cell level due to altered E_{GABA}, we conducted simulations using a compartmental model in the NEURON environment in which it was possible to vary the level of GABAergic and glutamatergic synaptic input and E_{GABA}. The results revealed that a change in E_{GABA} of as little as 5 mV is sufficient to significantly alter the input-output property of a neuron and thus its net excitability [48] (Fig. 2). It is particularly important to note that when E_{GABA} is below a certain value, the input-output curve remains below that which would be expected if GABAergic transmission were completely blocked. Thus, under such conditions, the upward shift in E_{GABA} (toward less negative potentials) causes net disinhibition, but GABAergic transmission continues to be inhibitory. Upon greater upward shifts in E_{GABA}, the input-output curve lies above that with no GABAergic transmission, and thus GABA transmission exerts a net excitatory action (Fig. 2).

The impact of this dual situation is that, depending on the degree of E_{GABA} shift, the ensuing disinhibition may be affected in an opposite manner by modulation of GABAergic transmission. For example, when GABA is excitatory, blocking $GABA_A$ receptors may counterbalance the hyperexcitability, although it must be kept in mind that the altered E_{GABA} is probably restricted to a specific population of neurons, and thus systemic blockage of $GABA_A$ receptors is likely to cause hyperexcitability of other subpopulations of neurons. This caveat is particularly true in the spinal

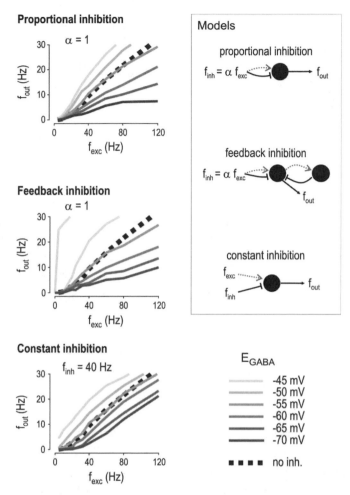

Fig. 2. Changing the reversal potential for GABA currents (E_{GABA}) significantly alters the input-output relationship and thus the excitability of neurons. Data are from a multicompartmental model neuron using NEURON simulation software [48]. The neuron had a resting membrane potential of −63 mV, realistic intrinsic membrane properties, and synaptic inputs based on data from [47], [16], and [20,42]. Different models of the relationship between excitation and inhibition were used: feedforward inhibition (where the frequency of inhibitory postsynaptic events was proportional to that of excitatory ones); feedback inhibition and constant inhibition (see insets). Note how, in each type of synaptic arrangements, slight changes in E_{GABA} caused a significant shift in the slope of the input-output curve. The thick dashed black line represents the case where $GABA_A$ transmission is blocked (no inhibition). When E_{GABA} is below a certain value, the input-output curve remains below that which would be expected if GABAergic transmission were completely blocked. Thus, under such conditions, the upward shift in E_{GABA} (toward less negative potentials) causes net disinhibition, but GABAergic transmission continues to be inhibitory. Upon greater upward shifts in E_{GABA}, the input-output curve lies above that with no GABAergic transmission, and thus GABA transmission exerts a net excitatory action. Modified from Prescott et al. [48].

dorsal horn, where presynaptic GABA$_A$-receptor-mediated inhibition is unlikely to be affected similarly to postsynaptic inhibition because KCC2 receptors are not expressed on sensory fibers. If GABA has a net excitatory action on dorsal horn neurons, while it remains inhibitory on primary afferents, the net effect of blocking GABA$_A$ receptors (e.g., with the antagonist bicuculline) is difficult to predict. In turn, potentiating GABAergic transmission (e.g., with allosteric modulators such as benzodiazepines) may paradoxically compound the hyperexcitability. On the other hand, with modest changes in E$_{GABA}$, GABA remains inhibitory; enhancement of GABAergic transmission may thus effectively counteract the hyperexcitability.

The outcome of drug treatments aimed at enhancing GABA$_A$-receptor function—benzodiazepines or barbiturates, for example—will depend on the degree of chloride accumulation in neurons and on the overall proportion of cells subject to net excitation by GABA [48]. In addition, the outcome will depend on the net balance of pre- versus postsynaptic inhibition. It is interesting to note, in this context, that recent evidence indicates that local spinal administration of benzodiazepines acting preferentially on the α$_2$ and α$_3$ subunits of the GABA$_A$ receptor are analgesic following peripheral nerve injury [31], suggesting that sufficient GABAergic inhibition may remain. However, a large proportion of these receptor subunits are on sensory terminals, and selective deletion of these subunits on primary afferents significantly attenuates benzodiazepine-mediated analgesia [31,78]. Thus, benzodiazepine-mediated analgesia in neuropathic pain may be mainly due to enhancement of inhibition on sensory terminals in the spinal cord. Overall, these findings illustrate how important it is to choose therapies not only on the basis of a disease mechanism, but also with regard to quantitative understanding of that mechanism [48].

In consistency with the above results, we also found that blocking chloride transport in control animals unmasked innocuous mechanical input to normally nociceptive-specific spinal lamina I projection neurons (Fig. 3) [30]. Impaired chloride extrusion is therefore a potentially sufficient substrate for the tactile allodynia (pain sensation in response to a

Fig. 3. Blockade of cation-chloride cotransport and local application of ATP-stimulated microglia unmask low-threshold input to normally selectively high-threshold lamina I projection neurons. (A) Schematic representation of the experimental setting to perform single-unit extracellular recordings from antidromically identified lamina I projection neurons. (B) Confirmation of a recording from a lamina I projection neuron.

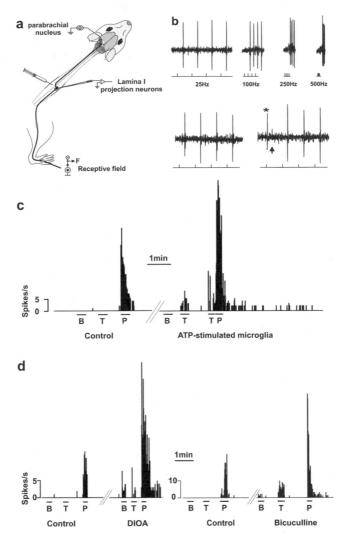

Top: Extracellular single-unit recordings from a lamina I neuron showing that the cell responds to every stimulus in a high-frequency train of antidromic stimuli (lower traces mark the stimulus) delivered from an electrode positioned in the lateral parabrachial nucleus. Bottom: Collision of the first of four antidromic action potentials (25 Hz) with an orthodromic action potential (*) occurring within the critical interval. The arrow points to the position where the first antidromic action potential would have occurred in the absence of the orthodromic action potential (as in the trace on the left). (C) Local spinal administration of ATP-stimulated microglia unmasked innocuous input to a normally nociceptive specific lamina I projection neuron (B = brush; T = touch; P = noxious pinch). (D) Local spinal administration of the cation-chloride cotransporter blocker [(dihydroindenyl)oxy]alkanoic acid (DIOA) or of the GABA$_A$ receptor antagonist bicuculline unmasked innocuous input to lamina I spinoparabrachial neurons that responded only to noxious pinch stimulation in control conditions. Modified from Keller et al. [30].

normally innocuous stimulus) that is characteristic of neuropathic pain. Because nociceptive relay neurons in spinal lamina I do not receive direct input from low-threshold afferents, the latter finding indicated that the disruption of inhibition by the impaired chloride transport in the superficial dorsal horn effectively unmasked indirect (most likely polysynaptic) connections between low-threshold mechanoreceptive afferents and these nociceptive relay neurons, akin to what occurs with local spinal blockade of $GABA_A$- and or glycine-receptor-mediated inhibition (Fig. 3) [68].

Loss of KCC2 as a Result of Intercellular Signaling Mechanisms

Importantly, the loss of KCC2 expression observed after peripheral nerve injury occurred in neurons intrinsic to the dorsal horn and therefore not in the directly injured neurons [16]. This finding indicated that, in contrast to the situation with other traumatic injuries [41,73], altered chloride homeostasis in spinal neurons after peripheral nerve injury involved a signaling mechanism between the injured afferents and dorsal horn neurons.

BDNF: A Signaling Molecule Controlling KCC2 Expression

Modulating ion gradients as a means to control the strength of synaptic transmission provides a novel perspective on synaptic plasticity. Indeed, changes in ion gradients, especially chloride gradients, have been well documented throughout development, but little consideration has been given until recently to the possibility that ion gradients could be actively modulated in adult tissue.

Initial demonstration of a potential intercellular signaling event modulating chloride homeostasis in adult tissue came from the observation that application of BDNF onto dissociated hippocampal cell cultures caused a selective shift in reversal potential of inhibitory postsynaptic currents (IPSCs) in a subpopulation of neurons [75]. Subsequent research showed that exposing hippocampal slice cultures to BDNF caused a downregulation of both KCC2 RNA and protein on a rapid time scale (within an hour), with a corresponding deficit in chloride extrusion capacity [52].

Kindling-induced epileptogenesis caused a concurrent upregulation of BDNF and downregulation of KCC2, with similar temporal profiles. In consistency with these original findings, we found that BDNF application onto adult spinal cord slices caused a depolarizing shift in E_{GABA}. In a subset of neurons, BDNF application even switched GABAergic currents into net excitatory events [15]. We then tested whether endogenous BDNF was responsible for the shift in E_{GABA} after nerve injury. For this, we either removed (or "mopped up") endogenous BDNF using a TrkB-Fc fusion protein [35,67] or blocked its binding to TrkB receptors using a function-blocking anti-TrkB antibody [5] in spinal slices taken from rats with peripheral nerve injury. We found that acute blockade of BDNF-TrkB signaling reversed the depolarizing shift in E_{GABA} [15].

These findings indicated (1) that endogenously released BDNF was causing the depolarizing shift in E_{GABA} and (2) that E_{GABA} is maintained at a depolarized level in dorsal horn neurons by tonically released BDNF at the spinal level after peripheral nerve injury. Thus, in the absence of TrkB receptor activity, chloride homeostasis maintains itself at its normal value. Maintenance of chloride homeostasis at a given level is thus an ongoing process that can be readily modulated to control the strength of $GABA_A$/glycine-receptor mediated transmission. Important for therapeutic considerations is the fact that chloride homeostasis was maintained after nerve injury at an altered level by a tonically released modulator, which indicates that impaired inhibition (disinhibition) could be reversed by drug treatment.

Intracellular Mechanisms Regulating KCC2 Activity

Two intracellular second messenger pathways have been identified by which BDNF-TrkB signaling controls KCC2 expression: the Shc/FRS-2 (src homology 2 domain-containing transforming protein/fibroblast growth factor receptor substrate 2) pathway and the phospholipase C-γ (PLCγ)-cyclic adenosine monophosphate response element-binding protein (CREB) pathway [53]. Interestingly, activation of both Shc and PLCγ cascades by TrkB causes a downregulation of KCC2, whereas activation of the Shc pathway in the absence of PLCγ activation leads to an upregulation of KCC2 [53]. This finding is particularly interesting because BDNF plays an important role in the ontogeny of chloride homeostasis by promoting the upregulation of KCC2 during the early postnatal period [2].

The bidirectional action of BDNF on KCC2 expression, depending on whether both Shc and PLCγ are involved, provides a potential mechanism for the divergent action of BDNF in early developmental stages compared to in adulthood (reminiscent of the opposite effects of BDNF on $GABA_A$-receptor trafficking in immature and adult brain tissue [39]). Thus, while BDNF signaling at early developmental stages appears to promote maturation of inhibition and thus a decrease in excitability, in adult tissue it promotes hyperexcitability by impairing and reversing inhibition. In other words, if BDNF secretion is involved in a repair response following nerve injury, a side effect of the action of the neurotrophin at the spinal level is to weaken the chloride extrusion capacity of the cell, yielding pain hypersensitivity. Other intracellular signaling pathways associated with TrkB activation, such as the protein kinase A pathway [50], may be involved in regulating the activity of KCC2 and perhaps that of other co-transporters [21], but this possibility remains to be studied more directly.

Microglia Control Neuronal Excitability by Altering Chloride Homeostasis

Active Sensors and Effectors in Normal and Pathological Conditions

Within the CNS, microglia and astrocytes represent two highly reactive intraparenchymal cell populations. Microglia represent the resident macrophages of the CNS. In normal conditions, they fulfill a constitutive surveillance function [22]. They acquire a different reactive profile—often termed "activation"—early in response to injury, infections, ischemia, brain tumors, or neurodegeneration. Activated microglia change from a ramified to ameboid morphology, proliferate, increase their expression of cell surface markers/receptors, migrate to areas of damage, become phagocytotic, and produce and release pro-inflammatory substances or cell-signaling mediators [15,18,22,23,32].

Multiple Sources and Multiple Phenotypes

Importantly, microglial activations are multidimensional. There are many different activational states, with various components expressed with different time-courses and intensities that depend on the stimulus that triggers activation [22]. Recent results have also revealed that nerve-injury-induced spinal microglial response can include not only activation of preexisting resident microglia, but also the generation of new microglia from proliferation [18] and from recruitment of peripheral monocytes [81]. Both resident and bone-marrow-derived microglia may be involved in the generation of neuronal hyperexcitability in the CNS. The ability of blood-borne monocytes to populate the CNS parenchyma and differentiate into microglia has been observed in adult animals, especially in certain special pathological conditions, although the exact conditions enabling CNS infiltration remain a subject of debate [63].

ATP-Stimulated Microglia Alter Neuronal E_{GABA}

While activated microglia are known to release a number of pro-inflammatory and signaling molecules, the direct mechanism by which microglia alter neuronal excitability in different pathological conditions has remained largely elusive. Peripheral nerve injury induces spinal microglial activation in several models of pain hypersensitivity [13,19,71,85]. After nerve injury, spinal activated microglia express de novo the $P2X_4$ receptor, and blockade of $P2X_4$ receptors reverses the tactile allodynia associated with the injury [71]. The finding by Tsuda et al. [71] that it is possible to administer locally, onto the spinal cord, ATP-stimulated microglia to cause tactile allodynia provided an ideal framework to test whether microglia may exert their action by altering neuronal E_{GABA} [15]. We indeed found that local spinal administration of ATP-stimulated microglia (unlike the administration of unstimulated microglia) caused a significant shift in E_{GABA} of superficial spinal dorsal horn neurons to more depolarized values and effectively unmasked low-threshold input to normally nociceptive-specific lamina I projection neurons. We obtained the same effects with nerve injury, pharmacological blockade of cation chloride cotransport, and blockade of $GABA_A$ receptors (Fig. 3) [30].

The fact that microglia caused a shift in E_{GABA} similar to that seen with BDNF administration suggested that microglia may act on the chloride gradient by releasing this neurotrophin [15]. Assays in microglial cultures indeed confirmed that ATP stimulation promotes the secretion of BDNF from microglia. More direct evidence that microglia signal directly to neurons via BDNF came from the finding that treatment of microglia with siRNA against BNDF prior to ATP stimulation and spinal administration prevented their behavioral effect and their effect on the chloride gradient [15]. The neurotrophin BDNF thus appears to be the direct mediator of microglia-neuron signaling, and alteration in neuronal chloride homeostasis appears to be a biophysical mechanism by which microglia can control neuronal excitability.

Ongoing Microglial Stimulation after Nerve Injury

The P2X-receptor antagonist TNP-ATP (at doses specific for $P2X_4$ receptors), when administered to spinal cord slices taken from rats that had received nerve injury, produced a shift in E_{GABA} toward more hyperpolarized values, thus effectively reversing the collapse in chloride gradient that characterizes neuropathic pain [15]. This finding indicates that the altered chloride homeostasis is maintained by continuous signaling from microglia in chronic pathological conditions, consistent with the observation of tonic spinal BDNF secretion in neuropathic animals.

Coupling of $P2X_4$ to BDNF

Enhanced spinal release of BDNF after peripheral nerve injury appears to be specifically linked to $P2X_4$-receptor activation by ATP. Indeed, in $P2X_4$ null mice, nerve injury failed to cause tactile allodynia, and application of ATP onto microglial cells failed to cause BDNF release [72]. Stimulation of $P2X_4$ causes an increase in expression and release of BDNF by microglia in culture, and this effect is dependent on p38 mitogen-activated protein kinase (MAPK) [70].

Microglia, Not Sensory Nerves, Are the Source of BDNF in Neuropathic Pain

We know that microglia release BDNF, but that does not necessarily mean that they represent the sole, or even the main, source of BDNF involved in KCC2 downregulation. In the spinal cord, for example, an important source of BDNF can be the terminals of peptidergic afferents, especially after peripheral inflammation [24,35,67]. The results of an interesting recent study demonstrate the likely source of BDNF after nerve injury or peripheral inflammation. The investigators reported that selective deletion of BDNF from small-diameter afferents effectively prevented tactile allodynia due to peripheral inflammation [83], consistent with findings that enhanced BDNF release occurs from small-diameter sensory afferents after peripheral inflammation [24,35,67]. Deletion of BDNF from peptidergic afferents had no effect on nerve injury-induced tactile allodynia, however, in consistency with the idea that BDNF originates from another source (e.g., microglia) in neuropathic pain conditions [15].

BDNF from Other Sources Affects KCC2 Expression

As mentioned above, after nerve injury, microglia appear to be the source of enhanced BDNF release, which causes a disruption of chloride homeostasis. In contrast, after peripheral inflammation, enhanced BDNF release occurs from small-diameter sensory fibers [24,35,67,83]. These findings have raised the question of whether enhanced BDNF release from different sources can similarly affect chloride homeostasis.

A recent study showed a downregulation of KCC2 in the spinal cord after peripheral inflammation [82], consistent with enhanced release of BDNF in the spinal cord from peptidergic sensory fibers [24,35,67,83]. KCC2 downregulation was prevented by pretreatment with K252a, consistent with the hypothesis that BDNF-TrkB signaling is responsible for the KCC2 downregulation.

In summary, regardless of the source of BDNF, neuronal or glial, activation of TrkB receptors by this neurotrophin appears to cause a disruption of chloride homeostasis. Thus, the latter mechanisms may represent the common pathway by which enhanced excitability occurs at the spinal level in chronic pain conditions involving enhanced BDNF expression [52,53].

What Activates Microglia?

While blockade/knockdown or knockout of $P2X_4$ receptors prevents the development of nerve-injury-induced tactile allodynia, neither of these interventions affects microglial activation [71,72]. Thus, other mechanisms, upstream of ATP signaling, must trigger microglial activation after injury.

Microglial Activation/Migration Is Spatially Defined and Depends on Intercellular Signaling

We and others have found that after peripheral nerve injury, microglial activation and migration occur in a spatially delimited area within the spinal cord parenchyma, essentially comprising the spinal territory occupied by the central terminals of injured afferents [7,79,81]. Yet, unlike the reaction seen after nerve injury, only a weak microglial reaction occurs within the spinal gray matter following rhizotomy (even though a strong activation occurs in the spinal dorsal funiculus) [55]. This finding suggests that although degeneration of central terminals is sufficient to elicit microglial activation, it does not account for the intraparenchymal response within the dorsal horn after peripheral nerve injury. Thus, in the latter case, microglial activation and chemotaxis must result from a local signaling mechanism between injured nerve terminals and microglia. Several potential candidate intercellular signaling cascades have been identified recently, as outlined below and summarized in Fig. 4.

Fractalkine to CX3CR1 Signaling

In the spinal cord dorsal horn, the chemokine fractalkine is expressed on neurons and sensory terminals, whereas its receptor, CX3CR1, is expressed primarily on microglia [74]. This chemokine is unique in that it is tethered to the extracellular surface of neurons and can be cleaved to form a diffusible signal [11]. Lysosomal cysteine protease cathepsin S (CatS), when expressed by activated spinal microglia, is responsible for the cleavage of neuronal transmembrane fractalkine into active soluble fractalkine [12]. After nerve injury, CatS-expressing activated microglia in spinal cord dorsal horn innervated by damaged fibers release CatS, which then liberates soluble fractalkine from afferent terminals and surrounding spinal neurons. The released fractalkine feeds back onto microglia cells via the CX3CR1 receptors to activate the p38 MAPK pathway. Both exogenous or endogenous fractalkine and CatS have pronociceptive effects, and inhibition of CatS enzymatic activity and neutralization of the CX3CR1 receptor reversed pain hypersensitivity in animals with nerve injury [6,38]. CatS-induced hyperalgesia is lost in CX3CR1 null mice [12].

Thus, while neurons are the source of fractalkine signaling to CX3CR1 on microglia, the initiating signal appears to be microglial CatS. Activated microglia may be signaling to other microglia via the cleavage of fractalkine on neurons. The concurrent increase in CatS expression by microglia and fractalkine by neurons could thus serve as a mechanism of amplification and coincidence detection. Because it is activated microglia that appear to release CatS, the release of CatS is unlikely to be the initiating mechanism for the activation of microglia. Another signaling mechanism probably triggers microglial activation, perhaps followed by an amplification of microglial activation and upregulation of p38 MAPK expression via CatS-fractalkine-CX3CR1 signaling (Fig. 4).

Matrix Metalloproteases

A recent study demonstrated that after nerve injury, matrix metalloproteinase (MMP)-9 is induced in dorsal root ganglion (DRG) sensory neurons within hours and returns to baseline 3 days after injury, whereas MMP-2 is induced in DRG satellite cells and in spinal astrocytes at later times (from days to weeks after injury) [28]. Although cellular distribution and temporal profile are different, both MMPs require a common molecular player, the cytokine interleukin (IL)-1β. MMP-9 induces neuropathic pain through IL-1β cleavage and microglial activation at early times, whereas MMP-2 maintains neuropathic pain through IL-1β cleavage and astrocyte activation at later times [28]. MMP-9 may thus be a good candidate as an initial trigger of microglial activation (Fig. 4).

MCP-1 to CCR2 Signaling

Monocyte chemoattractant protein-1 (MCP-1) is a member of the CC chemokine family (also termed CCL2). It specifically attracts and activates monocytes to sites of inflammation [33]. MCP-1 is upregulated in DRG sensory neurons by chronic constriction of the sciatic nerve [65,79]. The MCP-1 induced in DRG neurons is transported to their central terminals [79] and is released in the dorsal horn in response to electrical stimulation of sensory nerves [66]. Its receptor, CCR2, is upregulated in the spinal microglia after peripheral nerve injury, and transgenic mice lacking CCR2 do not develop tactile allodynia after nerve injury [1].

Both temporally and spatially, induction of MCP-1 in terminals of damaged sensory neurons correlates closely with the subsequent activation of surrounding spinal microglia [79]. This nerve-injury-induced spinal microglial activation is completely abolished in mice lacking CCR2 [81]. Local spinal injection of exogenous MCP-1 induces microglial activation, and this activation is lost in CCR2 knockout mice [81]. Together, these results implicate MCP-1 as a trigger for spinal microglial activation after peripheral nerve injury.

In addition to activation of microglia resident within the spinal cord, blood-borne monocytes/macrophages have the ability to infiltrate the spinal cord, to proliferate, and to differentiate into activated microglia [81]. MCP-1/CCR2 signaling is also involved in the neuron-to-monocytes/macrophages crosstalk from the CNS to the periphery, given that neutralization of MCP-1 at the spinal level prevented monocyte/macrophage infiltration after nerve injury [81]. Thus, both activation of resident microglia and infiltration of monocytes/macrophages appear to be due to a signaling mechanism within the spinal cord.

Other evidence implicates MCP-1/CCR2 in the recruitment of monocytes/macrophages and activated lymphocytes into the CNS in a

Fig. 4. Summary of the cascade of signaling events in the spinal cord leading to altered ⟶ chloride homeostasis following peripheral nerve injury or inflammation. See the text for a detailed description of the evidence implicating each of the signaling events depicted here. Briefly, following peripheral nerve injury, damaged sensory neurons upregulate the matrix metalloprotease MMP-9 [28] and the chemokine MCP-1 (also named CCL2 [79]). MMP-9 cleaves the cytokine IL-1β to activate microglia, while MCP-1 causes both microglial activation and chemotaxis of circulating monocytes via activation of the CCR2 receptor [1,81]. Stimulated monocytes infiltrate the spinal cord parenchyma and differentiate into activated microglia [81]. Activated microglia proliferate and release cathepsin S (CatS), which cleaves fractalkine tethered to the extracellular surface of neurons [12]. Cleaved fractalkine acts on CX3CR1 receptors on microglia to amplify microglial activation and upregulate p38 mitogen-activated protein kinase (MAPK) [27,86]. Activated microglia express de novo the $P2X_4$ receptors [71]. Selective stimulation of $P2X_4$ receptors by endogenous ATP causes the release of brain-derived neurotrophic factor (BDNF) in a p38 MAPK-dependent fashion [70,72]. In turn, BDNF acts on neuronal tyrosine kinase B (TrkB) receptors to downregulate the K^+-Cl^- cotransporter KCC2 in dorsal horn neurons [15,52,53]. After peripheral inflammation, enhanced BDNF release originates from sensory nerve terminals [82,83]. Regardless of the source of BDNF, the final common pathway appears to be a loss of KCC2 expression, causing an accumulation of resting intracellular Cl^- concentration and a decrease in Cl^- extrusion capacity. This alteration effectively impairs the efficacy of $GABA_A$- and glycine receptor-mediated transmission and, in extreme cases, changes the action of GABA and glycine into net excitation [14,15]. This event leads to a loss of spinal inhibition (disinhibition) and thus increases the excitability of dorsal horn neurons [30,48]. Modified from Zhang and De Koninck [80].

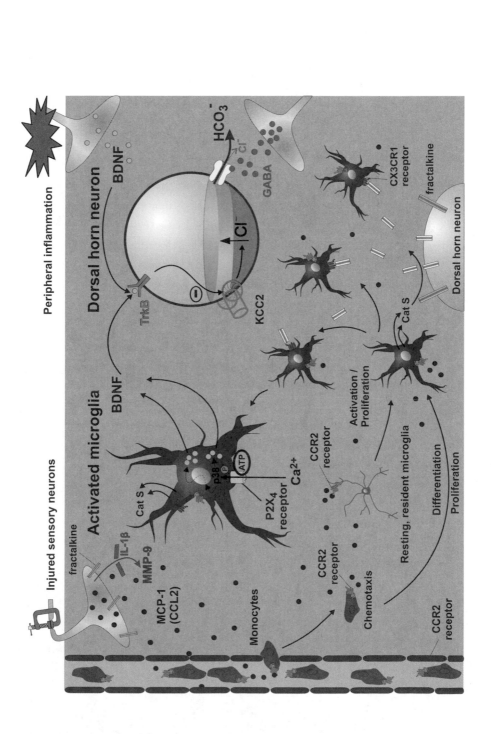

variety of inflammatory, infective, and traumatic conditions [25,29,51]. CCR2+ monocytes were identified as direct circulating precursors of microglia responsible for CNS infiltration [37]. A potential role of MCP-1 in the chemotaxis from the periphery to the CNS involves altering the expression of tight-junction-associated proteins in microvascular endothelial cells in the brain and spinal cord, thereby increasing the permeability of the blood-brain/spinal cord barrier [61,64] (Fig. 4).

Not only is MCP-1 a necessary mediator for spinal microglial activation, but its action is necessary for the development of mechanical allodynia. Indeed, mice lacking CCR2 do not develop pain hypersensitivity following nerve injury [81]. By selectively deleting central and peripheral CCR2, respectively, we found that either source of microglia—resident or blood-derived—was sufficient to cause pain hypersensitivity. Thus, infiltration of monocytes/macrophages into the CNS under pathological and or traumatic conditions may disrupt chloride homeostasis and alter neuronal excitability (Fig. 4).

Does Microglial Activation Always Disrupt Chloride Homeostasis?

As mentioned above, microglial activation is highly diverse and dynamic [22], and expression of $P2X_4$ receptors and secretion of BDNF occur only in specific conditions. Several other phenotypes have been observed in pathologies [3,22,44]. It thus remains to be determined whether the microglia are a source of enhanced BDNF in conditions other than pain induced by peripheral nerve injury.

Interestingly, a recent study showed a downregulation of KCC2 and a shift in E_{GABA} in the spinal dorsal horn following spinal cord injury [34]. This depolarizing shift in E_{GABA} effectively impaired $GABA_A$-receptor-mediated inhibition and caused normally subthreshold primary A- and C-fiber inputs to evoke action potentials in superficial dorsal horn neurons. Given the evidence of involvement of microglia in pain hypersensitivity after spinal cord injury [84], it is likely that, in this condition, downregulation of KCC2 is also caused by release of BDNF from microglia.

However, it remains to be determined whether BDNF-TrkB signaling is the only intercellular signaling pathway involved in disruption of neuronal chloride homeostasis. Another possibility to consider is whether

BDNF-TrkB signaling affects the activity of other cotransporters such as NKCC1. In several cases, NKCC1 and KCC2 appear to be regulated in an opposite manner by intracellular signaling pathways (one is upregulated when the other is downregulated) [17]. Thus, NKCC1 may be upregulated in response to activation of TrkB receptors, although a recent study reported no change in NKCC1 expression in the dorsal horn after peripheral inflammation, which enhanced spinal BDNF release [82].

Therapeutic Implications

The results of the studies outlined in this chapter open interesting avenues for therapeutic interventions. Drugs aimed at restoring normal chloride homeostasis may present advantages over current therapeutics strategies because they do not affect neuronal excitability directly, but rather modulate the efficacy of endogenous inhibition. Restoring endogenous inhibition rather than imposing inhibition (actively depressing excitability) may also yield more specific therapeutic treatments with less detrimental side effects [17].

The finding that normal expression of KCC2 is restored upon blocking BDNF-TrkB or ATP-P2X$_4$ signaling *after* the pathogenesis has developed, in the case of nerve-injury-induced pain hypersensitivity [15], is encouraging because it indicates that there may be targets by which to *restore* transporter function. Targeting BDNF-TrkB signaling directly may not be an attractive therapeutic option because this neurotrophin is involved in several functions throughout the CNS. Specifically preventing activated microglia from secreting BDNF—by targeting P2X$_4$ receptors, by altering p38-MAPK kinase signaling, or by preventing BDNF transcription selectively in microglia—may represent more promising strategies.

The identification of the complex cascade of events that lead to microglial activation also offers a wide array of novel therapeutic targets. However, because microglial activation is part of the normal immune reaction, preventing microglia from playing their role in the central inflammatory response to injury may be highly detrimental. Thus, the discovery of specific signaling mechanisms in which microglia participate under certain conditions of activation, and new understanding of selected downstream effector mechanisms such as chloride homeostasis, provide potential avenues to selectively control certain side effects of the central inflammatory response without affecting other aspects of neuroimmune function.

Acknowledgments

The author acknowledges support from the Canadian Institutes of Health (CIHR), the Natural Sciences and Engineering Research Council of Canada (NSERC), the Neuroscience Canada Foundation, the Ontario Neurotrauma Foundation, and the Krembil Foundation. The author is also a *Chercheur National* of the Fonds de la recherche en santé du Québec (FRSQ).

References

[1] Abbadie C, Lindia JA, Cumiskey AM, Peterson LB, Mudgett JS, Bayne EK, DeMartino JA, MacIntyre DE, Forrest MJ. Impaired neuropathic pain responses in mice lacking the chemokine receptor CCR2. Proc Natl Acad Sci USA 2003;100:7947–52.

[2] Aguado F, Carmona MA, Pozas E, Aguilo A, Martinez-Guijarro FJ, Alcantara S, Borrell V, Yuste R, Ibanez CF, Soriano E. BDNF regulates spontaneous correlated activity at early developmental stages by increasing synaptogenesis and expression of the K^+/Cl^- co-transporter KCC2. Development 2003;130:1267–80.

[3] Avignone E, Ulmann L, Levavasseur F, Rassendren F, Audinat E. Status epilepticus induces a particular microglial activation state characterized by enhanced purinergic signaling. J Neurosci 2008;28:9133–44.

[4] Baba H, Ji RR, Kohno T, Moore KA, Ataka T, Wakai A, Okamoto M, Woolf CJ. Removal of GABAergic inhibition facilitates polysynaptic A fiber-mediated excitatory transmission to the superficial spinal dorsal horn. Mol Cell Neurosci 2003;24:818–30.

[5] Balkowiec A, Katz DM. Activity-dependent release of endogenous brain-derived neurotrophic factor from primary sensory neurons detected by ELISA in situ. J Neurosci 2000;20:7417–23.

[6] Barclay J, Clark AK, Ganju P, Gentry C, Patel S, Wotherspoon G, Buxton F, Song C, Ullah J, Winter J, Fox A, Bevan S, Malcangio M. Role of the cysteine protease cathepsin S in neuropathic hyperalgesia. Pain 2007;130:225–34.

[7] Beggs S, Salter MW. Stereological and somatotopic analysis of the spinal microglial response to peripheral nerve injury. Brain Behav Immun 2007;21:624–33.

[8] Castro-Lopes JM, Malcangio M, Pan BH, Bowery NG. Complex changes of $GABA_A$ and $GABA_B$ receptor binding in the spinal cord dorsal horn following peripheral inflammation or neurectomy. Brain Res 1995;679:289–97.

[9] Castro-Lopes JM, Tavares I, Coimbra A. GABA decreases in the spinal cord dorsal horn after peripheral neurectomy. Brain Res 1993;620:287–91.

[10] Castro-Lopes JM, Tölle TR, Pan B, Zieglgänsberger W. Expression of GAD mRNA in spinal cord neurons of normal and monoarthritic rats. Brain Res Mol Brain Res 1994;26:169–76.

[11] Chapman GA, Moores K, Harrison D, Campbell CA, Stewart BR, Strijbos PJ. Fractalkine cleavage from neuronal membranes represents an acute event in the inflammatory response to excitotoxic brain damage. J Neurosci 2000;20:RC87.

[12] Clark AK, Yip PK, Grist J, Gentry C, Staniland AA, Marchand F, Dehvari M, Wotherspoon G, Winter J, Ullah J, Bevan S, Malcangio M. Inhibition of spinal microglial cathepsin S for the reversal of neuropathic pain. Proc Natl Acad Sci USA 2007;104:10655–60.

[13] Colburn RW, Rickman AJ, DeLeo JA. The effect of site and type of nerve injury on spinal glial activation and neuropathic pain behavior. Exp Neurol 1999;157:289–304.

[14] Cordero-Erausquin M, Coull JA, Boudreau D, Rolland M, De Koninck Y. Differential matura-
      tion of GABA action and anion reversal potential in spinal lamina I neurons; impact of chloride
      extrusion capacity. J Neurosci 2005;25:9613–23.
[15] Coull JA, Beggs S, Boudreau D, Boivin D, Tsuda M, Inoue K, Gravel C, Salter MW, De Koninck Y.
      BDNF from microglia causes the shift in neuronal anion gradient underlying neuropathic pain.
      Nature 2005;438:1017–21.
[16] Coull JA, Boudreau D, Bachand K, Prescott SA, Nault F, Sik A, De Koninck P, De Koninck Y.
      Trans-synaptic shift in anion gradient in spinal lamina I neurons as a mechanism of neuropathic
      pain. Nature 2003;424:938–42.
[17] De Koninck Y. Altered chloride homeostasis in neurological disorders: a new target. Curr Opin
      Pharmacol 2007;7:93–9.
[18] Echeverry S, Shi XQ, Zhang J. Characterization of cell proliferation in rat spinal cord following
      peripheral nerve injury and the relationship with neuropathic pain. Pain 2008;135:37–47.
[19] Fu KY, Light AR, Matsushima GK, Maixner W. Microglial reactions after subcutaneous formalin
      injection into the rat hind paw. Brain Res 1999;825:59–67.
[20] Furue H, Narikawa K, Kumamoto E, Yoshimura M. Responsiveness of rat substantia gelatinosa
      neurones to mechanical but not thermal stimuli revealed by in vivo patch-clamp recording. J
      Physiol (Lond) 1999;521:529–35.
[21] Gamba G. Molecular physiology and pathophysiology of electroneutral cation-chloride cotrans-
      porters. Physiol Rev 2005;85:423–93.
[22] Hanisch UK, Kettenmann H. Microglia: active sensor and versatile effector cells in the normal
      and pathologic brain. Nat Neurosci 2007;10:1387–94.
[23] Haynes SE, Hollopeter G, Yang G, Kurpius D, Dailey ME, Gan WB, Julius D. The P2Y12 receptor
      regulates microglial activation by extracellular nucleotides. Nat Neurosci 2006;9:1512–9.
[24] Heppenstall PA, Lewin GR. BDNF but not NT-4 is required for normal flexion reflex plasticity
      and function. Proc Natl Acad Sci USA 2001;98:8107–12.
[25] Huang DR, Wang J, Kivisakk P, Rollins BJ, Ransohoff RM. Absence of monocyte chemoattrac-
      tant protein 1 in mice leads to decreased local macrophage recruitment and antigen-specific T
      helper cell type 1 immune response in experimental autoimmune encephalomyelitis. J Exp Med
      2001;193:713–26.
[26] Ibuki T, Hama AT, Wang XT, Pappas GD, Sagen J. Loss of GABA-immunoreactivity in the spinal
      dorsal horn of rats with peripheral nerve injury and promotion of recovery by adrenal medullary
      grafts. Neuroscience 1997;76:845–58.
[27] Ji RR, Suter MR. p38 MAPK, microglial signaling, and neuropathic pain. Mol Pain 2007;3:33.
[28] Kawasaki Y, Xu ZZ, Wang X, Park JY, Zhuang ZY, Tan PH, Gao YJ, Roy K, Corfas G, Lo EH, Ji
      RR. Distinct roles of matrix metalloproteases in the early- and late-phase development of neuro-
      pathic pain. Nat Med 2008;14:331–6.
[29] Kelder W, McArthur JC, Nance-Sproson T, McClernon D, Griffin DE. Beta-chemokines MCP-1
      and RANTES are selectively increased in cerebrospinal fluid of patients with human immuno-
      deficiency virus-associated dementia. Ann Neurol 1998;44:831–5.
[30] Keller AF, Beggs S, Salter MW, De Koninck Y. Transformation of the output of spinal lamina
      I neurons after nerve injury and microglia stimulation underlying neuropathic pain. Mol Pain
      2007;3:27.
[31] Knabl J, Witschi R, Hosl K, Reinold H, Zeilhofer UB, Ahmadi S, Brockhaus J, Sergejeva M, Hess
      A, Brune K, Fritschy JM, Rudolph U, Mohler H, Zeilhofer HU. Reversal of pathological pain
      through specific spinal GABA$_A$ receptor subtypes. Nature 2008;451:330–4.
[32] Koizumi S, Shigemoto-Mogami Y, Nasu-Tada K, Shinozaki Y, Ohsawa K, Tsuda M, Joshi BV,
      Jacobson KA, Kohsaka S, Inoue K. UDP acting at P2Y6 receptors is a mediator of microglial
      phagocytosis. Nature 2007;446:1091–5.
[33] Leonard EJ, Skeel A, Yoshimura T. Biological aspects of monocyte chemoattractant protein-1
      (MCP-1). Adv Exp Med Biol 1991;305:57–64.
[34] Lu Y, Zheng J, Xiong L, Zimmermann M, Yang J. Spinal cord injury-induced attenuation of
      GABAergic inhibition in spinal dorsal horn circuits is associated with down-regulation of the
      chloride transporter KCC2 in rat. J Physiol 2008;586:5701–15.
[35] Mannion RJ, Costigan M, Decosterd I, Amaya F, Ma QP, Holstege JC, Ji RR, Acheson A, Lind-
      say RM, Wilkinson GA, Woolf CJ. Neurotrophins: peripherally and centrally acting modula-
      tors of tactile stimulus-induced inflammatory pain hypersensitivity. Proc Natl Acad Sci USA
      1999;96:9385–90.

[36] Marchand F, Perretti M, McMahon SB. Role of the immune system in chronic pain. Nat Rev Neurosci 2005;6:521–32.

[37] Mildner A, Schmidt H, Nitsche M, Merkler D, Hanisch UK, Mack M, Heikenwalder M, Bruck W, Priller J, Prinz M. Microglia in the adult brain arise from Ly-6ChiCCR2+ monocytes only under defined host conditions. Nat Neurosci 2007;10:1544–53.

[38] Milligan ED, Zapata V, Chacur M, Schoeniger D, Biedenkapp J, O'Connor KA, Verge GM, Chapman G, Green P, Foster AC, Naeve GS, Maier SF, Watkins LR. Evidence that exogenous and endogenous fractalkine can induce spinal nociceptive facilitation in rats. Eur J Neurosci 2004;20:2294–302.

[39] Mizoguchi Y, Ishibashi H, Nabekura J. The action of BDNF on $GABA_A$ currents changes from potentiating to suppressing during maturation of rat hippocampal CA1 pyramidal neurons. J Physiol 2003;548:703–9.

[40] Moore KA, Kohno T, Karchewski LA, Scholz J, Baba H, Woolf CJ. Partial peripheral nerve injury promotes a selective loss of GABAergic inhibition in the superficial dorsal horn of the spinal cord. J Neurosci 2002;22:6724–31.

[41] Nabekura J, Ueno T, Okabe A, Furuta A, Iwaki T, Shimizu-Okabe C, Fukuda A, Akaike N. Reduction of KCC2 expression and $GABA_A$ receptor-mediated excitation after in vivo axonal injury. J Neurosci 2002;22:4412–7.

[42] Narikawa K, Furue H, Kumamoto E, Yoshimura M. In vivo patch-clamp analysis of IPSCs evoked in rat substantia gelatinosa neurons by cutaneous mechanical stimulation. J Neurophysiol 2000;84:2171–4.

[43] Nguyen MD, Julien JP, Rivest S. Innate immunity: the missing link in neuroprotection and neurodegeneration? Nat Rev Neurosci 2002;3:216–27.

[44] Pocock JM, Kettenmann H. Neurotransmitter receptors on microglia. Trends Neurosci 2007;30:527–35.

[45] Polgar E, Gray S, Riddell JS, Todd AJ. Lack of evidence for significant neuronal loss in laminae I–III of the spinal dorsal horn of the rat in the chronic constriction injury model. Pain 2004;111:144–50.

[46] Polgar E, Hughes DI, Arham AZ, Todd AJ. Loss of neurons from laminas I-III of the spinal dorsal horn is not required for development of tactile allodynia in the spared nerve injury model of neuropathic pain. J Neurosci 2005;25:6658–66.

[47] Prescott SA, De Koninck Y. Four cell types with distinctive membrane properties and morphologies in lamina I of the spinal dorsal horn of the adult rat. J Physiol (Lond) 2002;539:817–36.

[48] Prescott SA, Sejnowski TJ, De Koninck Y. Reduction of anion reversal potential subverts the inhibitory control of firing rate in spinal lamina I neurons: a biophysical basis for neuropathic pain. Mol Pain 2006;2:32.

[49] Prince DA. Epileptogenic neurons and circuits. Adv Neurol 1999;79:665–84.

[50] Qiu J, Cai D, Filbin MT. A role for cAMP in regeneration during development and after injury. Prog Brain Res 2002;137:381–7.

[51] Rancan M, Otto VI, Hans VH, Gerlach I, Jork R, Trentz O, Kossmann T, Morganti-Kossmann MC. Upregulation of ICAM-1 and MCP-1 but not of MIP-2 and sensorimotor deficit in response to traumatic axonal injury in rats. J Neurosci Res 2001;63:438–46.

[52] Rivera C, Li H, Thomas-Crusells J, Lahtinen H, Viitanen T, Nanobashvili A, Kokaia Z, Airaksinen MS, Voipio J, Kaila K, Saarma M. BDNF-induced TrkB activation down-regulates the K^+-Cl^- cotransporter KCC2 and impairs neuronal Cl^- extrusion. J Cell Biol 2002;159:747–52.

[53] Rivera C, Voipio J, Thomas-Crusells J, Li H, Emri Z, Sipila S, Payne JA, Minichiello L, Saarma M, Kaila K. Mechanism of activity-dependent downregulation of the neuron-specific K-Cl cotransporter KCC2. J Neurosci 2004;24:4683–91.

[54] Rock RB, Gekker G, Aravalli RN, Hu S, Sheng WS, Peterson PK. Potentiation of HIV-1 expression in microglial cells by nicotine: involvement of transforming growth factor-beta1. J Neuroimmune Pharmacol 2008;3:143–9.

[55] Scholz J, Abele A, Marian C, Haussler A, Herbert TA, Woolf CJ, Tegeder I. Low-dose methotrexate reduces peripheral nerve injury-evoked spinal microglial activation and neuropathic pain behavior in rats. Pain 2008;138:130–42.

[56] Scholz J, Broom DC, Youn DH, Mills CD, Kohno T, Suter MR, Moore KA, Decosterd I, Coggeshall RE, Woolf CJ. Blocking caspase activity prevents transsynaptic neuronal apoptosis and the loss of inhibition in lamina II of the dorsal horn after peripheral nerve injury. J Neurosci 2005;25:7317–23.

[57] Sherman SE, Loomis CW. Morphine insensitive allodynia is produced by intrathecal strychnine in the lightly anesthetized rat. Pain 1994;56:17–29.

[58] Sherman SE, Luo L, Dostrovsky JO. Spinal strychnine alters response properties of nociceptive-specific neurons in rat medial thalamus. J Neurophysiol 1997;78:628–37.

[59] Sivilotti L, Woolf CJ. The contribution of $GABA_A$ and glycine receptors to central sensitization: disinhibition and touch-evoked allodynia in the spinal cord. J Neurophysiol 1994;72:169–79.

[60] Somers DL, Clemente FR. Dorsal horn synaptosomal content of aspartate, glutamate, glycine and GABA are differentially altered following chronic constriction injury to the rat sciatic nerve. Neurosci Lett 2002;323:171–4.

[61] Song L, Pachter JS. Monocyte chemoattractant protein-1 alters expression of tight junction-associated proteins in brain microvascular endothelial cells. Microvasc Res 2004;67:78–89.

[62] Sorkin LS, Puig S. Neuronal model of tactile allodynia produced by spinal strychnine: effects of excitatory amino acid receptor antagonists and a []-opiate receptor agonist. Pain 1996;68:283–92.

[63] Soulet D, Rivest S. Bone-marrow-derived microglia: myth or reality? Curr Opin Pharmacol 2008;8:508–18.

[64] Stamatovic SM, Keep RF, Kunkel SL, Andjelkovic AV. Potential role of MCP-1 in endothelial cell tight junction 'opening': signaling via Rho and Rho kinase. J Cell Sci 2003;116:4615–28.

[65] Tanaka T, Minami M, Nakagawa T, Satoh M. Enhanced production of monocyte chemoattractant protein-1 in the dorsal root ganglia in a rat model of neuropathic pain: possible involvement in the development of neuropathic pain. Neurosci Res 2004;48:463–9.

[66] Thacker MA, Clark AK, Bishop T, Grist J, Yip PK, Moon LD, Thompson SW, Marchand F, McMahon SB. CCL2 is a key mediator of microglia activation in neuropathic pain states. Eur J Pain 2008;Epub Jun 11.

[67] Thompson SW, Bennett DL, Kerr BJ, Bradbury EJ, McMahon SB. Brain-derived neurotrophic factor is an endogenous modulator of nociceptive responses in the spinal cord. Proc Natl Acad Sci USA 1999;96:7714–8.

[68] Torsney C, MacDermott AB. Disinhibition opens the gate to pathological pain signaling in superficial neurokinin 1 receptor-expressing neurons in rat spinal cord. J Neurosci 2006;26:1833–43.

[69] Toth Z, Hollrigel GS, Gorcs T, Soltesz I. Instantaneous perturbation of dentate interneuronal networks by a pressure wave-transient delivered to the neocortex. J Neurosci 1997;17:8106–17.

[70] Trang T, Beggs S, Wan X, Salter MW. P2X4-receptor mediated synthesis and release of brain-derived neurotrophic factor in microglia is dependent on calcium and p38-mitogen-activated protein kinase activation. J Neurosci 2009;29:3518–28.

[71] Tsuda M, Shigemoto-Mogami Y, Koizumi S, Mizokoshi A, Kohsaka S, Salter MW, Inoue K. P2X4 receptors induced in spinal microglia gate tactile allodynia after nerve injury. Nature 2003;424:778–83.

[72] Ulmann L, Hatcher JP, Hughes JP, Chaumont S, Green PJ, Conquet F, Buell GN, Reeve AJ, Chessell IP, Rassendren F. Up-regulation of P2X4 receptors in spinal microglia following peripheral nerve injury mediates BDNF release and neuropathic pain. J Neurosci 2008;28:11263–8.

[73] Van den Pol AN, Obrietan K, Chen G. Excitatory actions of GABA after neuronal trauma. J Neurosci 1996;16:4283–92.

[74] Verge GM, Milligan ED, Maier SF, Watkins LR, Naeve GS, Foster AC. Fractalkine (CX3CL1) and fractalkine receptor (CX3CR1) distribution in spinal cord and dorsal root ganglia under basal and neuropathic pain conditions. Eur J Neurosci 2004;20:1150–60.

[75] Wardle RA, Poo MM. Brain-derived neurotrophic factor modulation of GABAergic synapses by postsynaptic regulation of chloride transport. J Neurosci 2003;23:8722–32.

[76] Woolf CJ, Salter MW. Neuronal plasticity: increasing the gain in pain. Science 2000;288:1765–9.

[77] Yaksh TL. Behavioral and autonomic correlates of the tactile evoked allodynia produced by spinal glycine inhibition: effects of modulatory receptor systems and excitatory amino acid antagonists. Pain 1989;37:111–23.

[78] Zeilhofer HU. Synaptic disinhibition in inflammatory pain states. In: Gate control revisited: spinal disinhibition in inflammatory and neuropathic pain. Workshop presented at: 12th World Congress on Pain, Glasgow, 2008.

[79] Zhang J, De Koninck Y. Spatial and temporal relationship between monocyte chemoattractant protein-1 expression and spinal glial activation following peripheral nerve injury. J Neurochem 2006;97:772–83.

[80] Zhang J, De Koninck Y. Central neuroglial interactions in the pathophysiology of neuropathic pain. In: Mayer EA, Bushnell MC, editors. Functional pain syndromes: presentation and pathophysiology. Seattle: IASP Press; 2009. p. 319–36.

[81] Zhang J, Shi XQ, Echeverry S, Mogil JS, De Koninck Y, Rivest S. Expression of CCR2 in both resident and bone marrow-derived microglia plays a critical role in neuropathic pain. J Neurosci 2007;27:12396–406.

[82] Zhang W, Liu LY, Xu TL. Reduced potassium-chloride co-transporter expression in spinal cord dorsal horn neurons contributes to inflammatory pain hypersensitivity in rats. Neuroscience 2008;152:502–10.

[83] Zhao J, Seereeram A, Nassar MA, Levato A, Pezet S, Hathaway G, Morenilla-Palao C, Stirling C, Fitzgerald M, McMahon SB, Rios M, Wood JN. Nociceptor-derived brain-derived neurotrophic factor regulates acute and inflammatory but not neuropathic pain. Mol Cell Neurosci 2006;31:539–48.

[84] Zhao P, Waxman SG, Hains BC. Extracellular signal-regulated kinase-regulated microglia-neuron signaling by prostaglandin E_2 contributes to pain after spinal cord injury. J Neurosci 2007;27:2357–68.

[85] Zhuang ZY, Gerner P, Woolf CJ, Ji RR. ERK is sequentially activated in neurons, microglia, and astrocytes by spinal nerve ligation and contributes to mechanical allodynia in this neuropathic pain model. Pain 2005;114:149–59.

[86] Zhuang ZY, Kawasaki Y, Tan PH, Wen YR, Huang J, Ji RR. Role of the CX3CR1/p38 MAPK pathway in spinal microglia for the development of neuropathic pain following nerve injury-induced cleavage of fractalkine. Brain Behav Immun 2007;21:642–51.

Correspondence to: Yves De Koninck, PhD, Centre de recherche Robert-Giffard, Université Laval, 2601 Chemin de la Canardière, Québec, QC, Canada G1J 2G3. Email: yves.dekoninck@crulrg.ulaval.ca.

Traumatic Nerve Injury: Diagnosis, Recovery, and Risk Factors for Neuropathic Pain

Satu K. Jääskeläinen

Department of Clinical Neurophysiology, Turku University Hospital, Turku, Finland

Introduction to Traumatic Nerve Injury

Much of what we know today about traumatic nerve injury, and the neuropathic pain that frequently accompanies it, comes from clinical studies conducted during wartime. The first of these studies were the seminal works by Silas Weir Mitchell and his coworkers [31], published after the American Civil War. Mitchell coined the term "causalgia," from the Greek words *kausos* (heat) and *algos* (pain), to describe "the whole catalogue of terms vainly used to convey some idea of variety in torture" in patients with neuropathic pain, a common consequence of nerve wounds, which most of his patients called "aching pain" [31]. It was Mitchell who first noticed the spread of symptoms and signs in neuropathic pain patients to uninjured neighboring nerve territories or to other extremities, ipsilateral or contralateral to the initial injury. The First and Second World Wars resulted in more traumatic nerve injuries that were carefully investigated and followed in clinical studies, often after surgical nerve repair [40,44]. This material allowed a more detailed classification of nerve injuries according

Current Topics in Pain: 12th World Congress on Pain
edited by José Castro-Lopes
IASP Press, Seattle, © 2009

to the degree and type of damage to the large peripheral nerve fibers (α motor neurons and Aβ sensory afferents), with reference to neurophysiological characteristics and the patient's chances of making a functional recovery (Table I, Fig. 1).

Peripheral nerve injuries also arise in peacetime, causing major suffering and disability throughout the world due to functional impairment and pain. Traumatic peripheral nerve lesions are commonly caused

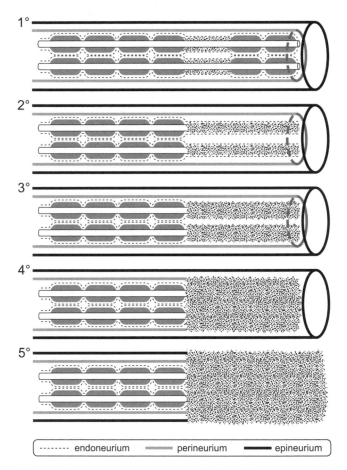

Fig. 1. Classification of traumatic nerve injuries. The five different degrees of nerve injury according to Sunderland [44] with increasing severity from 1 degree (pure demyelination) to 5 degrees (total nerve transection) are shown for a schematic peripheral nerve consisting of one nerve fascicle covered by the perineurium and including two myelinated nerve fibers, each covered by an endoneurial sheath. The differences in structural damage, functional alterations, and recovery process according to the degree of nerve injury are explained in Table I.

Table I
Classification of nerve injuries

Seddon [40]	Sunderland [44]	Structural	Functional	Recovery
Neurapraxia	1st degree	Injury to myelin and Schwann cells; ischemia	Conduction slowing; normal size of action potentials in neurography; blocking at lesion site	Excellent: up to 3–6 months
Axonotmesis	2nd degree	Axonal interruption; endoneurium intact; Wallerian degeneration distally; changes in cell body	No conduction in injured fibers, small action potentials, EMG: denervation, loss of motor units according to number of injured axons, mostly good axonal reinnervation in follow-up	Mostly good, depending upon distance; axonal sprouts grow 1–3 mm/day to correct targets
	3rd degree	Axonal and endoneurial interruption; perineurium intact; neuroma in continuity possible	No conduction in injured fibers, small to absent action potentials, conduction block at the site of neuroma; EMG: denervation, severe loss of motor units, collateral reinnervation, and poor to moderate axonal reinnervation in follow-up	Poor; axonal misdirection; incomplete axonal regeneration; surgery may be needed
	4th degree	Axonal, endoneurial, and perineurial interruption; epineurium intact; neuroma in continuity	No conduction in injured axons, EMG: severe to total loss of motor units, chronic denervation; there may be signs of collateral reinnervation, usually not of axonal reinnervation	Poor; axonal misdirection; spontaneous regeneration of little functional importance; surgery usually required
Neurotmesis	5th degree	Nerve transection: the entire nerve trunk is separated by a gap; neuroma-glioma formation	No conduction, total denervation, no signs of axonal reinnervation, but collateral reinnervation may occur	No recovery without surgical nerve repair; prognosis after surgery guarded or poor, depending on timing and distance

Source: Modified from Stewart [42] and Robinson [37].

by motor vehicle collisions, falls, gunshot wounds, and industrial accidents [37]. Even minor, rather superficial, lacerating injuries may cause severe nerve damage, especially to cutaneous sensory nerves. Nerves can be severely lacerated, stretched, or crushed in injuries involving bone dislocations and fractures. Especially susceptible are nerves traveling close to bony structures (e.g., the radial, ulnar, peroneal, sciatic, and inferior alveolar nerves).

Approximately 5% of patients at primary trauma centers have peripheral nerve injuries [33]. Traumatic peripheral neuropathies frequently arise in combination with severe multiple organ injuries. Fractures, brain damage, internal organ injuries, and severe disturbances of cardiovascular function require emergency treatment and take priority at the acute stage. Less obvious peripheral neuropathies and neuropathic pain may not be recognized early on, although they have a major impact on final functional recovery. Focal peripheral nerve injuries necessitate active rehabilitation, often with the aid of specific treatment for neuropathic pain. Recently, researchers have recognized that iatrogenic nerve injuries causing neuropathic pain play a major role in persistent, often disabling, postsurgical pain (for review, see [22]). Furthermore, iatrogenic nerve injuries caused by previous surgery, misdirected injections, diathermy, and radiation represent the leading causes of nerve repair surgery in many specialized tertiary centers [23,24,28].

Early recognition, appropriate diagnosis, accurate localization, and correct treatment of focal peripheral nerve lesions and neuropathic pain demand familiarity with the mechanisms, pathophysiology, and classification of peripheral nerve injuries. These are decisive factors that guide the clinician in choosing appropriate treatment and predicting functional recovery after traumatic nerve injury. Many accurate and sensitive neurophysiological, psychophysical, and neuroanatomical diagnostic methods are available today that can help the clinician determine the type and exact site of nerve injury and assess the risk for development of neuropathic pain [4,6,14,30,37,39,41,42,55]. These methods complement clinical neurological examination to improve diagnosis of peripheral neuropathy. This chapter will elucidate some aspects of their application in pain research and clinical practice. When used appropriately, these methods can aid in the timely treatment of traumatic nerve injury and neuropathic pain.

Anatomical and Neurophysiological Classification of Peripheral Nerve Injury

Nerve injuries can be anatomically and neurophysiologically character-ized as axonal and demyelinating [40,44,45] (Table I; Fig. 1). In practice, most traumatic peripheral nerve lesions are of mixed type, where different degrees of axonal and myelin damage coexist. Demyelination affects only the myelin sheath and Schwann cells that cover the myelinated Aα, Aβ, and Aδ nerve fibers; the basal lamina of Schwann cells remains intact, as do the other supporting structures. In axonal lesions, the nerve fibers within a nerve trunk lose their continuity, with or without damage to the endoneurial sheath (Table I; Fig. 1). The distal part of the severed axon is degraded by Schwann cells and macrophages during Wallerian degenera-tion that lasts for 7 to 11 days after injury [12]. During this period, the distal part of the nerve may still appear excitable in neurography exami-nation, but when Wallerian degeneration has finished, no action poten-tials can be elicited from the injured nerve fibers distal to the lesion [5]. Moreover, the proximal parts of the injured neurons undergo degenerative changes [12], and secondary changes occur via apoptotic and collateral sprouting mechanisms within the spinal cord and the dorsal root ganglion [12,48]. The degree of damage to the external supporting connective tissue and vascular structures of the nerve fibers (endoneurium, perineurium, and epineurium) has an additional impact on functional disability and prognosis for recovery, on the risk for neuroma formation and pain, and on the choice of optimal treatment (Table I; Fig. 1). The most severe nerve injury is total transection (neurotmesis), in which the entire nerve trunk is separated, with all axons and shielding connective tissue structures los-ing their continuity. The two nerve ends retract, leaving a gap between them, impeding spontaneous recovery and requiring nerve repair surgery [37,40,42,44,45].

Axonal injuries are often partial, involving only a subset of nerve fibers or fascicles within a peripheral nerve trunk. Selective fas-cicular lesions give rise to restricted, patchy motor and sensory deficits, which may hamper correct interpretation of the results and localiza-tion of the lesion, in both clinical neurological and neurophysiological examinations [42].

Nerve Injury Mechanism, Type of Nerve Fiber Damage, and Recovery

Compression is the main cause of demyelination, and large myelinated fibers are especially vulnerable to pressure. Ischemia may also induce demyelination. Demyelination caused by acute transitory compression usually heals completely within a few weeks to 4 months; generally it is not associated with neuropathic pain. Although clinical recovery is excellent after demyelination, conduction velocity at the site of the lesion does not completely return to normal because the newly formed Schwann cell-myelin units are more tightly packed, with more numerous nodes of Ranvier and shorter internodal distances, which slows down saltatory conduction in the myelinated nerve fibers [12,37,42].

Various trauma mechanisms may induce axonal damage, including laceration, stretching, ischemia, extreme heat (e.g., during diathermy), and crushing. Axonal lesions heal slowly via collateral and axonal reinnervation. Neurophysiological techniques show that the axons never fully recover compared to their pre-injury baseline, although functional recovery may be satisfactory after less severe injuries (Table I). Following an initial shock period, which may last up to 1 month, axonal sprouts start to grow from the proximal stump by 1–3 mm/day in an attempt to find their way to the distal end organs. If the endoneurial tube is intact, the sprouts are directed to the correct targets; the final recovery is usually good, if the distance between the lesion site and the innervated organ is not too long. The upper time limit for possible motor regeneration is approximately 1.5 years (corresponding to 51–153 cm), after which the axonal sprouts cannot make functionally adequate connections with the atrophied target muscles [37,45]. Sensory reinnervation may not have any strict time limits [17,37], but regeneration after nerve repair surgery may be worse for sensory nerves compared to motor nerves [23]. In addition, the capacity for sensory reinnervation varies widely among healthy subjects and can be influenced by diseases such as diabetes [36]. During collateral reinnervation, the neighboring intact nerve fibers produce collateral sprouts to take care of the nearby target organs that have lost their innervation [17,46].

In more severe axonal injuries (Sunderland's classes 3–5; see Table I and Fig. 1), functional recovery is at best moderate but often poor, and surgical exploration, resection of neuroma, and nerve repair surgery may be needed [12,24,34,37,42,44,45]. In addition, after these more severe axonal injuries, misdirection of the axonal sprouts through the wrong endoneurial tubes to incorrect target organs is the rule rather than the exception, leading to poor functional recovery. This aberrant regeneration leads to disturbed motor unit recruitment patterns, altered central reflex modulation, and distorted, erroneously located sensory perceptions, inducing peculiar and disabling symptoms at the chronic phase of recovery [43].

In practice, most of the traumatic nerve injuries are of a mixed type: some fascicles within a nerve trunk may be completely cut, while in others, the axons lose their continuity but the perineurium remains intact. Some fibers only undergo demyelination. These mixed lesions typically recover in stages: quick early improvement with remyelination by 4 months, followed by gradual improvement for up to 2 years along with axonal and collateral reinnervation [37,42,44].

Nerve Injury and Neuropathic Pain

Neuropathic pain occurring after peripheral nerve injury has been particularly related to partial axonal nerve damage, in both experimental and human studies [3]. The majority of the nerve fibers within the peripheral nerves are small myelinated Aδ and unmyelinated C fibers that are also more susceptible to mechanisms inducing axonal injury than to compression [7,29,37]. Injury to somatosensory small-fiber tracts is considered to be a prerequisite for the occurrence of neuropathic pain [6,22,19,52].

Crushing of the nerves, or stretching with ragged lacerations that disrupt the supporting connective tissue structures and the nerve's vascular supply, lead to neuropathic pain more frequently than injuries involving clean-cut incisions [15,27,37,47]. One reason may be that the injury-related neurotonic bursts of action potentials that usually occur with actual or threatened axonal damage happen much less frequently or not at all in sudden, clean-cut, "electrically silent" injuries [13]. Probably more importantly, damage to the supporting neural structures increases the risk for neuroma formation. Both stump neuromas after total nerve transection and neuromas-in-continuity after partial, fascicular lesions can induce positive sensory symptoms and signs (paresthesias and allodynia), along with neuropathic pain [27,42,44,45].

Neuropathic pain after peripheral nerve injury is a poorly recognized and underdiagnosed entity. Correct diagnosis may be delayed for up to 2.5 years [32]. In many cases, neuropathic pain is of iatrogenic origin [23,24,28], which should facilitate early recognition and treatment. However, the diagnosis of iatrogenic nerve injury is also delayed far beyond the optimal treatment period (within 6 months) in most patients [23,28]. This problem is attributed to difficulties in early recognition and clinical diagnosis of neuropathic pain, both at the primary care level [32] and at specialized clinics [23,28].

Diagnosis of Peripheral Neuropathy and Neuropathic Pain

History and clinical examination form the basis of the diagnosis of peripheral nerve injuries and neuropathic pain. Clinical examination findings guide the choice of additional investigations with more sensitive and specific diagnostic methods that are often needed to confirm the diagnosis, to localize the lesion, and to assess the type and profile of nerve fiber damage as well as the efficiency of regeneration. These additional tests include neurophysiological investigations with electroneuromyography (ENMG); recordings using somatosensory evoked potentials (SEPs), laser-evoked potentials (LEPs), and contact heat evoked potentials (CHEPs); reflex studies; quantitative sensory testing (QST) of tactile, nociceptive, and thermal modalities; and measurement of intraepidermal and subepidermal nerve fiber densities in skin and mucosal biopsies [4,6,8,14,25,37,39,41,42,54]. Structural imaging with new magnetic resonance imaging (MRI) techniques has a growing role in the diagnosis of traumatic peripheral nerve lesions. At present, this type of imaging is mainly used in the diagnosis of radicular and plexus lesions and before explorative surgery to reveal hematomas and neuromas and to show the extent of scarring [42].

When conducting a clinical examination for suspected neuropathic pain, the clinician should keep in mind that although pain is a common symptom of focal peripheral nerve injuries, it has poor localizing value regarding the site of the neuroanatomical lesion. Distribution of motor and sensory deficits and paresthesias gives a much more accurate topographic level diagnosis in focal peripheral neuropathies [42]. Clinical neurological examination does not allow classification of the type of nerve damage or accurate assessment of the severity of peripheral nerve injury. This information is a prerequisite for reliable prognosis of recovery and appraisal of the treatments needed. For example, after a severe nerve injury with total loss of axonal continuity, clinical examination reveals findings similar to those of complete focal conduction block. However, these two injury types have completely different prognoses and need different treatment approaches (exploratory surgery with nerve repair versus waiting for an excellent prospect of spontaneous recovery) [37,42]. Similarly, in clinical examination, partial axonal lesions cannot be differentiated from partial demyelination during the first 4 months after injury. In addition, it may be impossible to verify old, incompletely healed, or minor acute partial nerve injuries with the rather crude clinical tests available [9,10,14,16,19,56].

Neurophysiological examination is invaluable in the diagnosis of traumatic neuropathy and neuropathic pain. ENMG, including neurography of sensory, motor, and mixed nerves, and needle electromyography (EMG) of the muscles reveals the type, degree, location, and age of a peripheral nerve lesion involving large myelinated fibers. After demyelination, nerve conduction velocity slows down, but the size of the response remains within normal limits. Needle EMG does not show any spontaneous denervation activity within the muscles innervated by the injured nerve. In axonal neuropathy, response size diminishes, nerve conduction velocity remains within normal limits, and EMG shows signs of denervation and loss of motor units according to the extent of nerve fiber damage. In focal nerve lesions, the exact site of injury or compression can sometimes be localized to within 1 cm (e.g., ulnar nerve entrapment at the elbow, focal neuroma, or nerve tumor). Recovery can also be assessed with ENMG, which enables the separate detection of axonal and collateral reinnervation long before there is clear clinical evidence for improved function [25,37,42].

Clinical neurophysiological and psychophysical tests (QST, which is also often performed in clinical neurophysiology laboratories) offer sensitive and objective tools for determining the type and extent of damage to sensory fibers, including small $A\delta$ and C fibers. Thermal QST, LEPs, and recently, CHEP recordings enable in vivo assessment of the four main classes of small fibers mediating innocuous (cool, warm) and noxious (cold, heat pain) thermal sensory information. These methods provide diagnostic efficacy superior to clinical examination in the diagnosis and follow-up of functional status of peripheral small fibers or the anterolateral spinothalamic tract after injury. When combined with skin biopsy for quantification of intraepidermal nerve fiber density (IENFD), neurophysiological examination provides a means for both topographic-level diagnosis of small-fiber dysfunction and assessment of the various functional phenomena related to neuropathy, nerve regeneration, and neuropathic pain. Both the negative (hypoesthesia, anesthesia) and positive (paresthesia, allodynia, hyperesthesia, abnormal spread, aftersensations, wind-up) symptoms and signs related to sensory neuropathy can be evaluated in detail during the neurophysiological and psychophysical investigation [4,6,14,30,39,43].

Surgical Nerve Injury in the Study of Peripheral Neuropathy and Neuropathic Pain

Chronic postsurgical pain (defined as pain lasting more than 3 months), unfortunately common, is currently considered to be neuropathic pain secondary to iatrogenic nerve injury. The incidence of persistent postsurgical pain is higher after procedures carrying a high risk of nerve injury. Due to the anatomical circumstances and surgical techniques applied, the incidence of chronic pain is especially high—around 50%—after limb amputation, coronary artery bypass surgery, and thoracotomy [22].

Surgery may thus offer models for the study of chronic pain in humans, including neuropathic pain [35]. There is evidence that QST [1,11] and neurophysiological investigations [2] improve the recognition of neuropathy and neuropathic pain after surgery. It is clear that not all patients with postoperative neuropathy develop neuropathic pain, but without exact knowledge about the pathophysiological mechanism and type of injury, the injury-related risk factors of postoperative pain cannot be fully clarified.

Intraoperative neurophysiological monitoring (IOM) is routinely used in many centers during various neurosurgical, otological, and orthopedic surgical procedures to prevent iatrogenic nervous system injury and postoperative neurological morbidity. During IOM, standard neurophysiological recordings (ENMG, evoked potentials, or electroencephalography) are performed continuously in the operating room. Signs of impending nerve injury such as neurotonic discharges or decrease in response amplitude, indicating axonal damage, are immediately reported to the surgeon, who will change the operating strategy accordingly to prevent any further damage to nervous tissue [13]. Repeated neurophysiological recordings have been used to investigate the risk stages and surgical events leading to nerve injury during mandibular surgery [18] and thoracotomy [38]; however, without continuous monitoring, the findings remain suggestive. These studies have shown that long or forceful compression with retractors, causing ischemia, and nerve crush may be especially likely to lead to the development of neuropathic pain. In addition, IOM is used in nerve repair surgery to identify nerve tissue among scar formation and to assess the continuity of the nerve fascicles within the lesion site [24,26,27].

Iatrogenic Trigeminal Nerve Injury: A Human Model for Sensory Neuropathy, Recovery, and Neuropathic Pain

In a recent series of studies with a prospective 1-year follow-up design, bilateral sagittal split osteotomy of the mandible (BSSO) was used as a human model for the study of perioperative traumatic neuropathy, postsurgical nerve regeneration, and development of neuropathic pain [20,21,49,50,51]. This model and study design additionally enabled evaluation of the diagnostic efficacy of various tests for sensory neuropathy. A new intraoperative neurophysiological monitoring technique based on neurography of the inferior alveolar nerve (IAN) was developed to prevent surgical nerve damage during BSSO [18,21]. This technique allowed accurate on-line detection, classification, and grading of nerve injury. Potential iatrogenic sensory nerve damage was evaluated by comparing the results of IAN neurography, blink reflex (a trigeminal brainstem reflex), thermal (cool, warm, heat and cold pain) and tactile sensory detection thresholds, and a thorough, standardized clinical sensory examination at five time points for 1 year after surgery to the individual baseline values before surgery in 20 healthy subjects (40 nerves at risk).

Different degrees of IAN damage occurred in connection with BSSO in 95% of the nerves at risk [49,50]. However, macroscopic events and inspection during BSSO did not suffice for reliable detection and classification of intraoperative IAN injury; even visibly intact nerves could have suffered severe axonal injury [18,21,49]. During BSSO, the most frequent type of nerve injury (found in 52% of the nerves at risk) was demyelination due to compression of the neurovascular bundle with retractors during medial mucosal opening. Partial axonal nerve damage due to laceration, stretch, or ischemia was found in 38% of the nerves. In primarily demyelinating injuries, secondary axonal damage occurred in 15% of the nerves. There were no total nerve transections, probably because intraoperative monitoring allowed timely prevention of these most severe lacerating injuries [21,49].

Sensory recovery depended on the type of injury. Most of the demyelinating injuries recovered via remyelination back to normal baseline condition during the first 4 months, but after axonal lesions, both subjective and neurophysiological recovery was only moderate and most often (in 80% of cases) incomplete [20,51]. In addition to axonal regeneration, very late sensory recovery may occur via collateral reinnervation from the neighboring intact nerve distributions, even years after the initial injury [17].

Considering the diagnostic value of different tests for IAN neuropathy (see Table II), neurophysiological recordings in combination with quantitative testing of innocuous warm and cool detection thresholds increased diagnostic sensitivity at the early postoperative examinations by up to >90% compared to the lower 30–40% sensitivity of clinical sensory tests [51]. The quantitative neurophysiological and psychophysical tests also correlated better with the subjective sensory disturbances at both the early and late stages of follow-up compared to clinical sensory examination (Table II) [20,51]. Hypoesthesia to cooling and warming at the acute stage was compatible with axonal injury and predicted poor recovery at 1 year, whereas heat pain detection threshold was not a reliable indicator of peripheral neuropathy (with 40% sensitivity at the early postoperative stage, but only 13% at 1-year follow-up). Contrary to neurophysiological recordings and innocuous thermal detection thresholds, heat pain detection did not correlate with intraoperative nerve injury or subjective sensory symptoms in early postoperative tests. This finding is probably due to high interindividual variation in pain detection thresholds, which leads to wide normal reference limits that reduce the diagnostic value of pain detection thresholds. One year after BSSO, sensory alteration was still present in 38% of the IAN distributions. This finding could be verified with a combination of neurography and cool and warm detection tests in nearly all nerve distributions (93%), but with clinical sensory examination, it could be verified in only one (7%) [20,51].

Table II
Clinical, quantitative sensory, and neurophysiological tests in the diagnosis of inferior alveolar nerve (IAN) neuropathy

Test	Sensitivity (%) at 2 weeks / 1 year	Specificity (%) at 2 weeks / 1 year
Brush stroke direction	40 / 0	89 / 100
Sharp/blunt discrimination	40 / 0	89 / 100
Warm/cold discrimination	44 / 7	100 / 100
Grating orientation discrimination	59 / 27	73 / 88
Tactile detection threshold	58 / 33	56 / 88
Cool detection threshold	64 / 40	100 / 88
Warm detection threshold	50 / 47	100 / 92
Heat pain detection threshold	43 / 13	100 / 96
Blink reflex of the mental nerve	59 / 27	60 / 100
Neurography of the IAN	88 / 82	55 / 100

Source: Modified from Teerijoki-Oksa et al. [50,51].
Note: When the diagnostic values were calculated at 2 weeks, the end result of intraoperative neurophysiological monitoring (IOM) was considered the gold standard for neuropathy; at 1 year, the gold standard consisted of IOM result combined with subjective report of sensory alteration.

In this prospective study on BSSO, overall occurrence of neuropathic pain at 1 year was 5%, which is similar to the overall estimated incidence of neuropathic pain after traumatic and iatrogenic nerve injuries [22,27]. Neuropathic pain occurred only after partial axonal lesions, and its incidence in the group with axonal injuries was 13% [20]. Notably, the clinical sensory examination was normal, as was heat pain detection, in patients with neuropathic pain 1 year after severe axonal nerve injury that had been verified macroscopically and by intraoperative neurophysiological monitoring. Abnormal findings in thermal QST for cool and warm detection and neurography were able to confirm the correct diagnosis of neuropathic pain even at this late stage. The risk for neuropathic pain may be greater after slight to moderate axonal damage than after severe axonal loss [11,55]. This is also true in the trigeminal distribution because the sensory action potential amplitudes of the inferior alveolar nerve are higher in neuropathic patients with pain compared to those without pain [19]. Older age (>30 years) and female gender may additionally increase the risk of neuropathic pain after trigeminal nerve injury [19,20].

Spread of pain outside the involved neuropathic distribution is common and was acknowledged in the early works by Mitchell [31]. It may be less well recognized that the negative signs may also spread outside the initially involved nerve territory, for example to a homologous area in the contralateral upper extremity after unilateral nerve injury [53]. In the trigeminal distribution, the spread of negative signs has been shown to occur in the form of bilateral thermal hypoesthesia after unilateral nerve injury [19]. This phenomenon may be related to central plasticity in the trigeminal system and is specifically associated with the occurrence of neuropathic pain [19]. This finding indicates that the contralateral homologous area cannot be used as a normal reference point in clinical sensory examination or QST. There is a need for proper reference values and also for normal differences between the two sides of the body when QST is applied in clinical practice [39].

All phenomena related to changes in the central nervous system after peripheral nerve injury complicate the clinical diagnosis of neuropathic pain, especially at the chronic stages (>6 months after injury), when routine clinical sensory examination may easily fail to demonstrate the underlying neuropathy due to its low diagnostic sensitivity (Table II). The neurophysiological tests used in this prospective study on surgical IAN injury have also been applied to the study of potential neurogenic mechanisms in the clinically less well-defined idiopathic orofacial pain conditions [9,10,16]. The tests have revealed subgroups with different profiles of large or small nerve-fiber deficits and dysfunction among patients suffering from burning mouth syndrome and atypical facial pain. Although by definition their clinical examination is normal, in the majority of these patients, neurophysiological and psychophysical signs clearly indicate various degrees of neuropathic involvement at different levels of the trigeminal system [9,10,16]. The frequent finding of thermal hypoesthesia to cool or warm in burning mouth syndrome patients [9] has been confirmed, by measuring IENFD, to be due to focal peripheral small-fiber neuropathy of the tongue mucosa [41].

Conclusions

Iatrogenic nerve injuries are frequent, but only some of them give rise to neuropathic pain. When surgical nerve injury is used in the study of human neuropathic pain, ENMG-based intraoperative monitoring methods provide the most powerful means to document and classify potential iatrogenic nerve injury. Combined with macroscopic observations and information of the causal mechanism, IOM enables detailed analysis of the injury-related factors contributing to the incidence of postsurgical neuropathic pain. At the same time, it allows prevention of severe axonal nerve injury and reduces postsurgical morbidity and persistent pain. In our prospective study, neuropathic pain was associated with severe but partial laceration of the nerve trunk (partial axonal injury), which may be associated with aberrant axonal regeneration and formation of fascicular neuromas in-continuity. Other injury-related factors increasing the risk for pain included damage to small Aδ and C fibers. Additional injury to large Aβ afferents was also present, but a lesser degree of permanent damage (or more efficient reinnervation) of these fibers may be associated with a higher risk of neuropathic pain.

While the purely demyelinating injuries healed by 6 months, sensory recovery was incomplete at 1 year after most cases of axonal injury. The neuropathic etiology of the subjective symptoms could, in most cases, only be confirmed with thermal QST and neurography at later times. All the large- and small-fiber tests showed recovery at approximately the same rate; the higher incidence of abnormalities in the large-fiber test at 1 year is due to the ability of short-segment neurography to document stable sequelae of old injuries.

Both positive and negative signs such as neuropathic pain and thermal hypoesthesia may spread extrasegmentally and to the contralateral side after unilateral nerve injury, which in combination with restricted partial fascicular lesions complicates interpretation of clinical examination. These phenomena also challenge the rigid definition of neuropathic pain of peripheral origin as a condition in which the signs have to conform to the classical innervation territories of peripheral nervous system structures.

Fig. 2 presents a flow chart of the diagnostic steps for investigation of traumatic nerve injuries. The main findings in human focal neuropathy with or without pain are those of motor and sensory deficits: decreased or absent tendon reflexes, muscle weakness, and hypoesthesia/anesthesia. In patients with trigeminal neuropathy, positive signs such as hyperesthesia and allodynia seem to be rare, as has been reported for other human nerve injuries [1]. Thus, the main focus in the investigation of suspected peripheral neuropathic pain should be the search for negative symptoms and signs compatible with deficits in the somatosensory system. Clinical sensory examination, even when performed in a highly standardized manner, shows poor sensitivity at chronic stages of recovery (>6 months after injury), which severely limits its value in the diagnosis of neuropathic pain in old, partial nerve injuries. In addition, QST for heat pain detection is an insensitive diagnostic tool as regards human neuropathy and neuropathic pain at the chronic stage, whereas cool and warm detection tests moderately improve diagnostic accuracy at both the early and late stages of recovery after axonal nerve injury. Neurography has the best diagnostic value at both the acute and chronic stages after injury, and it correlates well with both intraoperative events and subjective sensory alteration. The good diagnostic value is probably due to the ability of ENMG to verify both demyelination and axonal nerve damage, while investigations for small-fiber function are mainly sensitive to axonal injuries. ENMG examination can thus be recommended for patients with suspected peripheral neuropathy and neuropathic pain as a first-line additional investigation whenever available. Thermal QST for detection of warm and cool hypoesthesia and LEP, CHEP, and IENFD from skin biopsy complement one other in the diagnosis of axonal and small-fiber damage, especially in nerve distributions not easily reached with ENMG techniques and in pure small-fiber neuropathies.

With the aid of a detailed clinical neurophysiological examination, including QST and skin biopsy, the diagnostic work-up of individual patients can be significantly improved, which is especially important in

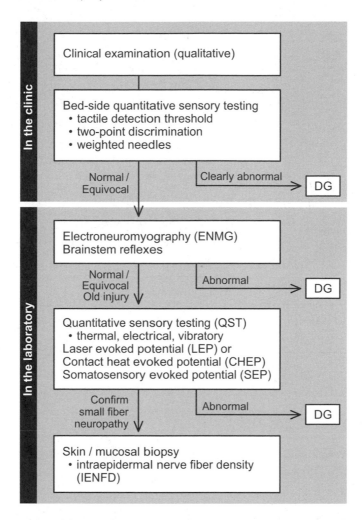

Fig. 2. Diagnostic steps for traumatic nerve injury. It is important that in the clinical examination, more than just qualitative tests should be applied in the diagnostic work-up. The results of the tests should be accurately described in the patient records, with special attention to negative signs such as tactile and thermal hypoesthesia or hypoalgesia, which are more specific to neuropathy than are positive signs such as allodynia or hyperesthesia. Some of the quantitative sensory tests can easily be included in a chair or bedside examination, whereas others are better performed in dedicated laboratories with expertise in clinical neurophysiology and reference values. Traumatic and especially iatrogenic nerve injuries that may lead to litigation require initial early examination with laboratory tests such as electroneuromyography (ENMG), thermal quantitative sensory testing (QST), or evoked potential recordings. In the case of symptoms and signs indicating predominant small-fiber damage but normal findings in ENMG and QST, skin biopsy should be considered at the early stages after injury. All these tests complement each other in the diagnosis of peripheral nerve injury, and rational combinations during the first 4 months after injury give the best diagnostic accuracy. DG = diagnosis.

traumatic and iatrogenic nerve injuries, which often lead to litigation. In these cases, objective and quantitative diagnostic tools should be used at the acute stage after injury when the tests have the best diagnostic value; at late stages, such as during litigation, their diagnostic accuracy may not suffice for correct diagnosis. If sufficiently sensitive diagnostic tools are not used in time, reimbursement and correct treatment may be unnecessarily delayed or denied to patients with chronic neuropathic pain after trauma or invasive medical procedures. In the study of peripheral neuropathy, treatment effects in neuropathic pain patients, and genetic risk factors for neuropathic pain, multiple diagnostic tools (clinical, neurophysiological, QST, and IENFD techniques) should be systematically used in combination because in many cases, the presence or absence of a peripheral neuropathy cannot be reliably determined with a single test. These additional laboratory investigations should also be included in the protocols when defining neuropathic pain for clinical and research purposes because there is clearly a continuum of peripheral neuropathic conditions ranging from clear-cut, clinically evident nerve lesions to neurophysiologically or neuroanatomically definite neuropathies, in which the results of clinical examination are equivocal or totally normal.

Acknowledgments

This study was supported by grants from the Sigrid Jusélius Foundation and the Finnish Medical Foundation.

References

[1]   Aasvang EK, Brandsborg B, Christensen B, Jensen TS, Kehlet H. Neurophysiological characterization of postherniotomy pain. Pain 2008;137:173–81.

[2]   Benedetti F, Vighetti S, Ricco C, Amanzio M, Bergamasco L, Casadio C, Cianci R, Giobbe R, Oliaro A, Bergamasco B, Maggi G. Neurophysiologic assessment of nerve impairment in posterolateral and muscle-sparing thoracotomy. J Thorac Cardiovasc Surg 1998;115:841–7.

[3]   Campbell JN. Nerve lesions and generation of pain. Muscle Nerve 2001;24:1261–73.

[4]   Chao C-C, Hsieh S-C, Tseng M-T, Chang Y-C, Hsieh ST. Patterns of contact heat evoked potentials (CHEP) in neuropathy with skin denervation: correlation of CHEP amplitude with intraepidermal nerve fiber density. Clin Neurophysiol 2008;119:653–61.

[5]   Chaudry V, Cornblath DR. Wallerian degeneration in human nerves: serial electrophysiological studies. Muscle Nerve 1992;15:687–93.

[6]   Cruccu G, Anand P, Attal N, Garcia-Larrea L, Haanpää M, Jorum E, Serra J. EFNS guidelines on neuropathic pain assessment. Eur J Neurol 2004;11:153–62.

[7]   Cruccu G, Inghilleri M, Fraioli B, Guidetti B, Manfredi M. Neurophysiologic assessment of trigeminal function after surgery for trigeminal neuralgia. Neurology 1987;37:631–8.

[8] England JD, Gronseth GS, Franklin G, Miller RG, Asbury AK, Carter GT, Cohen JA, Fisher MA, Howard JF, Kinsella LJ, et al. Distal symmetric polyneuropathy: a definition for clinical research. Report of the American Academy of Neurology, the American Association of Electrodiagnostic Medicine, and the American Academy of Physical Medicine and Rehabilitation. Neurology 2005;64:199–207.

[9] Forssell H, Jääskeläinen SK, Tenovuo O, Hinkka S. Sensory dysfunction in burning mouth syndrome. Pain 2002;99:41–7.

[10] Forssell H, Tenovuo O, Silvoniemi P, Jääskeläinen SK. Differences and similarities between atypical facial pain and neuropathic trigeminal pain. Neurology 2007;69:1451–9.

[11] Gottrup H, Andersen J, Arendt-Nielsen L, Jensen TS. Psychophysical examination in patients with post-mastectomy pain. Pain 2000;87:275–84.

[12] Hall S. The re-sponse to injury in the peripheral nervous system. J Bone Joint Surg (Br) 2005;87B:1309–19.

[13] Harper CM, Daube JR. Facial nerve electromyography and other cranial nerve monitoring. J Clin Neurophysiol 1998;15:206–16.

[14] Jääskeläinen SK. Clinical neurophysiology and quantitative sensory testing in the investigation of orofacial pain and sensory function. J Orofac Pain 2004;18:85–107.

[15] Jääskeläinen SK, Peltola JK. Clinical application of the blink reflex with stimulation of the mental nerve in lesions of the inferior alveolar nerve. Neurology 1994;44:2356–61.

[16] Jääskeläinen SK, Forssell H, Tenovuo O. Electrophysiological testing of the trigeminofacial system: aid in the diagnosis of atypical facial pain. Pain 1999;80:191–200.

[17] Jääskeläinen SK, Peltola JK. Electrophysiological evidence for extremely late sensory collateral reinnervation in man. Neurology 1996;46:1703–5.

[18] Jääskeläinen SK, Peltola JK, Forssell K, Vähätalo K. Evaluating the function of the inferior alveolar nerve during mandibular sagittal split osteotomy with repeated nerve conduction tests. J Oral Maxillofac Surg 1995;53:269–79.

[19] Jääskeläinen SK, Teerijoki-Oksa T, Forssell H. Neurophysiologic and quantitative sensory testing in the diagnosis of trigeminal neuropathy and neuropathic pain. Pain 2005;117:349–57.

[20] Jääskeläinen SK, Teerijoki-Oksa T, Forssell K, Virtanen A, Forssell H. Sensory regeneration following intraoperatively verified trigeminal nerve injury. Neurology 2004;62:1951–7.

[21] Jääskeläinen SK, Teerijoki-Oksa T, Forssell K, Vähätalo K, Peltola J, Forssell H. Intraoperative monitoring of the inferior alveolar nerve during mandibular sagittal split osteotomy. Muscle Nerve 2000;23:368–75.

[22] Kehlet H, Jensen TS, Woolf C. Persistent postsurgical pain: risk factors and prevention. Lancet 2006;367:1618–25.

[23] Khan R, Birch R. Iatropathic injuries of peripheral nerves. J Bone Joint Surg 2001;83B:1145–8.

[24] Kim DH, Kline DG. Surgical outcome for intra- end extrapelvic femoral nerve lesions. J Neurosurg 1995;83:783–90.

[25] Kimura J. Electrodiagnosis in diseases of the nerve and muscle: principles and practice. New York: Oxford University Press; 2001.

[26] Kline DG. Timing for exploration of nerve lesions and evaluation of the neuroma-in-continuity. Clin Orthoped Rel Res 1982;163:42–9.

[27] Kline DG, Hudson AR. Nerve injuries. Philadelphia: Saunders; 1995.

[28] Kretschmer T, Antoniadis G, Braun V, Rath SA, Richter H-P. Evaluation of iatrogenic lesions in 722 surgically treated cases of peripheral nerve trauma. J Neurosurg 2001;94:901–12.

[29] Lacomis D. Small-fiber neuropathy. Muscle Nerve 2002;26:173–88.

[30] Løseth S, Lindal S, Stålberg E, Mellgren SI. Intraepidermal nerve fibre density, quantitative sensory testing and nerve conduction studies in a patient material with symptoms and signs of sensory polyneuropathy. Eur J Neurol 2006;13:105–11.

[31] Mitchell SW, Morehouse GR, Keen WW. Gunshot wounds and other injuries of nerves. Philadelphia: Lippincott; 1864. p.100–11.

[32] Neuropathic Pain Network, Pfizer Inc. Global neuropathic pain survey. Harris Interactive; 2007.

[33] Noble J, Munro CA, Prasad VSSV, Midha R. Analysis of upper and lower extremity peripheral nerve injuries in a population of patients with multiple injuries. J Trauma 1998;45:116–22.

[34] Omer GE. Results of untreated peripheral nerve injuries. Clin Orthop Rel Res 1982;163:15–9.

[35] Perkins FM, Gopal A. Postsurgical chronic pain: a model for investigating the origins of chronic pain. Tech Reg Anesth Pain Manag 2003;7:122–6.

[36] Polydefkis M, Hauer P, Sheth S, Sirdofsky M, Griffin JW, McArthur JC. The time course of epidermal nerve fibre regeneration: studies in normal controls and in people with diabetes, with and without neuropathy. Brain 2004;127:1606–15.
[37] Robinson LR. Traumatic injury to peripheral nerves. Muscle Nerve 2000;23:863–73.
[38] Rogers ML, Henderson L, Mahajan RP, Duffy JP. Preliminary findings in the neurophysiological assessment of intercostal nerve injury during thoracotomy. Eur J Cardiothorac Surg 2002;21:298–301.
[39] Rolke R, Baron R, Maier C, Tölle TR, Treede RD, Beyer A, Binder A, Birbaumer N, Birklein F, Bötefür IC, et al. Quantitative sensory testing in the German Research Network on Neuropathic Pain (DFNS): standardized protocol and reference values. Pain 2006;123:231–43.
[40] Seddon HJ. Three types of nerve injury. Brain 1943;66:236–88.
[41] Sommer C, Lauria G. Skin biopsy in the management of peripheral neuropathy. Lancet Neurol 2007;6:632–42.
[42] Stewart JD. Focal peripheral neuropathies, 3rd ed. Philadelphia: Lippincott Williams & Wilkins; 2000.
[43] Sumner AJ. Aberrant reinnervation. Muscle Nerve 1990;13:801–3.
[44] Sunderland S. A classification of peripheral nerve injuries producing loss of function. Brain 1951;74:491–516.
[45] Sunderland S. The anatomy and physiology of nerve injury. Muscle Nerve 1990;13:771–84.
[46] Sunderland S. Factors complicating the evaluation of sensory function in nerve injuries. In: Sunderland S. Nerves and nerve injuries, 2nd ed. Edinburgh: Churchill Livingstone; 1978. p. 362–5.
[47] Sunderland S, McArthur R, Nam DA. Repair of a transected sciatic nerve. A study of nerve regeneration and functional recovery. J Bone Joint Surg 1993;75A:911–4.
[48] Tandrup T, Woolf CJ, Coggeshall RE. Delayed loss of small dorsal root ganglion cells after transection of the rat sciatic nerve. J Comp Neurol 2000;422:172–80.
[49] Teerijoki-Oksa T, Jääskeläinen SK, Forssell K, Forssell H, Vähätalo K, Tammisalo T, Virtanen A. Risk factors of nerve injury during mandibular sagittal split osteotomy. Int J Oral Maxillofac Surg 2002;31:33–9.
[50] Teerijoki-Oksa T, Jääskeläinen S, Forssell K, Virtanen A, Forssell H. An evaluation of clinical and electrophysiologic tests in nerve injury diagnosis after mandibular sagittal split osteotomy. Int J Oral Maxillofac Surg 2003;32:15–23.
[51] Teerijoki-Oksa T, Jääskeläinen SK, Forssell K, Virtanen A, Forssell H. Recovery of nerve injury after mandibular sagittal split osteotomy. Diagnostic value of clinical and electrophysiologic tests in the follow-up. Int J Oral Maxillofac Surg 2004;33:134–40.
[52] Treede R-D, Jensen TS, Campbell JN, Cruccu G, Dostrovsky JO, Griffin JW, Hansson P, Hughes R, Nurmikko T, Serra J. Neuropathic pain. Redefinition and a grading system for clinical and research purposes. Neurology 2008;70:1630–5.
[53] Wahren LK, Torebjörk E, Nyström B. Quantitative sensory testing before and after regional guanethidine block in patients with neuralgia in the hand. Pain 1991;16:23–30.
[54] Yarnitsky D, Granot M. Quantitative sensory testing. In: Cervero F, Jensen TS, editors. Handbook of clinical neurology, Vol. 81. Pain. Amsterdam: Elsevier; 2006. p. 397–409.
[55] Yoon YW, Dong H, Arends JJ, Jacquin MF. Mechanical and cold allodynia in a rat spinal cord contusion model. Somatosens Mot Res 2004;21:25–31.
[56] Zuniga JR, Meyer RA, Gregg JM, Miloro M, Davis L. The accuracy of clinical neurosensory testing for nerve injury diagnosis. J Oral Maxillofac Surg 1998;56:2–8.

Correspondence to: Satu K. Jääskeläinen, MD, PhD, Department of Clinical Neurophysiology, Turku University Hospital, Postal Box 52, FIN-20521 Turku, Finland. Email: satu.jaaskelainen@tyks.fi.

Moving Pain Genetics into the Genome-Wide Association Era

Mitchell B. Max

Departments of Anesthesiology and Medicine, University of Pittsburgh, Pittsburgh, Pennsylvania, USA

Over the past year, the leading medical journals and the newspapers' front pages have reported weekly discoveries of novel mediators of diabetes; breast, prostate, and lung cancer; Crohn's disease; macular degeneration; obesity; sudden cardiac death; multiple sclerosis; and many other diseases—all the results of a new method called genome-wide association studies (GWAS). These studies, and the preparatory work of cataloging human genetic variation, represent a multibillion dollar research investment.

Unfortunately, pain researchers are not yet sharing in this bounty. Approximately 400 GWAS will have been published by the end of 2009, and although pain treatment represents 10–20% of medical activities and costs [11], it is a safe bet that none of these studies will concern pain, in that I am unaware of any investigator who has yet been funded to carry out such a study.

This chapter will discuss why genome-wide association studies may greatly advance pain research and treatment, and how we pain researchers can "join the party." Readers who seek a more extensive introduction to human pain genetics can consult other recent reviews [5,9,11,14].

First, I must define what we mean by *association study* and *genome-wide association study.*

An association study is perhaps the simplest analysis that a geneticist can do. The investigator compares the frequency or average magnitude of a trait in individuals with one form of a gene, compared to individuals with other gene variants, or looks at the relative distribution of the alleles in individuals with a disease compared to controls without the disease. Most commonly, this comparison is carried out in unrelated individuals. This analysis is essentially the same procedure that we do when analyzing the effects of an active versus a control treatment on a disorder, or the effects of any epidemiological variable on a disorder, using methods such as *t* tests, contingency tables, analysis of variance, or regression analysis. Geneticists call this type of study an *association study* to distinguish it from the more traditional within-family analysis methods, such as pedigree or sib-pair analyses.

In the past, most association studies were done at one gene locus at a time. Much of the recent progress in human pain genetics is represented by such single-gene studies of *COMT, GCH1, IL6, MC1R, OPRM1,* and genes responsible for metabolizing analgesic drugs. Such studies are termed *candidate gene studies,* because the investigator has relied upon prior evidence to select the genes as candidates for human pain mediators. A stimulus to change the reliance on candidate gene studies occurred when Risch and Merikangas [23] calculated that by increasing sample size by only a factor of eight, the investigator keeps the statistical power constant while increasing the number of independent loci tested from one to 1 million! If this seems improbable, consider a case where one does a clinical trial in 100 patients and gets a P value of 0.05. If one then repeated the same trial seven more times and obtained the same result, the possibility of getting this result by chance alone is $(0.05)^8$, a P value so small that it could remain significant after correction for 1 million independent tests.

Risch and Merikangas [23] speculated that one could adequately test every common variant in the genome with these million tests, even though there are 3 billion base pairs in the human genome. The Human Genome Project soon proved them correct, in that there are only about 10 million common one-base variants, or *single nucleotide polymorphisms* (SNPs). Moreover, present-day human populations each arose relatively recently from a few founder individuals in Africa, Europe, and Asia, and the DNA of these founders is still being passed down in chunks, or *haplotype blocks*, in which tens or hundreds of these SNPs are inherited together. Therefore, one only needs to genotype a subset of these—500,000 to a million—and one can infer the genotype of the other SNPs on the haplotype block. This theoretical model spurred biotechnology companies to develop inexpensive "GWAS chips," making the current cost of these scans less than $500 per individual. It should be noted, however, that structural variants (e.g., copy number variants) account for a considerable percentage of human genetic variation [12].

Potential Value of Genome-Wide Association Studies

How might genome-wide association studies of pain facilitate pain research and treatment? (Table I). First, they can identify entirely novel mediators of disease. Traditional hypothesis-driven research tends to be limited to a small group of molecules determined by classic experiments a few generations old. For example, Belfer et al. [2] searched the pain basic science literature in 2002 and could find only about 250 molecules mentioned. In contrast, genomic or proteomic methods can find novel molecules arising from the 20,000 genes that traditional research has ignored. A strong finding in GWAS can revolutionize the basic and clinical research in a disease. For example, the recent GWAS findings that several members of the interleukin family are each implicated in Crohn's disease [1] and multiple sclerosis [21] have given a new focus to all immunological research on these disorders.

Table I
What genome-wide association studies might do for pain research

Identify novel mediators of pain beyond the few hundred molecules extensively discussed in the neurobiology literature.

Prioritize among the many existing pain targets for physiological studies and drug development *with human data*.

Extract up to 50% of the variance from studies of nongenetic factors that affect pain, sharpening studies of nongenetic contributors to pain.

Understand pain risks, mechanisms, and treatments of individual patients.

Better classify pain disorders.

GWAS can help to focus ongoing programs of drug development. Most drug companies interested in analgesics are faced with a choice of dozens of potential targets. Traditionally, they have relied on animal models of pain for most of the development phase, adding human data only after the investment of tens of millions of dollars. Although animal experiments were excellent guides in the development of spinal opioids, adrenergic agonists, and omega-conotoxins [24], they inaccurately predicted efficacy in the development of several systemically administered drugs, including neurokinin-1 receptor antagonists, glycine-site NMDA antagonists, and sodium channel antagonists [8,29,30]. Although GWAS are too new to have a track record in establishing proof of principle for new drugs, the demonstration that a polymorphism (that is, the presence of at least two versions of a gene) affected the severity of pain would imply that this pathway was a necessary mediator of human pain. Armed with this knowledge, a drug company might choose to invest in development of this class of drugs instead of classes without such evidence. This approach is not necessarily applicable to all potential analgesic classes, however. If there are no common variants of the genes that affect the function of the target pathway, association studies will not be informative.

Although my passion for the GWAS approach is based on these potential boosts to analgesic discovery, such studies can have other benefits. The elucidation of genetic factors that affect the risk of pain in certain conditions will decrease the error variance in studies of non-genetic factors that affect pain. For example, Slade et al. [26] reported that the genotype at the *COMT* gene and several psychological variables independently contributed to the risk of developing temporomandibular disorder, and the testing of each made the contribution of the other clearer. Expressed another way, putting together knowledge of genetic variables with other types of variables could make possible a more individualized approach to diagnosis, prognosis, and treatment, which could be called "personalized medicine." Finally, GWAS in multiple pain conditions could improve the rationale for classifying pain disorders, just as comparative genomics has become a new arbiter of classification of biological species. This technique would help to create an algorithm for inferring the response of many disorders to a treatment, given clinical data from a smaller subset.

Based on findings from the first hundred or so GWAS, can we predict which of these goals might be realized? Not with any certainty, because the patterns of findings have varied across the common diseases, depending upon their "genetic architecture"—how the total heritability of the disease is divided among the common variants in the genome. Table II shows, for example, that common genes with relatively large effects on risk have been replicated in Alzheimer's disease, Crohn's disease, and macular degeneration. In such cases, genetic tests for these variants may help to predict risk or identify important differences of disease biology in individual patients. In contrast, GWAS in diseases such as diabetes and lipid disorders have been a tremendous success, but the effects of each variant have been small. For example, 10 replicated variants associated with a risk of type II diabetes explain only about 5% of the population risk for the disease [25]. Because 40,000 cases have been studied already, it is unlikely that common gene variants of larger effect have been missed. If pain turns out to be like diabetes, genotyping for these SNPs will explain only a small amount of the risk or individualized biology of the disorder. On the other hand, discovery of a SNP with small but definite effects on a medical phenotype may prove a principle

Table II
"Genetic architecture" varies among diseases

Replicate Evidence for Association with Common Variants in GWAS	
Strong	Weak to None
Alzheimer's disease	Schizophrenia
Diabetes (type II)	Unipolar depression
Crohn's disease	Hypertension
Cancer: breast, prostate, lung	
Macular degeneration	
Multiple sclerosis	
Many others	

Size (Relative Risk) of Effect of Replicated Common Variants	
Very Large (Need <1,000 Patients)	Small (Need 5,000–10,000 Patients)
Alzheimer's disease: APOE e4	Height
Crohn's disease: NOD2	Most lipid, diabetes, and obesity
Macular degeneration	genes, and most other disease genes

that allows development of a much stronger treatment. Imagine, for example, that we did not know about opioid analgesics, but observed the type of very small effect on pain sensitivity that some investigators have reported with common variants in the μ-opioid receptor gene [7]. The effect is small because the two variants have only a slight difference on opioid receptor function, yet this knowledge might lead pharmacologists to make powerful opioids with powerful effects on the opioid receptors, sufficient to relieve severe pain.

However, GWAS have not been successful in every disease. Psychiatric disorders have been the most frustrating. Twin studies have suggested high levels of heritability of schizophrenia and bipolar illness, yet GWAS have not yet persuasively replicated any loci [4]. Unipolar disorder has been even more unrevealing. Psychiatric researchers, puzzled by this paradox, have suggested several explanations: there is variability and uncertainty in how psychiatric illnesses are defined; diverse brain systems may give rise to the defining symptoms; study participants have diverse environmental exposures. Similar difficulties might be experienced in trying to study pains that develop in the absence of tissue injury. One could argue that some types of pain—particularly those caused by a rather uniform peripheral injury—avoid these liabilities. Clinical drug trials show that standard pain measures are quite sensitive to modest biochemical effects; pain is mediated by a well-characterized set of peripheral nerve and spinal cord systems; and pains caused by a uniform peripheral injury therefore have very similar environmental influences.

Sample Size Required for Genome-Wide Association Studies

Fig. 1 shows the sample size required to test 500,000 SNPs in a GWAS. The graph shows two factors that affect N. First, the frequency of the SNPs, as shown on the x-axis: N would be minimized if one were to study SNPs that are evenly divided between their two forms, but because the average frequency of SNPs is 10–15%, larger cohorts are required. An even more powerful driver of N, illustrated by the multiple curves, is the size of the effect one wishes to detect. As in any clinical trial or epidemiological study, large increases in N are required to lower the detection threshold. An allele that increases the risk of severe pain by 80%—that is, a relative risk (RR) of 1.8—can be detected in a study of fewer than one thousand cases and controls. Unfortunately, only a minority of replicated SNPs from GWAS have had such a large effect. More commonly, RR values have been 1.2 or less, and therefore the effect is only detected with studies of 10,000 or more individuals [13].

Given that it may cost several hundred to several thousand dollars to phenotype each patient, depending upon the type of study, the issue of effect size is crucial. Part of this is beyond the investigator's control—the magnitude of the differential effect on cell biochemistry produced by various SNPs cannot be changed. On the other hand, RR values may be dramatically enhanced by thoughtful choice of the phenotype to maximize the homogeneity of the population and the impact of environmental factors on the phenotype. For example, the relative risks of most alleles that

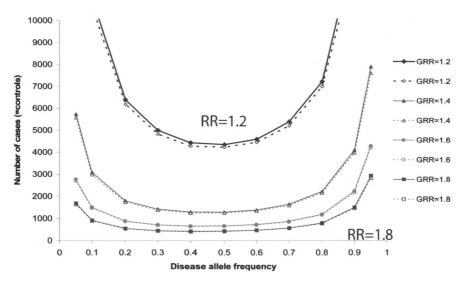

Fig. 1. Required number of cases and controls for whole-genome association study. The number of controls and cases required to detect varying disease allele frequencies and genotypic relative risks (GRRs or more simply, RRs) with 80% power is shown for a genome-wide association study of 500,000 independent single nucleotide polymorphisms (SNPs). To correct for this number of comparisons and maintain a P value of 0.05, one must reach a nominal P value of 1×10^{-7} or less. A multiplicative model was assumed; i.e., the relative risk for a homozygote equals the square of the relative risk for a heterozygote. Numbers were adjusted for a mean $r^2 = 0.97$, implying a close correlation between the SNP on the array and the common disease allele. Modified with permission from Macmillan Publishers Ltd.: Nature Protocols [32].

influence breast cancer in the entire population are very small, largely because breast cancer can arise through the influence of many endogenous and environmental factors. However, when investigators limited their phenotypes to families with multiple individuals developing breast cancer prior to age 40, the relative risks conferred by the *BRCA1* and *BRCA2* genes were greatly enlarged [28]. Similarly, the identification of nongenetic factors and their inclusion in the statistical analysis decreases heterogeneity and increases relative risk. Thoughtful choice of phenotypes may also improve the chances of finding pain genes. For example, although I am somewhat pessimistic about replicating genetic effects that contribute to multisomatoform disorders such as fibromyalgia, irritable bowel syndrome, or temporomandibular disorder, perhaps effect sizes will be higher in the more homogenous subset of patients who amplify experimental pain stimuli.

Choice of Pain Phenotype for Genome-Wide Association Studies

Table III lists four classes of pain conditions that might be chosen for GWAS. Some might argue that the current overriding consideration is to prove that genetic studies of humans will yield replicable targets. Such proof will open the coffers for studies of more complex phenotypes. This view would argue for studies of experimental pain stimuli, because the tight control of the environment—including the painful stimuli—would tend to increase the RR of any relevant allele, while the low cost of recruiting subjects makes it feasible to study thousands of individuals.

However, researchers have always questioned to what degree the results from experimental pain studies can be generalized to clinical pain studies. It seems obvious that experimental pain stimuli that do not damage tissue or cause the deep-seated emotional changes associated with disease-related pain will exclude the unique neurochemistry related to those processes. On the other hand, similar peripheral and spinal neurons signal experimental and pathological pain, so it is plausible that chemical modulators of experimental pain may also affect disease-related pain. In order to prove this, however, we need studies in disease-related pain.

Table III
Human pain models

Type of Pain	Typical N for Drug RCT
Human pain, laboratory-induced	10–15
Human acute surgical pain	20–50
Human chronic pain from uniform lesion (osteoarthritis, post-shingles pain, diabetic neuropathy, bone metastases)	50–100
Human chronic pain without clear causative lesion (fibromyalgia, temporomandibular disorder, idiopathic low back pain, chronic tension-type headache, irritable bowel syndrome, interstitial cystitis)	>100–200

Note: Homogeneous causes and controlled environment have permitted smaller sample size in randomized treatment trials; this principle should carry over into genetic studies. RCT = randomized controlled trial.

Table III orders three types of clinical pain conditions according to their homogeneity and apparent sensitivity in clinical analgesic trials. Acute surgical pain is the closest to experimental pain in power. Studies of chronic pain conditions caused by definite structural lesions generally require larger sample sizes, partly because the inciting stimulus and the outpatient environment are more heterogeneous. Studies of idiopathic pain disorders might be the least sensitive to the effects of gene variants, according to this argument. On the other hand, my epidemiologist colleague Walter Stewart argued in our recent review [11] that the vast economic and public health impact of these conditions made them important targets for GWAS.

Regardless of which category of pain phenotype one prefers, statistical and budgetary realities suggest that it will be challenging to recruit enough patients in chronic pain studies to detect relative risks in the 1.2 range until investigators devise medical record systems that routinely collect the relevant diagnostic and pain data, perhaps combined with prospective collection of DNA as part of medical care. In the short term, we may be identifying a large proportion of "pain genes" through studies of experimental and acute surgical pain and testing a small number of genetic variants with high power in chronic pain cohorts. GWAS in chronic pain may also pick up novel loci if they have moderate to high relative risk values.

How Pain Researchers Can Better Compete for Funding for Genome-Wide Studies

The success of the GWAS approach has created new difficulties. Everyone wants to apply these methods in their own disease, but with costs of many millions of dollars per study, most applications must be rejected. Pain genomics grants are often judged in competition with genomics grants from other diseases, and they suffer several disadvantages. First, the 10–20-year lead time that has accrued to genetic investigators in many common diseases provides much greater proof-of-principle and methodological validation to our competitors' proposals. Second, many grants are rated for innovation. One might think that it might be an advantage to adapt the best of proven methods from other diseases to pain, but this approach may be viewed as "not innovative."

To overcome these disadvantages, pain researchers should first try to influence funding agencies to consider pain genomics grants as competing only against each other, and judged by reviewers familiar with pain research. U.S. investigators have pressed their case by rigorously counting the number of National Institutes of Health grants devoted to pain, and showing that the current system has put pain research at a disadvantage [3]. Second, clinical pain researchers should increase their coordination, for example, picking several conditions for targets of GWAS and working together to decide on the phenotype and optimizing the methods of assessing any nongenetic variables that may contribute to the pain outcome. This cooperation is crucial, because an important current criterion for the awarding of GWAS grants is the availability of well-characterized replication cohorts with the same phenotype. Third, pain researchers should study the current shortcomings of GWAS in other diseases and seek to leap ahead of them. Current reviews of GWAS suggest that there has been a "rush to quantity," with too little attention to crucial issues such as measurement of environmental exposures or heterogeneity of the disease process.

Because many reviewers of pain genetics grants may be unfamiliar with pain research, applicants should succinctly dispel the impression that many scientific generalists have that pain is a hopelessly complex subjective phenomenon. The reproducibility of analgesic clinical trial results in modest-sized samples in 20,000 published studies over 60 years can be stressed, as well as the more recent demonstration that a range of pain traits are strongly heritable in mice [10,16] and in human twin pairs [19,20].

My basic science colleagues have pointed out that pain genomics demands new types of collaborative work between clinicians and basic scientists. A simple example is the comparison of human and animal studies demonstrated in the investigation of the effects of *COMT* [6,18] and *GCH1* [27] on pain, and the effects of *MC1R* on both pain and analgesia [15,17]. To take another example, GWAS experts in other diseases have pondered the source of the large proportion of genetic variance suggested by twin studies, yet unexplained by a handful of replicated individual genes. Many speculate that gene-gene and gene-environment interactions make up much of this variance. However, the investigation of human gene-gene interactions, for example, is in its infancy [22], and may be too speculative for grant reviewers. If studies of gene-gene interactions in animal models were to show that this factor is an important contributor to pain variability in mammals, it would give a boost to analogous clinical proposals.

There is also a growing consensus that a new generation of methods should get beyond single types of molecular studies in single species and integrate genotype-phenotype association studies with mRNA and protein expression studies in the relevant cell types in both animal models and humans. Initial investigations in lipid disorders and obesity [31] have suggested that these approaches are more sensitive in identifying important disease pathways than just waiting for overwhelmingly significant hits on single molecules.

Successful pain genomics efforts will require large numbers of collaborating researchers with expertise not yet found in the pain field. Epidemiology and genetics are the two most obvious such disciplines [11]. Molecular biology, computational neuroscience, statistics, and medical informatics will be other areas in which we need to find collaborators.

A final point is that we cannot rely upon the wisdom of governmental funding agencies alone to ensure that meritorious pain GWAS proposals are funded. There is a decades-old consensus among science administrators that laissez-faire competition among proposals relating to diverse diseases often elicits the best science. However, reviewers from other disease areas are rarely aware of the vast unmet public health needs of pain, and given that epidemiology is the weakest area of clinical pain research, we are at a disadvantage in convincing them otherwise. In contrast, the pharmaceutical and biotechnology sectors are well aware of the unsatisfied market needs in pain. At present, they spend at least 10 times as much on pain research as governmental agencies. Because they will be major beneficiaries of better identification of analgesic targets, drug companies may be essential funders, cofunders, or policy advocates for moving pain genetics into the GWAS era.

References

[1]   Barrett JC, Hansoul S, Nicolae DL, Cho JH, Duerr RH, Rioux JD, Brant SR, Silverberg MS, Taylor KD, Barmada MM, et al. Genome-wide association defines more than 30 distinct susceptibility loci for Crohn's disease. Nat Genet 2008;40:955–62.

[2]   Belfer I, Wu T, Kingman A, Krishnaraju RK, Goldman D, Max MB. Candidate gene studies of human pain mechanisms: a method for optimizing choice of polymorphisms and sample size. Anesthesiology 2004;100:1562–72.

[3]   Bradshaw DH, Nakamura Y, Chapman CR. National Institutes of Health grant awards for pain, nausea, and dyspnea research: an assessment of funding patterns in 2003. J Pain 2004;6:277–93.

[4]   Burmeister M, McInnis MG, Zollner S. Psychiatric genetics: progress amid controversy. Nat Rev Genet 2008;9:527–40.

[5]   Diatchenko L, Nackley AG, Tchivileva IE, Shabalina SA, Maixner W. Genetic architecture of human pain perception. Trends Genet 2007;23:605–13.

[6]   Diatchenko L, Slade GD, Nackley AG, Bhalang K, Sigurdsson A, Belfer I, Goldman D, Xu K, Shabalina SA, Shagin D, et al. Genetic basis for individual variations in pain perception and the development of a chronic pain condition. Hum Mol Genet 2005;14:135–43.

[7]   Fillingim RB, Kaplan L, Staud R, Ness TJ, Glover TL, Campbell CM, Mogil JS, Wallace MR. The A118G single nucleotide polymorphism of the μ-opioid receptor gene (*OPRM1*) is associated with pressure pain sensitivity in humans. J Pain 2005;6:159–67.

[8]   Hill R. NK1 (substance P) receptor antagonists—why are they not analgesic in humans? Trends Pharmacol Sci 2000;21:244–6.

[9]   LaCroix-Fralish ML, Mogil JS. Progress in genetic studies of pain and analgesia. Annu Rev Pharmacol Toxicol 2009;49:97–121.

[10] Lariviere WR, Wilson SG, Laughlin TM, Kokayeff A, West EE, Adhikari SM, Wan Y, Mogil JS. Heritability of nociception. III. Genetic relationships among commonly used assays of nociception and hypersensitivity. Pain 2002;97:75–86.

[11] Max MB, Stewart WF. The molecular epidemiology of pain: a new discipline for drug discovery. Nat Rev Drug Discov 2008;7:647–58.

[12] McCaroll SA, Altshuler DM. Copy-number variation and association studies of human disease. Nat Genet 2007;39(Suppl 7):S37–42.

[13] McCarthy MI, Abecasis GR, Cardon LR, Goldstein DB, Little J, Ioannidis JPA, Hirschhorn JN. Genome-wide association studies for complex traits: consensus, uncertainty and challenges. Nat Rev Genet 2008;9:356–69.

[14] Mogil JS, Max MB. The genetics of pain. In: Koltzenburg M, McMahon SB, editors. Wall and Melzack's textbook of pain. London: Elsevier Churchill Livingstone; 2006. pp 159–74.

[15] Mogil JS, Ritchie J, Smith SB, Strasburg K, Kaplan L, Wallace MR, Romberg RR, Bijl H, Sarton EY, Fillingim RB, Dahan A. Melanocortin-1 receptor gene variants affect pain and ☐-opioid analgesia in mice and humans. J Med Genet 2005;42:583–7.

[16] Mogil JS, Wilson SG, Bon K, Lee SE, Chung K, Raber P, Pieper JO, Hain HS, Belknap JK, Hubert L, et al. Heritability of nociception. I. Responses of eleven inbred mouse strains on twelve measures of nociception. Pain 1999;80:67–82.
[17] Mogil JS, Wilson SG, Chesler EJ, Rankin AL, Nemmani KVS, Lariviere WR, Groce MK, Wallace MR, Kaplan L, Staud R, et al. The melanocortin-1 receptor gene mediates female-specific mechanisms of analgesia in mice and humans. Proc Natl Acad Sci USA 2003;100:4867–72.
[18] Nackley AG, Tan KS, Fecho K, Flood P, Diatchenko L, Maixner W. Catechol-O-methyltransferase inhibition increases pain sensitivity through activation of both β_2- and β_3-adrenergic receptors. Pain 2007;128:199–208.
[19] Nielsen CS, Stubhaug A, Price DD, Vassend O, Czajkowski N, Harris JR. Individual differences in pain sensitivity: genetic and environmental contributions. Pain 2008;136:21–9.
[20] Norbury TA, MacGregor AJ, Urwin J, Spector TD, McMahon SB. Heritability of responses to painful stimuli in women: a classical twin study. Brain 2007;130:3041–9.
[21] Oksenberg JR, Baranzini SE, Sawcer S, Hauser SL. The genetics of multiple sclerosis: SNPs to pathways to pathogenesis. Nat Rev Genet 2008;9:516–26.
[22] Pattin KA, Moore JH. Exploiting the proteome to improve the genome-wide genetic analysis of epistasis in common human diseases. Hum Genet 2008;124:19–29.
[23] Risch N, Merikangas K. The future of genetic studies of complex human diseases. Science 1996;273:1516–7.
[24] Schug SA, Saunders D, Kurowski I, Paech MJ. Neuraxial drug administration: a review of treatment options for anaesthesia and analgesia. CNS Drugs 2006;20:917–33.
[25] Scott LJ, Mohlke KL, Bonnycastle LL, Willer CJ, Li Y, Duren WL, Erdos MR, Stringham HM, Chines PS, Jackson AU, et al. A genome-wide association study of type 2 diabetes in Finns detects multiple susceptibility variants. Science 2007;316:1341–5.
[26] Slade GD, Diatchenko L, Bhalang K, Sigurdsson A, Fillingim RB, Belfer I, Max MB, Goldman D, Maixner W. Influence of psychological factors on risk of temporomandibular disorders. J Dent Res 2007;86:1120–5.
[27] Tegeder I, Costigan M, Griffin RS, Abele A, Belfer I, Schmidt H, Ehnert C, Nejim J, Marian C, Scholz J, et al. GTP cyclohydrolase and tetrahydrobiopterin regulate pain sensitivity and persistence. Nat Med 2006;12:1269–77.
[28] Turnbull C, Rahman N. Genetic predisposition to breast cancer: past, present, and future. Annu Rev Genomics Hum Genet 2008;9:321–45.
[29] Wallace MS, Rowbotham M, Bennett GJ, Jensen TS, Pladna R, Quessy S. A multicenter, double-blind, randomized, placebo-controlled crossover evaluation of a short course of 4030W92 in patients with chronic neuropathic pain. J Pain 2002;2:227–33.
[30] Wallace MS, Rowbotham M, Katz NP, Dworkin RH, Dotson RM, Galer BS, Rauck RL, Backonja M, Quessy SN, Meisner PD. A randomized, double-blind, placebo-controlled trial of a glycine antagonist in neuropathic pain. Neurology 2002;59:1694–1700.
[31] Zhu J, Zhang B, Schadt EE. A systems biology approach to drug discovery. Adv Genet 2008;60:603–35.
[32] Zondervan KT, Cardon LR. Designing candidate gene and genome-wide case-control association studies. Nat Protocols 2007;2:2492–501.

Correspondence to: Jeffrey S. Mogil, PhD, Department of Psychology and Alan Edwards Centre for Research on Pain, 1205 Dr. Penfield Avenue, Montreal, Quebec, Canada H3A 1B1. Tel: 1-514-398-6085; email: jeffrey.mogil@mcgill.ca.

11

External Validity of Randomized Controlled Trials: General Principles and Lessons from Trials in Neuropathic Pain

Peter M. Rothwell[a] and C. Peter N. Watson[b]

[a]University Department of Clinical Neurology, John Radcliffe Hospital, Headington, Oxford, United Kingdom; [b]Department of Medicine, University of Toronto, Toronto, Ontario, Canada

Randomized controlled trials (RCTs) and systematic reviews are the most reliable methods of determining the effects of treatment. However, to be clinically useful the results must be relevant to routine clinical practice; this is generally termed *external validity, applicability,* or *generalizability.* The beneficial effects of some interventions, such as lowering blood pressure in chronic uncontrolled hypertension, have been shown to be generalizable to the vast majority of patients and settings, but the effects of other interventions can largely depend on factors such as the characteristics of the patient, the method of application of the intervention, and the setting of treatment. How these factors are taken into account in the design and performance of an RCT and in the reporting of the results can have a major impact on external validity. In this chapter, we will first review some of the most important determinants of the external validity of RCTs in general. We will then use the same principles to determine the external validity of trials of drugs used to treat neuropathic pain.

RCTs must be internally valid (i.e., their design and conduct must eliminate the possibility of bias), but to be clinically useful the result must also be relevant to a definable group of patients in a particular clinical setting (i.e., they must be externally valid). Lack of external validity is the most frequent criticism by clinicians of RCTs, systematic reviews, and guidelines, and it is one explanation for the widespread underuse in routine practice of many treatments that have been shown to be beneficial in trials and are recommended in guidelines [45]. Yet medical journals, funding agencies, ethics committees, the pharmaceutical industry, and governmental regulators seem to give external validity a low priority. Admittedly, whereas the determinants of internal validity are intuitive and can generally be worked out from first principles, understanding of the determinants of the external validity of an RCT requires clinical rather than statistical expertise and often depends on a detailed understanding of the particular clinical condition under study and its management in routine clinical practice. However, reliable judgements about the external validity of RCTs are essential if treatments are to be used correctly in as many patients as possible in routine clinical practice.

The results of an RCT will never be relevant to all patients and all settings, but they should be designed and reported in a way that allows clinicians to judge to whom the results can reasonably be applied. Table I lists some of the important potential determinants of external validity, each of which is reviewed briefly below. Many of the considerations will only be relevant in certain types of trial, for certain interventions, or in certain clinical settings, but they can each sometimes undermine external validity. Moreover, the list is not exhaustive and requires more detailed annotation and explanation than in possible in this short review.

Some of the issues that determine external validity are relevant to the distinction between pragmatic trials and explanatory trials [64], but it would be wrong to assume that pragmatic trials always have greater external validity than explanatory trials. For example, broad eligibility criteria, limited collection of baseline data, and inclusion of centers with a range of expertise and differing patient populations have many advantages, but they can also make it very difficult to generalize the overall average effect of treatment to a particular clinical setting.

Table I

Issues that can affect external validity that should be addressed in reports of
randomized controlled trials or systematic reviews and be considered by clinicians

Setting of the Trial
Health care system
Country
Recruitment from primary, secondary, or tertiary care
Selection of participating centers and clinicians

Selection of Patients
Methods of prerandomization diagnosis and investigation
Eligibility and exclusion criteria
Placebo run-in period
Treatment run-in period
"Enrichment" strategies
Ratio of randomized to eligible nonrandomized patients in participating centers
Proportion of patients who declined randomization

Characteristics of Randomized Patients
Baseline clinical characteristics
Racial group
Uniformity of underlying pathology
Stage in the natural history of the disease
Severity of disease
Comorbidity
Absolute risks of a poor outcome in the control group

Differences between the Trial Protocol and Routine Practice
Trial intervention
Timing of treatment
Appropriateness/relevance of the control intervention
Adequacy of non-trial treatment, both intended and actual
Prohibition of certain non-trial treatments
Therapeutic or diagnostic advances since the trial was performed

Outcome Measures and Follow-up
Clinical relevance of surrogate outcomes
Clinical relevance, validity, and reproducibility of complex scales
Effect of intervention on most relevant components of composite outcomes
Who measured the outcome
Use of patient-centered outcomes
Frequency of follow-up
Adequacy of the length of follow-up

Adverse Effects of Treatment
Completeness of reporting of relevant adverse effects
Rates of discontinuation of treatment
Selection of trial centers and/or clinicians on the basis of skill or experience
Exclusion of patients at risk of complications
Exclusion of patients who experienced adverse effects during a run-in period
Intensity of trial safety procedures

Source: Adapted from Rothwell [45].

Determinants of External Validity of Trials

The Setting of the Trial

A detailed understanding of the setting in which a trial is performed, including any peculiarities of the health care system in particular counties, can be essential in judging external validity. The potential impact of differences between health care systems is illustrated by an analysis of the results of the European Carotid Surgery Trial (ECST) [11], an RCT of endarterectomy for recently symptomatic carotid stenosis. In this trial, national differences in the speed with which patients were investigated resulted in very different treatment effects in different health care systems [45], due to the shortness of the time window for effective prevention of stroke. Similar differences in performance between health care systems will exist for other conditions, and there is, of course, the broader issue of how trials conducted in the developed world apply in the developing world. Moreover, other differences between countries in the methods of diagnosis and management of disease, which can be substantial, or important racial differences in pathology and natural history of disease, also affect the external validity of RCTs. A good example is the heterogeneity of results of trials of the BCG vaccine in prevention of tuberculosis, with a progressive loss of efficacy ($P < 0.0001$) with decreasing latitude [12].

How centers and clinicians were selected to participate in trials is seldom reported, but this factor can also have important implications for external validity. For example, the Asymptomatic Carotid Atherosclerosis Study (ACAS) of endarterectomy for asymptomatic carotid stenosis only accepted surgeons with an excellent safety record, rejecting 40% of applicants initially, and subsequently barring from further participation those who had adverse operative outcomes in the trial. The benefit from surgery in ACAS was due in major part to the consequently low operative risk [1]. A meta-analysis of 46 surgical case series that published operative risks during the 5 years after ACAS found operative mortality to be eight times higher and the risk of stroke and death to be about three times higher [45]. Trials should not include centers that do not have the competence to treat patients safely, but selection should not be so exclusive that the results cannot be generalized to routine clinical practice.

Selection and Exclusion of Patients

Concern is often expressed about highly selective trial eligibility criteria, but there are often several earlier stages of selection that are rarely recorded or reported but can be more problematic. For example, consider a trial of a new blood pressure-lowering drug, which like most such trials is performed in a hospital clinic. Fewer than 10% of patients with hypertension are managed in hospital clinics, and this group will differ from those managed in primary care. Moreover, only one of the 10 physicians who see hypertensive patients in this particular hospital is taking part in the trial, and this physician mainly sees young patients with resistant hypertension. Thus, even before any consideration of eligibility or exclusion criteria, potential recruits are already extremely unrepresentative of patients in the local community. It is essential, therefore, that where possible trials record and report the pathways to recruitment.

Patients are then further selected according to trial eligibility criteria. Some RCTs exclude women, and many exclude the elderly and/or patients with common comorbidities. One review of 214 drug trials in acute myocardial infarction found that over 60% excluded patients aged over 75 years [20], despite the fact that over 50% of myocardial infarctions occur in this older age group. A review of 41 RCTs from the U.S. National Institutes of Health found an average exclusion rate of 73% [6], but rates can be much higher. One study of the eligibility criteria for an acute stroke treatment trial found that of the small proportion of patients admitted to hospital sufficiently quickly to be suitable for treatment, 96% were ineligible based on the various other exclusion criteria [25]. One center in another acute stroke trial had to screen 192 patients over 2 years to find an eligible patient [29]. Yet, highly selective recruitment is not inevitable. The GISSI-1 trial of thrombolysis for acute myocardial infarction, for example, recruited 90% of patients admitted within 12 hours of the event with a definite diagnosis and no contraindications [19].

Strict eligibility criteria can limit the external validity of RCTs, but physicians should at least be able to select similar patients for treatment in routine practice. Unfortunately, however, reporting of trial eligibility criteria is frequently inadequate. A review of trials leading to clinical alerts by the U.S. National Institutes of Health revealed that of an average of 31 eligibility criteria, only 63% were published in the main trial report and only 19% in the clinical alert [52]. Inadequate reporting is also a major problem in secondary publications, such as systematic reviews and clinical guidelines, where the need for a succinct message does not usually allow detailed consideration of the eligibility and exclusion criteria or other determinants of external validity

Prerandomization run-in periods are also often used to select or exclude patients. In a placebo run-in, all eligible patients receive placebo, and those who are poorly compliant are excluded. There can be good reasons for doing this, but high rates of exclusion will reduce external validity. Active treatment run-in periods in which patients who have adverse events or show signs that treatment may be ineffective are excluded are more likely to undermine external validity. For example, two RCTs of carvedilol, a vasodilatory beta-blocker, in chronic heart failure excluded 6% and 9% of eligible patients in treatment run-in periods, mainly because of worsening heart failure and other adverse events, some of which were fatal [45]. In both trials, the complication rates in the subsequent randomized phase were much lower than in the run-in phase.

Trials also sometimes actively recruit patients who are likely to respond well to treatment (often termed "enrichment"). For example, some trials of antipsychotic drugs have selectively recruited patients who had a good response to antipsychotics previously [45]. Other trials have excluded nonresponders in a run-in phase. One RCT of a cholinesterase inhibitor, tacrine, in Alzheimer's disease recruited 632 patients to a 6-week "enrichment" phase in which they were randomized to different doses of tacrine versus placebo [8]. After a washout-period, only the 215 (34%) patients who had a measured improvement on tacrine in the "enrichment" phase were randomized to tacrine (at their best dose) versus placebo in the main phase of the trial. External validity is clearly undermined here.

Characteristics of Randomized Patients

Even in large pragmatic trials with very few exclusion criteria, recruitment of less than 10% of potentially eligible patients in participating centers is common. Those patients who are recruited generally differ from those who are eligible but not recruited in terms of age, sex, race, severity of disease, educational status, social class, and place of residence. The outcome in patients included in RCTs is also usually better than those not participating in trials, often markedly so, not because of better treatment but because of a better baseline prognosis. Trial reports usually include the baseline clinical characteristics of randomized patients, and so it is argued that clinicians can assess external validity by comparison with their patients. However, recorded baseline clinical characteristics often say very little about the real make-up of the trial population, and they can sometimes be misleading. For example, although the baseline clinical characteristics of the patients randomized to warfarin in two RCTs of secondary prevention of stroke were almost identical, the risk of intracranial hemorrhage on warfarin was 19 times higher ($P < 0.0001$) in the SPIRIT trial than in the EAFT trial, even after adjustment for differences in baseline clinical characteristics and the intensity of anticoagulation [16]. In judging external validity, an understanding of how patients were referred, investigated, and diagnosed (i.e., their pathway to recruitment) as well as how they were subsequently selected and excluded is often very much more informative than a list of baseline characteristics.

The Intervention, Control Treatment, and Pretrial or Nontrial Management

External validity can also be affected if trials have protocols that differ from usual clinical practice. For example, prior to randomization in the RCTs of endarterectomy for symptomatic carotid stenosis, patients had to be diagnosed by a neurologist and have conventional arterial angiography, neither of which are routine in many centers. The trial intervention itself may also differ from that used in current practice, such as in the formulation and bioavailability of a drug, or the type of anesthetic used for an operation. The same can be true of the treatment in the control group in a trial, which may use a particularly low dose of the comparator drug or fall short of best current practice in some other way. External validity can also be undermined by too stringent limitations on the use nontrial treatments. Any prohibition of nontrial treatments should be reported in the main trial publications along with details of relevant nontrial treatments that were used. The timing of many interventions is also critical and should be reported when relevant.

Outcome Measures and Follow-up

The external validity of an RCT also depends on whether the outcomes were clinically relevant. Many trials use "surrogate" outcomes, usually biological or imaging markers that are thought to be indirect measures of the effect of treatment on clinical outcomes. However, as well as being of questionable clinical relevance, surrogate outcomes are often misleading. There are many examples of treatments that had a major beneficial effect on a surrogate outcome, which had been shown to be correlated with a relevant clinical outcome in observational studies, but where the treatments proved ineffective or harmful in subsequent large RCTs that used these same clinical outcomes (Table II) [45].

Table II
Examples where trials based on surrogate outcomes proved to be misleading predictors of the effect of treatment on clinical outcomes in subsequent trials

Treatment	Condition	Surrogate Outcome	Clinical Outcome
Fluoride	Osteoporosis	Increase in bone density	Major increase in fractures
Antiarrhythmic drugs	Post-myocardial infarction	Reduction in ECG abnormalities	Increased mortality
Beta-interferon	Multiple sclerosis	70% reduction in new lesions on brain MRI	No convincing effect on disability
Milrinone and epoprostenol	Heart failure	Improved exercise tolerance	Increased mortality
Ibopamine	Heart failure	Improved ejection fraction	Increased mortality and heart rate variability

Note: See Rothwell [45] for more details.

Complex scales, often made up of arbitrary combinations of symptoms and clinical signs, are also problematic. A review of 196 RCTs in rheumatoid arthritis identified more than 70 different outcome scales [17]. More worryingly, a review of 2,000 RCTs in schizophrenia identified 640 scales, many of which were devised for the particular RCT and had no supporting data on validity or reliability, but which were more likely to show statistically significant treatment effects than established scales [33]. Moreover, the clinical meaning of apparent treatment effects (e.g., a 2.7-point mean reduction in a 100-point outcome scale made up of various symptoms and signs) is usually impossible to discern. Simple clinical outcomes usually have the most external validity, but even then only if they reflect the priorities of patients. For example, patients with epilepsy are much more interested in the proportion of individuals rendered free of seizures in RCTs of anticonvulsants than they are in changes in mean seizure frequency. Who actually measured the outcome can also be important. For example, the recorded operative risk of stroke due to carotid endarterectomy is highly dependent on whether patients were assessed by a surgeon or a neurologist [46].

Many trials combine events in their primary outcome measure. This practice can produce a useful measure of the overall effect of treatment on all the relevant outcomes, and it usually affords greater statistical power, but the outcome that is most important to a particular patient may be affected differently by treatment than the combined outcome. Composite outcomes also sometimes combine events of very different severity, and treatment effects can be driven by the least important outcome, which is often the most frequent. Equally problematic is the composite of definite clinical events and episodes of hospitalization. The fact that a patient is in an RCT will probably affect the likelihood of hospitalization, and it will certainly vary between different health care systems.

Another major problem for the external validity of RCTs is an inadequate duration of treatment and/or follow-up. For example, although patients with refractory epilepsy or migraine require treatment for many years, most RCTs of new drugs look at the effect of treatment for only a few weeks [67]. Whether initial response is a good predictor of long-term benefit is unknown. The same problem has been identified in RCTs in schizophrenia, with fewer than 50% of trials having more than 6 weeks of follow-up and only 20% following patients for longer than 6 months [63]. The contrast between beneficial effects of treatments in short-term RCTs and the less encouraging experience of long-term treatment in clinical practice has also been highlighted by clinicians treating patients with rheumatoid arthritis [40].

Adverse Effects of Treatment

Reporting of adverse effects of treatment in RCTs and systematic reviews is often poor. In a review of 192 pharmaceutical trials, less than a third had adequate reporting of adverse clinical events or laboratory toxicology [23]. Treatment discontinuation rates provide some guide to tolerability, but pharmaceutical trials often use eligibility criteria and run-in periods to exclude patients who might be prone to adverse effects.

Clinicians are usually most concerned about external validity of RCTs of potentially dangerous treatments. Complications of medial interventions are a leading cause of death in developed countries. Risks can be overestimated in RCTs, particularly during the introduction of new treatments when trials are often done in patients with very severe disease, but stringent selection of patients, confinement to specialist centers, and intensive safety monitoring usually lead to lower risks than in routine clinical practice. RCTs of warfarin in nonrheumatic atrial fibrillation are a good example. All trials reported benefit with warfarin, but complication rates were much lower than in routine practice, and consequent doubts about external validity are partly to blame for major underprescribing of warfarin, particularly in the elderly [45].

Systematic Review of the External Validity of Trials in Neuropathic Pain

The literature contains a large and increasing number of placebo-controlled RCTs in neuropathic pain, but many are pharmaceutical industry trials simply showing an effect of a new drug over placebo, with no comparative data with a standard therapy or information regarding the clinical meaningfulness of the new agent in ordinary practice. Neuropathic pain can be roughly divided into peripheral and central neuropathic pain. Peripheral neuropathic pain problems include a variety of painful generalized neuropathies and also mononeuropathies such as traumatic injury due to accidents or surgery, painful diabetic neuropathy (PDN), postherpetic neuralgia (PHN), phantom limb pain, and others. The central pain problems include central poststroke pain, spinal cord injury pain, syringomyelia, and multiple sclerosis. The RCTs of different oral analgesics in these conditions can be mainly divided into antidepressants, anticonvulsants, and opioids, and most trials have studied these drugs using PDN and PHN as experimental models. These conditions were chosen because they are relatively common compared to other varieties of neuropathic pain and reasonably uniform and stable if subjects are appropriately recruited and carefully chosen. The extensive use of these two disorders can be a problem in terms of generalizability to other less common types of nerve injury pain. Clinicians treating these patients know that despite our best therapy, most patients are incompletely relieved of pain, and many are unable to tolerate the adverse effects of these drugs.

It is relatively easy for the pharmaceutical industry to meet the requirements for the approval of a new drug by submitting two RCTs showing a difference over placebo. Continuing this economically driven approach may simply continue to generate "me too" drugs, as has occurred with the statins, triptans, and many others, which is of limited help pragmatically for clinicians struggling with these patients who need to know if a new drug effect is clinically meaningful and any better than the standard of therapy. The placebo-controlled trial also offers little from an explanatory point of view in terms of tailoring treatment to pathophysiological mechanisms and addressing the question as to whether the new drug works in a different group than the old drug. There are therefore significant problems with these trials, which provide barriers to better pain management. These problems include the lack of comparative studies (enabling us to determine if a new drug is any better than the standard of therapy and possibly whether it works in a different subgroup), the lack of data in trial reports regarding clinical meaningfulness (how many patients obtain a satisfactory response and have tolerable side effects), and whether the results are relevant to clinical practice.

A systematic review was carried out by searching PubMed, Medline, and the Cochrane database for RCTs of analgesics (oral antidepressants, anticonvulsants, and opioids) in neuropathic pain and also by searching for the terms "postherpetic neuralgia" and "painful diabetic neuropathy" (since these are the most common conditions used for clinical trials in neuropathic pain) and for terms such as "central pain," "phantom limb pain," and other specific types of neuropathic pains [68]. The review searched for trials published in adults in English from 1966 to 2005. The search excluded the neuropathic pain conditions of trigeminal neuralgia and complex regional pain syndrome type II (causalgia). Reference lists of retrieved articles were searched as well, and investigators in this area were contacted. Of particular interest were comparative trials within an analgesic class and of different analgesics in neuropathic pain.

External validity was rated by the checklist in Table I. Trials were evaluated according to the quality criteria of Jadad [24]; to be included, they were required to score at least 3 out of 5 on this rating scale. A maximum score of 5 indicated that the RCT was randomized and double-blind, accounted for withdrawals, and described the methods of blinding and randomization. We required that all trials fulfilled the first three criteria (and thus scored 3), but many scored 4 or 5. Trials were determined to be enriched if (a) previous treatment with the trial drug or a similar drug resulted in exclusion, (b) patients having adverse events from the study drug prior to the treatment were excluded, or (c) nonresponders to the drug were excluded. Measures of clinical meaningfulness such as effect size, percentage of patients with 50% or greater improvement, and number need to treat (NNT) [7,30], number needed to harm (NNH) [7,30] and number needed to quit (NNQ) figures were sought as a means of comparison of efficacy and safety.

Forty-nine RCTs (meeting the criteria described above) were identified of antidepressants, anticonvulsants, and opioids in peripheral and central neuropathic pain. Six of the studies were comparative trials of different analgesics [14,18,26,31,38,41], and 6 compared different antidepressants [36,56,60,66,70,71]. Of the analgesics used in the trials, 26 were antidepressants, 17 were anticonvulsants, and 9 were opioids (some RCTs involved more than one drug). A total of 40 of the 49 trials were carried out in PHN, in PDN, or in both disorders. Forty-four of the 49 were favorable for the study drug. Of the antidepressant trials, 7 were in PHN [18,27,37,41,70–72], 13 were in PDN [28,34–36,38,47,57–62,66], and 7 were in other types of neuropathic pain [5,21,26,31,51,53,56] (HIV neuropathy 2, "neuropathic pain" 2, central pain 1, spinal cord injury 1, and cisplatinum neuropathy 1). Anticonvulsant trials involved gabapentin (7) [2,3,14,39,42,48], pregabalin (6) [9,13,32,43,44,50], lamotrigine (3) [10,54,65], and carbamazepine (1) [31]. There were 9 opioid RCTs [4,14,15,22,49,55,69,73], with one trial using two different opioids (tramadol 3, oxycodone 3, methadone 1, morphine 2, and levorphanol 1).

The Setting of the Trial

The RCTs were carried out in 12 countries, including the United States (26), Denmark (8), Canada (6), two in each of Finland, Germany, Sweden, and the United Kingdom, and one in each of Australia, India, Israel, and Spain. Some trials were carried out in more than one country. Patients were recruited in 16 trials from advertisements or primary care, 10 were from a neurology or diabetic clinic population (secondary care), 3 were from a pain clinic (tertiary), and 8 were from a mixed primary/secondary setting. In 15 studies the source of patients was not stated.

Selection and Exclusion of Patients

In 20 RCTs the diagnosis of neuropathic pain was not precisely determined and lacked a description in the methods section; there was no documentation of pain in a nerve territory, of descriptors typical of neuropathic pain, of physical findings, or of ancillary testing such as electromyography or nerve conduction studies supporting nerve injury. A statement of only "neuropathic pain" was not considered adequate. Eligibility criteria ranged from 2 to 19, with a median of 4, and no criteria stated in 2 trials. Exclusion criteria ranged from 1 to 19, with a median of 7 and a range of 1–19, and no criteria stated in 3 trials. Run-ins with placebo or drug were used in two trials to select those to be included. Study enrichment was present if participants were excluded if they had an adverse event or were nonresponsive to the study drug or to previous use of the study drug or a closely related drug (e.g., gabapentin in pregabalin studies). Sixteen trials were determined to involve this form of selection. Nineteen trials stated the number of individuals screened, 23 stated the ratio of randomized to eligible subjects, and 14 documented those who declined randomization.

Characteristics of Randomized Patients

Basic demographics of the study population were stated in 49 trials, although racial subgroups were not stated in 32 trials. In 21 trials it was determined that the disorder studied lacked uniformity in that different types of neuropathic pain or different types of neuropathy within a given category, such as PDN, were studied. In 34 trials it was not clear as to the stage of the disorder in terms of pain because the duration of the pain was not characterized or was judged to be less than optimum, i.e., 1 month's duration or less. In 19 trials, pain severity was not stated in the inclusion criteria or was mild or not described as being daily pain of moderate severity. Comorbidities were stated in 3 trials. The absolute risk in the control group appeared clear in 32 reports (the disorder was clearly chronic and severe because of the pain intensity and duration and therefore unlikely to improve with time).

The Intervention, Control Treatment, and Pretrial or Nontrial Management

The trial intervention was deemed appropriate in 42 trials, and the timing of the treatment appeared satisfactory in 36. The control group was thought appropriate or relevant in 43. Prohibition of nontrial treatments, including standard drugs used in neuropathic pain, often requiring prestudy drug withdrawal, occurred in 22 trials.

Outcome Measures and Follow-up

Surrogate outcomes were used in 6 trials and were judged problematic since they included numbness, paresthesia, and sleep components and did not use a clear pain rating scale. A clear statement of who measured outcomes was found in only 7 trials. Patient-centered outcomes were not found in any study. Clinic follow-up frequency was a median of 2 weeks (range 1–15 weeks) and did not include telephone contact. Median duration of follow-up was 8 weeks (range 5–20 weeks). A measure of clinical meaningfulness was reported in 21 trials, most commonly as number needed to treat (NNT) (9), or 50% or better pain relief (9). Clinical meaningfulness was good-to-excellent (based on pain relief, satisfaction, adverse effect tolerability, and satisfaction) in 3 trials and 30% improvement in 1 trial. Number-needed-to-harm (NNH) and number-needed-to-quit (NNQ) figures were given in one RCT. An effect size was reported in one study. A quality-of-life measure was used in 21 trials (the most common was the SF36), and satisfaction with pain relief was reported in 3 trials. Twenty-three reports stated that the study used an intent-to-treat analysis.

Adverse Effects of Treatment

Adverse effects were reported in 46 of the 49 trials. Rates of discontinuation of treatment were reported in all because this was a requirement of the RCT rating scale used. Selection of the trial center/clinicians was reported in 3 studies, although this information may have been inferred in many of the trials. Exclusion of patients at risk of complications occurred in 32 trials. No trial excluded patients at risk of adverse effects occurring during a run-in period. Trial safety procedures were considered adequate in 43 trials. An open-ended recording of adverse effects was used in 33 studies and a checklist in 3 studies. Satisfaction with the tolerability of adverse effects was reported in 2 studies.

Implications for Future Trials in Neuropathic Pain

Only 6 of the 49 trials in the systematic review were comparative trials of different analgesics, and these were non-industry-sponsored studies. It is important to conduct comparative trials with standard therapies to determine if a new drug is worthwhile, in terms of better pain relief and fewer side effects, and to determine if some patients respond to one drug and not the other. Those who participate in industry-funded studies should argue for comparative trials, and if a study is done they should insist on an independent data analysis and on its publication. Internet trial registries will help, but there is still no guarantee of the publication of unfavorable studies.

PHN and PDN were the subject of 40/49 (80%) of the studies; therefore, it is unknown how effective antidepressants, anticonvulsants, and opioids are in the many other neuropathic pain conditions seen in clinical practice (it is a clinical impression that neuropathic conditions such as central poststroke pain and incisional neuralgias after aortocoronary bypass and mastectomy are more intractable to pharmacotherapy). Thus, it appears important to carry out trials in other neuropathic pain conditions to determine the generalizability of these results.

All the trials in PHN and PDN in the systematic review showed that the experimental treatment was effective. Six out of 13 trials in the "other" neuropathic pain category were negative trials. This finding raises the possibility that neuropathic pain conditions respond differently to oral analgesics. It is also possible that only favorable trials were reported in the first two conditions. Therefore, these data argue for the study of a uniform population (which only occurred in approximately half of the studies), rather than a mixture of neuropathic pain conditions or of different neuropathies in the same condition, such as with diabetic neuropathy.

In approximately one-third of trials reviewed, the pain severity that was included was mild, of short duration, and not clearly occurring on a daily basis. One-third of trials had more than six inclusion criteria, indicating that these trials were probably performed in quite selected groups. This was particularly the case with RCTs in PDN, which calls into question the generalizability of the treatment effect in those trial populations. The number of exclusion criteria (median 7, range 1–19) also suggests considerable selection in many of the trials. Clinical meaningfulness figures such as NNT and NNH derived from RCTs with a large number of exclusion criteria will not be applicable to clinical practice, and results will not be as good.

Given that several trials excluded patients previously treated with the study or similar drug or patients not responding to the study drug, an enriched enrollment type of population may have been entered into these trials (i.e., patients who are more likely to respond). This was particularly true of the pregabalin and gabapentin trials. With pregabalin, since gabapentin is a very similar drug and had been available for some time prior to these trials, this approach could have resulted in considerable selection bias, and although this issue was mentioned, the numbers were not given, making it impossible to determine the effect of this exclusion criterion.

Clinical characteristics were stated in most trials, but notably absent was an indication of the proportion of different races. In a significant proportion it was not clear whether the disorder was a uniform condition, in other words one type of neuropathic pain or one type of neuropathy in a pain condition such as diabetes (e.g., the subgroup of painful symmetrical distal sensory neuropathy rather than all diabetic neuropathies). It may be important to study uniform conditions rather than a variety of neuropathic pain conditions because of the possible variability in responsivity. More data are needed in neuropathic pain conditions other than PHN and PDN (particularly in central pain such as poststroke pain, multiple sclerosis, and spinal cord injury; and peripheral neuropathic pain such as phantom pain and postsurgical nerve injury pain after mastectomy, thoracotomy, and coronary bypass surgery) in view of the negative trials or the lesser effect that appears in some neuropathic pain conditions.

In a proportion of trials, patients with mild pain were accepted, or it was not clear as to the pain severity, whether the pain occurred daily, or what the duration of the pain was. This lack of appropriate eligibility criteria or their reporting can be problematic for RCTs, and it is important to choose patients with a fairly chronic stable pain state of moderate daily pain for at least 3 months in order to limit the number of patients required in the trial. This consideration is of special importance for cross-over studies, where a period effect from natural resolution may be fatal to analysis of the results.

More than 50% of trials prohibited the use of other drugs known to relieve neuropathic pain. Unless patients on stable doses of these drugs, but with inadequate relief, are included in trials it may not be possible to determine whether a synergistic or additive effect occurs with a new treatment. Clinical practice now shows a trend to treat many patients with polypharmacy, and trials of this approach are currently underway. Responsive patients may also be selected out if they cannot tolerate withdrawal of these agents during a run-in period.

A few studies used surrogate scales to rate pain, which included other symptoms and parameters; however, the majority did use reliable and valid pain rating scales and pain relief rating scales. Many trials (21/45 = 57%) did not include a quality-of-life outcome or use an intent-to-treat analysis (26/49 = 53%). Few used a satisfaction rating regarding pain relief, adverse effects, or both. None utilized a patient-centered outcome measure.

All the trials were relatively short (weeks), and only two trials reported long-term follow-up. This extended follow-up should be possible with trial completers, and in this way adverse events that occur over time and long-term efficacy can be evaluated.

Adverse events were reported in most instances. The most common means of determining adverse events was by open-ended questions, which carries the risk of underreporting of adverse events. It would seem reasonable that a modified checklist of the most common symptoms with an additional category of "other side effects" should yield a more accurate assessment. Additionally, only two trials asked the patients if they were satisfied with their treatment, and none specifically asked the question as to whether they were satisfied with the pain relief and the tolerability of the adverse effects.

Table III
Recommendations for improving the external validity of future randomized
controlled trials of treatments for neuropathic pain

More comparative trials of different analgesics.

Further studies in NP conditions other than PHN and PDN.

Publishing unfavorable (negative) trials.

The study of uniform NP conditions.

Recruiting subjects by advertising and from primary care who more closely resemble clinical practice patients than secondary or tertiary source individuals.

Making the diagnostic criteria for a condition clear (it is not adequate to state "postherpetic neuralgia" or "diabetic neuropathy" without being more precise as to the definition).

Making exclusion criteria reasonable and keeping them to a minimum.

Discouraging the enrichment of studies.

The recording of "subjects screened," "the correct diagnosis/ineligible," and "eligible/declined" in a "flow through the trial" figure.

The recording of the racial origins of subjects.

Including patients with at least moderate pain on a daily basis for a period of 3 months or more.

Having as an outcome a means for the clinician and regulatory body of determining clinical meaningfulness, such as NNT, NNH, NNQ, as a part of every trial.

Having rating scales that specifically evaluate pain and pain relief by a reliable and valid means rather than a surrogate or complex scale.

Including as an outcome a quality-of-life measure to improve the determination of utility to clinical practice.

Using an intent-to-treat analysis as this more closely resembles clinical experience.

Having extended follow-up of study patients to determine long-term adverse effect tolerability and efficacy and the occurrence of late-occurring, significant, unusual adverse events.

The adverse event reporting should include at least a limited checklist of the more common side effects of the drug with "another category" to pick up other side effects, in order to more completely evaluate safety.

It seems reasonable to include a question asking if the patient was satisfied with the pain relief and the tolerability of the adverse events (if present).

Scientists participating with industry can improve external validity by arguing for comparative studies with a standard therapy, by insisting in a role in study design and in having access to and performing analysis of the data. They should write the article arising from the research themselves to avoid an industry spin on the results. There should be an insistence on the publication of all studies, even if unfavorable.

Abbreviations: NNH = number needed to harm, NNT = number needed to treat, NNQ = number needed to quit, NP = neuropathic pain, PDN = painful diabetic neuropathy, PHN = postherpetic neuralgia.

Thus, there were major shortcomings in the external validity of RCTs of treatments for neuropathic pain. Table III lists some recommendations that would help to address this important issue and improve the clinical usefulness of future trials.

Conclusions

Some RCTs have excellent external validity, but many do not, particularly some of those performed by the pharmaceutical industry. Yet, researchers, funding agencies, ethics committees, medical journals, and governmental regulators all neglect proper consideration of external validity. Judgment is left to clinicians, but reporting of the determinants of external validity in trial publications, and particularly in secondary reports and clinical guidelines, is rarely adequate, and much relevant information is never published. Trials cannot be expected to produce results that are directly relevant to all patients and all settings, but to be externally valid they should at least be designed and reported in a way that allows clinicians to judge to whom they can reasonably be applied.

References

[1]   Asymptomatic Carotid Atherosclerosis Study Group. Carotid endarterectomy for patients with asymptomatic internal carotid artery stenosis. JAMA 1995; 273:1421–8.
[2]   Backonja M, Beydoun A, Edwards KR. Gabapentin for the symptomatic treatment of painful neuropathy in patients with diabetes mellitus. JAMA 1998;280:1831–6.
[3]   Bone M, Critchley P, Buggy DJ. Gabapentin in post-amputation phantom limb pain: a randomized, double-blind, cross-over study. Reg Anesth Pain Med 2002;27:481–6.
[4]   Boureau F, Legallicier P, Kabir-Ahmadi M. Tramadol in postherpetic neuralgia: a randomized, double-blind, placebo-controlled trial. Pain 2003;104:323–31.
[5]   Cardenas DD, Warms CA, Turner JA, Marshall H, Brooke MM, Loeser JD. Efficacy of amitriptyline for relief of pain in spinal cord injury: results of a randomized controlled trial. Pain 2002;96:365–73.
[6]   Charleson ME, Horwitz RI. Applying results of randomised trials to clinical practice: impact of losses before randomisation. BMJ 1984;289:1281–4.
[7]   Cook RJ, Sackett DL. The number needed to treat: a clinically useful measure of treatment effect. BMJ 1995;310:452–4.
[8]   Davis KL, Thal LJ, Gamzu ER, Davis CS, Woolson RF, Gracon SI, Drachman DA, Schneider LS, Whitehouse PJ, Hoover TM, et al.; Tacrine Collaborative Study Group. A double-blind, placebo-controlled multicenter study of tacrine for Alzheimer's disease. N Engl J Med 1992;321:406–12.
[9]   Dworkin RH, Corbin AE, Young JP. Pregabalin for the treatment of postherpetic neuralgia. Neurology 2003;60:1274–83.
[10] Eisenberg E, Lurie Y, Braker C, Daoud D, Ishay A. Lamotrigine reduces painful diabetic neuropathy Neurology 2001;57:167–73.
[11] European Carotid Surgery Trialists' Collaborative Group. Randomised trial of endarterectomy for recently symptomatic carotid stenosis: final results of the MRC European Carotid Surgery Trial (ECST). Lancet 1998;351:1379–87.

[12] Fine PEM. Variation in protection by BCG: implications of and for heterologous immunity. Lancet 1995;346:1339–45.

[13] Freynhagen R, Strojek K, Griesing T, Whalen E, Balkenohl M. Efficacy of pregabalin in neuropathic pain evaluated in a 12 week, randomized, double blind, multicentre, placebo-controlled trial of flexible and fixed-dose regimens. Pain 2005;115:254–63.

[14] Gilron I, Bailey JM, Tu D, Holden RR, Weaver DF, Houlden RL. Morphine, gabapentin, or their combination for neuropathic pain. N Engl J Med 2005;352:1324–34.

[15] Gimbel JS, Richards P, Portenoy RK. Controlled-release oxycodone for pain in diabetic neuropathy: a randomized controlled trial. Neurology 2003;60:927–34.

[16] Gorter JW; Stroke Prevention in Reversible Ischaemia Trial (SPIRIT) and European Atrial Fibrillation Trial (EAFT) groups. Major bleeding during anticoagulation after cerebral ischaemia: patterns and risk factors. Neurology 1999;53:1319–27.

[17] Gøtzsche PC. Methodology and overt and hidden bias in reports of 196 double-blind trials of nonsteroidal antiinflammatory drugs in rheumatoid arthritis. Control Clin Trials 1989;10:31–56.

[18] Graff-Radford SB, Shaw LR, Naliboff BN. Amitriptyline and fluphenazine in postherpetic neuralgia. Clin J Pain 2000;16:188–92.

[19] Gruppo Italiano per lo Studio della Streptochinasi nell'Infarto Miocardico (GISSI). Effectiveness of intravenous thrombolytic treatment in acute myocardial infarction. Lancet 1986;1:397–402.

[20] Gurwitz JH, Col NF, Avorn J. The exclusion of elderly and women from clinical trials in acute myocardial infarction. JAMA 1992;268:1417–22.

[21] Hammack JE, Michalak JC, Loprinzi CL, Sloan JA, Novotny PJ, Soori GS, Tirona MT, Rowland KM Jr, Stella PJ, Johnson JA. Phase III evaluation of nortriptyline for alleviation of symptoms of cis-platinum-induced peripheral neuropathy. Pain 2002;91:195–203.

[22] Harati Y, Gooch C, Swenson M, Edelman S, Greene D, Raskin P, Donofrio P, Cornblath D, Sachdeo R, Siu CO, Kamin M. Double-blind randomized trial of tramadol for the treatment of the pain of diabetic neuropathy. Neurology 1998;50:1842–6.

[23] Ioannidis JP, Contopoulos-Ioannidis DG. Reporting of safety data from randomised trials. Lancet 1998;352:1752–3.

[24] Jadad AR, Moore A, Carroll D, et al. Assessing the reports of randomized clinical trials: Is blinding necessary? Control Clin Trials 2001;17:1–12.

[25] Jørgensen HS, Nakayama H, Kammersgaard LP, Raaschou HO, Olsen TS. Predicted impact of intravenous thrombolysis on prognosis of general population of stroke patients: simulation model. BMJ 1999;319:288–9.

[26] Kieburtz K, Simpson D, Yiannoutsos C, Max MB, Hall CD, Ellis RJ, Marra CM, McKendall R, Singer E, Dal Pan GJ, et al. A randomized trial of amitriptyline and mexiletine for painful neuropathy in HIV infection. AIDS Clinical Trial Group 242 Protocol Team. Neurology 1998;51:1682–8.

[27] Kishore-Kumar R, Max MB, Schafer SC, Gaughan AM, Smoller B, Gracely RH, Dubner R. Desipramine relieves postherpetic neuralgia. Clin Pharmacol Ther 1990;47:305–12.

[28] Kvinesdal B, Molin J, Frøland A, Gram LF. Imipramine treatment of painful diabetic neuropathy. JAMA 1984;251:1727–30.

[29] LaRue LJ, Alter M, Traven ND, Sterman AB, Sobel E, Kleiner J. Acute stroke therapy trials: problems in patient accrual. Stroke 1988;19:950–4.

[30] Laupacis A, Sackett DL, Robarts RS. An assessment of clinically useful measures of the consequences of treatment. N Engl J Med 1988;318:1728–33.

[31] Leijon G, Boivie J. Central post-stroke pain: a controlled trial of amitriptyline and carbamazepine. Pain 1989;36:27–36.

[32] Lesser H, Sharma U, LaMoreaux L, Poole RM. Pregabalin relieves symptoms of painful diabetic neuropathy a randomized controlled trial. Neurology 2004;63:2104–19.

[33] Marshall M, Lockwood A, Bradley C, Adams C, Joy C, Fenton M. Unpublished rating scales: a major source of bias in randomised controlled trials of treatments for schizophrenia? Br J Psychiatry 2000;176:249–52.

[34] Max MB, Culnane M, Schafer SC, Gracely RH, Walther DJ, Smoller B, Dubner R. Amitriptyline relieves diabetic neuropathy pain in patients with normal or depressed mood. Neurology 1987;37:589–96.

[35] Max MB, Kishore-Kumar R, Schafer SC, Meister B, Gracely RH, Smoller B, Dubner R. Efficacy of desipramine in painful diabetic neuropathy: a placebo-controlled trial. Pain 1991;45:3–9.

[36] Max MB, Lynch SA, Muir J, Shoaf SE, Smoller B, Dubner R. Effects of desipramine, amitriptyline, and fluoxetine on pain in diabetic neuropathy. N Engl J Med 1992;326:1250–6.

[37] Max MB, Schafer SC, Culnane M, Smoller B, Dubner R, Gracely R. Amitriptyline but not lorazepam relieves postherpetic neuralgia. Neurology 1988;38:1427–37.

[38] Morello CM, Leckband SG, Stoner CP, Moorhouse DF, Sahagian GA. Randomized double-blind study comparing the efficacy of gabapentin with amitriptyline on diabetic peripheral neuropathy pain. Arch Intern Med 1999;159:1931–7.

[39] Pandey CK, Bose N, Garg G, Singh N, Baronia A, Agarwal A, Singh PK, Singh U. Gabapentin for the treatment of pain in Guillain-Barré syndrome: a double-blind, placebo-controlled, crossover study. Anesth Analg 2002;95:1719–23.

[40] Pincus T. Rheumatoid arthritis: disappointing long-term outcomes despite successful short-term clinical trials. J Clin Epidemiol 1998;41:1037–41.

[41] Raja SN, Haythornthwaite JA, Pappagallo M, Clark MR, Travison TG, Sabeen S, Royall RM, Max MB. Opioids versus antidepressants in postherpetic neuralgia: a placebo-controlled study. Pain 2002;94:215–24.

[42] Rice ASC, Maton S; Postherpetic Neuralgia Study Group. Gabapentin in postherpetic neuralgia: a randomized, double blind, placebo controlled trial. Pain 2001;94:2001:215–24.

[43] Richter RW, Portenoy R, Sharma U, Lamoreaux L, Bockbrader H, Knapp LE. Relief of painful diabetic peripheral neuropathy with pregabalin: a randomized, placebo-controlled trial. J Pain 2005;6:253–60.

[44] Rosenstock J, Tuchman M, LaMoreaux L, Sharma U. Pregabalin for the treatment of painful diabetic peripheral neuropathy: a double-blind, placebo-controlled trial. Pain 2004;110:628–38.

[45] Rothwell PM. External validity of randomised controlled trials: to whom do the results of this trial apply? Lancet 2005;365:82–93.

[46] Rothwell PM, Warlow CP. Is self-audit reliable? Lancet 1995;346:1623.

[47] Rowbotham MC, Goli G, Kunz NR, Lei D. Venlafaxine extended release in the treatment of painful diabetic neuropathy: a double-blind, placebo-controlled study. Pain 2004;110:697–706.

[48] Rowbotham M, Harden N, Stacey B, Bernstein P, Magnus-Miller L. Gabapentin for the treatment of postherpetic neuralgia: a randomized controlled trial. JAMA 1998;280:1837–42.

[49] Rowbotham MC, Twilling L, Davies PS, Reisner L, Taylor K, Mohr D. Oral opioid therapy for chronic peripheral and central neuropathic pain. N Engl J Med 2003;13:1223–32.

[50] Sabatowski R, Gálvez R, Cherry DA, Jacquot F, Vincent E, Maisonobe P, Versavel M. Pregabalin reduces pain and improves sleep and mood disturbances in patients with postherpetic neuralgia: results of a randomized, placebo-controlled clinical trial. Pain 2004;109:26–35.

[51] Semenchuk MR, Shennan S, Davis B. Double-blind, randomized trial of bupropion SR for the treatment of neuropathic pain. Neurology 2001;57:1583–8.

[52] Shapiro SH, Weijer C, Freedman B. Reporting the study populations of clinical trials. Clear transmission or static on the line? J Clin Epidemiol 2000;53:973–9.

[53] Shlay JC, Chaloner K, Max MB, Flaws B, Reichelderfer P, Wentworth D, Hillman S, Brizz B, Cohn DL. Acupuncture and amitriptyline for pain due to HIV-related peripheral neuropathy: a randomized controlled trial. Terry Beirn Community Programs for Clinical Research on AIDS. JAMA 1998;280:1590–5.

[54] Simpson DM, McArthur JC, Olney R, Clifford D, So Y, Ross D, Baird BJ, Barrett P, Hammer AE; Lamotrigine HIV Neuropathy Study Team. Lamotrigine for HIV-associated painful sensory neuropathies: a placebo-controlled trial. Neurology 2003; 60:1508–14.

[55] Sindrup SH, Andersen G, Madsen C, Smith T, Brøsen K, Jensen TS. Tramadol relieves pain and allodynia in polyneuropathy; a randomized, double-blind, controlled trial. Pain 1999;83:85–90.

[56] Sindrup SH, Bach FW, Madsen C, Gram LF, Jensen TS. Venlafaxine versus imipramine in painful polyneuropathy: a randomized controlled trial. Neurology 2003;60:1284–9.

[57] Sindrup SH, Bjerre U, Dejgaard A, Brøsen K, Aaes-Jørgensen T, Gram LF. The selective serotonin reuptake inhibitor citalopram relieves the symptoms of diabetic neuropathy. Clin Pharmacol Ther 1992;52:547–52.

[58] Sindrup SH, Ejlertsen B, Frøland A, Sindrup EH, Brøsen K, Gram LF. Imipramine treatment in diabetic neuropathy: relief of subjective symptoms without changes in peripheral and autonomic nerve function. Eur J Clin Pharmacol 1989;37:151–3.

[59] Sindrup SH, Gram LF, Brøsen K, Eshøj O, Mogensen EF. The selective serotonin reuptake inhibitor paroxetine is effective in the treatment of diabetic neuropathy symptoms. Pain 1990;42:135–44.

[60] Sindrup SH, Gram LF, Skjold T, Grodum E, Brøsen K, Beck-Nielsen H. Clomipramine vs desipramine vs placebo in the treatment of diabetic neuropathy symptoms: a double-blind, crossover study. Br J Clin Pharmacol 1990;30:683–91.

[61] Sindrup SH, Grodum E, Gram LF, Beck-Nielsen H. Concentration-response relationship in paroxetine treatment of diabetic neuropathy symptoms: a patient-blinded dose escalation study. Ther Drug Monit 1991;13:408–14.

[62] Sindrup SH, Tuxen C, Gram LF. Lack of effect of mianserin on the symptoms of diabetic neuropathy. Eur J Clin Pharmacol 1992;43:251–5.

[63] Thornley B, Adams CE. Content and quality of 2000 controlled trials in schizophrenia over 50 years. BMJ 1998;317:1181–4.

[64] Tunis SR, Stryer DB, Clancy CM. Practical clinical trials: increasing the value of clinical research for decision making in clinical and health policy. JAMA 2003;290:1624–32.

[65] Vestergaard K, Andersen G, Gottrup H, Kristensen BT, Jensen TS. Lamotrigine for central post-stroke pain: a randomized controlled trial. Neurology 2001:56:184–9.

[66] Vrethem M, Boivie J, Arnqvist H, Holmgren H, Lindström T, Thorell LH. A comparison of amitriptyline and maprotiline in the treatment of painful diabetic neuropathy in diabetics and non-diabetics. Clin J Pain 1997;12:313–23.

[67] Walker MC, Sander JW. Difficulties in extrapolating from clinical trial data to clinical practice: the case of antiepileptic drugs. Neurology 1997;49:333–7.

[68] Watson CPN. External validity of pharmaceutical trials in neuropathic pain. In: Rothwell PM, editor. Treating individuals: from randomized trials to personalized medicine. Elsevier: The Lancet; 2007. p. 121–131.

[69] Watson CPN, Babul N. Oxycodone relieves neuropathic pain: a randomized trial in postherpetic neuralgia. Neurology 1998;50:1837–41.

[70] Watson CPN, Chipman M, Reed K. Amitriptyline versus nortriptyline in postherpetic neuralgia. Neurology 1998;51:1166–71.

[71] Watson CPN, Chipman M, Reed K, Evans RJ, Birkett N. Amitriptyline versus maprotiline in postherpetic neuralgia: a randomized, double-blind, crossover trial. Pain 1992;48:29–36.

[72] Watson CPN, Evans RJ, Reed K, Merskey H, Goldsmith I, Warsh J. Amitriptyline versus placebo in postherpetic neuralgia. Neurology 1982;32:671–3.

[73] Watson CPN, Moulin D, Watt-Watson J, Gordon A, Eisenhoffer J. Controlled-release oxycodone relieves neuropathic pain: a randomized controlled trial in painful diabetic neuropathy. Pain 2003;105;71–8.

Correspondence to: Prof. Peter M. Rothwell, MD, PhD, University Department of Clinical Neurology, Level 6, West Wing, John Radcliffe Hospital, Headington, Oxford OX3 9DU, United Kingdom. Email: peter.rothwell@clneuro.ox.ac.uk.

Extinction of Pain Memories: Importance for the Treatment of Chronic Pain

Herta Flor

Department of Cognitive and Clinical Neuroscience, Central Institute of Mental Health, University of Heidelberg, Mannheim, Germany

Chronic pain is determined to a large extent by learning and memory processes. This chapter reviews the contribution of implicit memory processes and shows that the extinction rather than the acquisition of aversive memory traces may be the crucial variable for pain chronicity. These pain memory traces are related to site-specific as well as general changes in the central nervous system and the periphery that enhance pain perception. The extinction of pain-related memory traces is difficult because extinction is fairly specific and does not easily generalize. Moreover, extinction necessitates the acquisition of a new memory trace that is fragile and can be disturbed by aversive experience. Chronic pain treatment must involve the extinction of these aversive memory traces and at the same time focus on the relearning of positive (appetitive) associations. Behavioral approaches, stimulation, pharmacological interventions targeting maladaptive learning, or a combination of these methods can be effective treatment options. Strategies for the prevention of chronic pain must also take these learning processes into account.

Current Topics in Pain: 12th World Congress on Pain
edited by José Castro-Lopes
IASP Press, Seattle, © 2009

Learning Processes in Chronic Pain

Recent scientific evidence suggests that chronic pain is largely determined by learning processes that are accompanied by plastic changes at multiple levels of the nervous system [2,20,25,62]. A fundamental distinction can be made between implicit (or nondeclarative) and explicit (or declarative) memory processes. Implicit memory processes refer to changes in behavior that develop—often unconsciously—as a consequence of experience. They involve nonassociative learning processes such as habituation and sensitization, as well as associative processes such as operant and respondent conditioning. Explicit learning usually refers to semantic and episodic memory processes that rely on the conscious reproduction of an encoded memory item. These memory processes also involve different brain structures and neuronal networks and may interact differentially in health and disease states [53]. For example, explicit memory depends heavily on intact hippocampal structures, whereas some types of implicit emotional memory require an intact amygdala or striatum. (For a review of explicit memory, see [19].) Although both types of learning and memory processes are important in chronic pain, implicit learning processes may be more pronounced because pain has a high biological relevance, which suggests that fast automatic processes may be important. Because implicit learning processes change an individual's behavior without his or her conscious awareness, they may be especially difficult to extinguish [20].

We may therefore assume that (a) the extinction or "unlearning," rather than the acquisition, of pain memories is the main problem in chronic pain; (b) central and peripheral memories are closely interwoven, and both need to be addressed; and (c) treatment can be viewed as extinction and relearning, and therefore it must be based on learning principles.

Sensitization

Sensitization refers to a nonassociative learning process in which the repeated application of a stimulus leads to an increased response that can be described on the physiological level, where it is usually referred to as "central sensitization" [e.g., 36], or on the psychological level, where it is commonly described as "perceptual sensitization" [e.g., 41]. The counterpart of sensitization is the process of habituation, in which repeated stimulation leads to a reduction of the response to the stimulus, which can also be described on a physiological or behavioral level.

In a number of chronic pain syndromes, perceptual sensitization has been observed, accompanied by enhanced activation in the central nervous system. For example, patients with fibromyalgia syndrome or with chronic back pain may demonstrate enhanced perception of tonic painful stimuli or repetitive painful stimulation [41,68]. An important factor in the development of perceptual sensitization may be previous painful experience that leaves memory traces in the central nervous system. For example, Hermann et al. [33; C. Hermann et al., unpublished data] investigated the consequences of early painful experience related to painful burns in the first years of life or related to perinatal medical procedures necessitated by preterm birth or other birth-related complications. Such experiences can lead to massive perceptual sensitization, as assessed by responses to a tonic heat stimulus when the children are of school age (see Fig. 1a,b). Perceptual sensitization is also seen in enhanced activation of pain-related brain regions, a finding that has also been reported in patients with fibromyalgia or chronic back pain [e.g., 28,29,30], as well as in those with neuropathic pain syndromes [47,50].

Operant Learning

Fordyce's [26] description of the role of operant factors in chronic pain suggests that when an individual is exposed to a stimulus that causes tissue damage, the immediate response is withdrawal and an attempt to escape from painful sensations. Withdrawal may be accomplished by avoiding activity believed to cause or exacerbate pain, by seeking help to reduce symptoms, and so forth. These behaviors are observable and, consequently, are subject to the principles of operant conditioning, i.e., they respond to contingencies of reward and punishment. The operant view proposes that acute "pain behavior," such as limping to protect a wounded limb and prevent additional nociceptive input, may come under the control of external contingencies of reinforcement and thus may develop into a chronic pain problem. Pain behavior (e.g., complaining and inactivity) may receive direct positive reinforcement by attention from a spouse or health care provider. Pain behavior may also be maintained by the escape from noxious stimulation by taking drugs or resting, or by avoiding undesirable

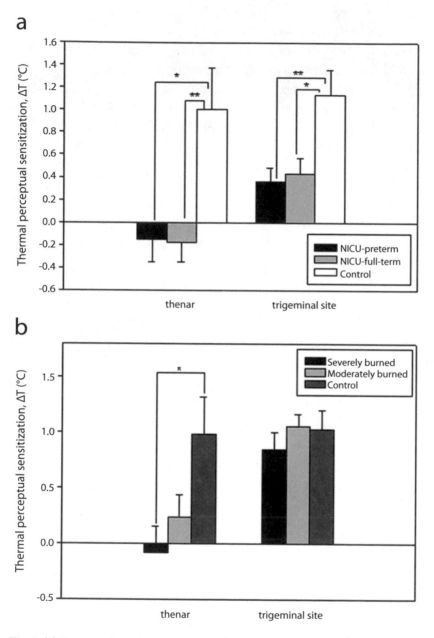

Fig. 1. (a) Perceptual sensitization to tonic heat stimulation (mean and standard error of the mean) for preterm (NICU-preterm) and full-term neonates (NICU-full-term) undergoing treatment in the neonatal intensive care unit (NICU) and controls (**$P < 0.01$, *$P < 0.05$, Tukey's post-test) [33]. (b) Perceptual sensitization to tonic heat stimulation (mean and standard error of the mean) for severely burned children, moderately burned

activities such as work (negative reinforcement). In addition, "well behavior" (e.g., activity and work) may not be sufficiently reinforcing, and the more rewarding pain behaviors may, therefore, be maintained by lack of reinforcement of healthy behaviors. The pain behavior originally elicited by somatic factors may come to occur, totally or in part, in response to reinforcing environmental events. Because of the consequences of specific behavioral responses, pain behaviors may persist long after the resolution or significant reduction of the initial cause of pain.

The operant conditioning model does not concern itself with the initial cause of pain. Rather, it considers pain as an internal subjective experience that may be maintained even after the initial physical basis of the pain has resolved. Operant conditioning can lead to increased inactivity and disability, and it also plays an important role in increases in medication levels because the intake of medication—especially on a p.r.n. basis when pain levels are high—may be viewed as a consequence of a negative reinforcement process (a negative consequence, the pain, is removed by medication intake). Not only observable pain behaviors but also verbal expressions of pain and physiological variables may be subject to the contingencies of reinforcement.

For example, Flor et al. [24] showed that monetary and social reinforcement of acute pain ratings can lead to an increase or reduction of self-reported pain levels, depending on the direction of the reinforced response. This response was equally well acquired by chronic pain patients and healthy controls and did not yield any differences in central brain responses (somatosensory evoked potentials recorded by an electroencephalogram [EEG]). However, when reinforcement was withdrawn, only the healthy controls downregulated their pain ratings and their brain response (following the normal habituation curves). The

children, and control children (*$P < 0.05$, Tukey's post-test) [77]. Thermal perceptual sensitization was assessed using a modified procedure reported by Kleinböhl et al. [41]. First, subjects increased the temperature until pain threshold was reached (T1). The temperature was then held constant for 30 seconds, with the participants not being informed that temperature remained unchanged. At the end of stimulation, participants were asked to readjust the temperature by lowering, increasing, or leaving it such that it just felt painful (T2). Perceptual sensitization is defined as $\Delta T = T2 - T1$. Negative ΔT values indicate perceptual sensitization, whereas positive ΔT values indicate habituation. Thermal perceptual sensitization was defined as the mean ΔT of three experimental trials. Stimulation was applied to the hand (thenar surface) and the face (trigeminal site).

chronic pain patients, however, maintained elevated pain responses, which were reflected in elevated brain potentials, during extinction. The patients were unaware of the altered pain processing and lack of extinction. Becker et al. [7] recently showed that implicit operant learning can also take place when a behavior-contingent reduction or increase in pain is used as a reinforcing stimulus and when behavioral adjustments of pain perception are used rather than verbal ratings or EEG measures (see Fig. 2).

Respondent and Social Learning Mechanisms

Given that the experience of pain is a very important biological stimulus, it is immediately evident that both operant and respondent (Pavlovian)

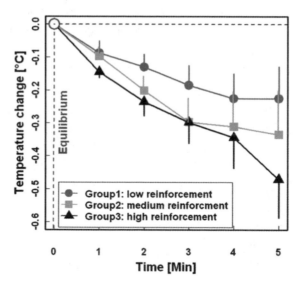

Fig. 2. Learning curves during operant heat-pain titration, given as self-adjusted temperature change from an individual equilibrium temperature (45.5–46.2°C) for groups receiving different magnitudes of reinforcement ("low reinforcement" group, $N = 13$, temperature change < 0.16°C; "medium reinforcement" group, $N = 11$, temperature change approximately 0.23°C; "high reinforcement" group, $N = 12$, temperature change > 0.45°C). Minute-to-minute mean time courses of the three groups are shown [7]. Each participant performed four trials of 8 minutes' duration. The subjects had to keep a memorized sensation constant against a gradual rise of temperature by pressing either of two keys for up- or downregulation. Up- and down-responses were differentially reinforced by temperature decreases or increases. ΔT: temperature change reinforcement. Operant training resulted in temperature decreases, indicating sensitization in a dose-dependent manner.

conditioning might play an important role when pain is experienced repeatedly, as is the case in the transition from acute to chronic pain [46].
In the typical classical conditioning paradigm, a previously neutral variable (which later becomes the conditioned stimulus), when paired with
a biologically significant stimulus (the unconditioned stimulus), comes
to elicit a conditioned response that resembles the response to the unconditioned stimulus (the unconditioned response). For example, if a
certain movement has been associated with pain, just thinking about
the movement may be enough to elicit fear and muscle tension (previously elicited by pain) and may then motivate avoidance behavior. Once
an acute pain problem exists, fear of motor activities that the patient
expects to result in pain may develop and motivate avoidance of activity.
Nonoccurrence of pain is a powerful reinforcer for reduction of activity,
and thus the original respondent conditioning may be followed by an
operant learning process whereby the nociceptive stimuli and the associated responses need no longer be present for the avoidance behavior
to occur.

In acute pain states, it may be useful to reduce movement, and
consequently avoid pain, to accelerate the healing process. Pain related
to sustained muscle contractions might, however, also be conceptualized as an unconditioned stimulus in cases that did not involve acute
injury. Sympathetic activation and tension increases might be viewed as
unconditioned responses that could elicit more pain, and conditioning
might proceed in the same fashion as outlined above. Thus, although
the original association between pain and pain-related stimuli results
in anxiety regarding these stimuli, over time the expectation of pain
related to activity may lead to avoidance of adaptive behaviors, even if
the nociceptive stimuli and the related sympathetic activation are no
longer present. Fear of pain and activity may become conditioned to an
expanding number of situations. Avoided activities may involve simple
motor behaviors, but also work, leisure, and sexual activity. In addition
to the avoidance learning, pain may be exacerbated and maintained in
these potentially pain-increasing situations due to the anxiety-related
sympathetic activation and increased muscle tension that may occur
both in anticipation of pain and as a consequence of pain. Thus, psychological factors may directly affect nociceptive stimulation and need

not be viewed merely as reactions to pain. Vlaeyen and Linton [73] have documented that fear avoidance is a major predictor of chronic pain and disability.

Aversive emotional conditioning with painful stimuli as the unconditioned stimulus is exaggerated in chronic pain patients, particularly in the site that is relevant for the specific type of pain [64]. This site-specificity of peripheral changes associated with pain-related memory traces is important because there may be a local aggravating factor that is, however, triggered by central changes. The incredible site-specificity of pain-related responses was shown by Avenanti et al. [3], who used transcranial magnetic stimulation to test the activation of the motor cortex in healthy humans in response to viewing painful stimulation applied to others. Subjects viewed short videos in which a needle penetrated the skin of a hand, the hand was touched with a cotton swab, or the skin of a tomato was penetrated by a needle. The muscle that received the painful stimulation on the video and an adjacent control muscle were used to record motor-evoked potentials (MEPs) elicited by transcranial magnetic stimulation. The magnitude of the MEPs is directly proportional to the cortical excitability induced by the experimental manipulation. Avenanti et al. showed a significant suppression of MEPs at the site that was shown to be painfully stimulated in the video, but not at the control site. Moreover, the degree of response suppression and the perceived intensity (but not unpleasantness) of the perceived pain were highly correlated, suggesting that this reaction is a somatosensory response to pain perceived in others. This response has not been tested in chronic pain patients, who generally show enhanced MEPs (see below). Craig [14] has emphasized that viewing pain in others and responding to it is a major learning factor related to pain. He confirmed the role of social learning for pain processing, a factor that has so far received insufficient attention. Empathy for pain [67] is a prerequisite for social learning, but social learning goes beyond emotional involvement in other people's pain.

Although the important role of these learning processes for chronic pain was formulated in the 1970s and 1980s, researchers in the neurosciences have only recently examined the mechanisms of these learning processes and made it possible to study their central mechanisms.

Central Changes Related to Learning and Memory Processes

Site-Specific Changes

The increase or decrease of sensory input into the brain leads to adaptive changes in the primary sensory and motor areas. For example, in patients with amputations, the map in the primary somatosensory cortex changes in such a manner that input from neighboring areas occupies the region that formerly received input from the amputated limb [e.g., 23]. These changes are mirrored in the motor cortex [e.g. 39]. Interestingly, reorganizational changes were found in amputees with phantom limb pain, but not in amputees without pain. These findings suggest that nociceptive input may contribute to the changes observed and that the persisting pain might also be a consequence of the plastic changes that occur. In several studies in human upper-extremity amputees, displacement of the representation of the lips in the primary motor and somatosensory cortex was positively correlated with the intensity of phantom limb pain, and it was not found in pain-free amputees or healthy controls. Also, in the patients with phantom limb pain, but not in the pain-free amputees, the imagined movement of the phantom hand activated the neighboring face area [47]. Such coactivation is probably due to the high overlap of the hand, arm, and mouth representations.

Similar observations were made in patients with complex regional pain syndrome (CRPS). In these patients, the representation of the affected hand tended to be smaller compared to that of the unaffected hand, and the individual digit representations had moved closer together [e.g., 37,50]. The extent of the pathological changes in the cortical representations correlated with the intensity of pain [37,66], but the changes were also related to a degradation of sensibility in the affected hand.

Increased behaviorally relevant input related to non-neuropathic pain also leads to changes in the cortical map [21,28,29,30]. For example, Flor et al. [21] reported a close association between pain chronicity and enhanced excitability and expansion of the back representation in the primary somatosensory cortex in patients with non-neuropathic back pain. The back representation had expanded and shifted toward the leg representation to an extent dependent on the length of time the pain

had persisted. Similar changes were reported by Giesecke et al. [28] using functional magnetic resonance imaging. Representations of painful
stimulation were also greatly enhanced in patients with fibromyalgia, who
showed more areas of the brain responding to painful stimulation of a
standard value and also higher activation intensities [29,30].

Hyperexcitability and Chronic Pain

In addition to cortical reorganization, general cortical hyperexcitability has
been observed in chronic neuropathic pain syndromes [9,12,18,40,43,66].
For example, Larbig et al. [43] presented pain-relevant and pain-irrelevant
words and found enhanced late visual potential amplitudes of the EEG to
all words in amputees with phantom limb pain but not in amputees without pain or in healthy controls. Karl et al. [40] reported significantly higher
P300 amplitudes in amputees with pain compared to amputees without
pain and healthy controls in a visual oddball paradigm. This finding suggests a higher magnitude of nonspecific cortical excitability in amputees
with pain and reduced excitability in amputees without pain. Schwenkreis
et al. [66] found a significant reduction of intracortical inhibition in both
hemispheres in patients with CRPS compared to healthy control subjects.
In upper- and lower-limb amputees, transcranial magnetic stimulation
studies demonstrated elevated excitability of the motor system at the site
ipsilateral to the stump [12,18]. Motor evoked potentials were elicited at
lower intensities in muscles immediately proximal to the site of amputation compared to the homologous muscle on the unaffected side. Transcranial magnetic stimulation also recruited a higher percentage of the
motor neuron pool in the muscle on the side of the stump than on the unaffected side. These results suggest an increase in excitability of the motor
system projecting to the muscle immediately above the amputation. Cortical hyperexcitability was also reported by Tinazzi et al. [71] in patients
with right primary trigeminal neuralgia and no clinical signs of trigeminal
deafferentation.

Activation in Areas Associated with the Affective
and Cognitive Processing of Pain

More recent evidence has focused on the affective and cognitive processing of pain and on how this processing might be altered in chronic pain.

For example, a study by Witting et al. [76] examined the brain correlates of allodynia in patients with allodynia related to neuropathic pain. In this positron emission tomography study, the authors observed that allodynia was related to enhanced ipsilateral insular and orbitofrontal activation as well as to a lack of contralateral primary somatosensory cortex activation. They explained this finding in terms of a stronger emotional load and higher computational demands in the processing of a mixed sensation of brush and pain. Orbitofrontal activation is probably related to mechanisms of descending pain modulation, but it might also be involved in anticipatory anxiety related to pain. Similarly, in trigeminal neuralgia, allodynia activated not only areas in the primary sensory pathway but also the basal ganglia and the frontal cortex [6]. Schweinhardt et al. [65] also observed a relationship between allodynia and caudal insular activity in pain patients.

In amputees, Willoch et al. [75] used hypnosis to induce painful phantom sensations and observed activation in areas such as the insula and the anterior cingulate cortex, regions that have been identified as important in the processing of affective pain components. However, the influence of the effort to create a specific sensation in the hypnotic state cannot be controlled for in this type of study. In a study that varied both acute and chronic pain intensity simultaneously, the investigators observed that chronic pain intensity covaried with prefrontal activation, whereas acute pain intensity changes covaried with insular activation. These results suggest different processing modes for acute and habitual pain [4].

The Influence of Learning on Pain Representation in the Brain

It is important to note that the neural signature of pain can be altered by learning and memory processes. In an ongoing study, my colleagues and I are investigating the influence of signaled or unsignaled pain on the processing of pain in the brain. Two groups of healthy persons received painful stimulation and simple graphic stimuli over the course of 10 days and underwent the same repetitive painful stimulation on test days before and after the training sessions. In one group, one graphic symbol signaled a painful stimulus, while another symbol signaled no stimulus (a differential delay conditioning paradigm). In the other group, the same type and number of painful and visual stimuli were given in random order. The brain's responses to pain before stimulation training were no different between the groups. After the 10 days of training, the brain activation patterns of the two groups were significantly different: the group with the history of signaled pain showed more activation in the amygdala, dorsolateral prefrontal cortex, and striatum, along with higher pain tolerance, whereas the group with the unpredictable stimulus experienced lower pain tolerance and showed more activation in the anterior cingulate cortex, hippocampus, and periaqueductal gray (see Fig. 3).

Albanese et al. [1] showed that learning and memory tasks related to discrimination of stimuli alter the somatosensory and insular cortex, and Diesch and Flor [16] documented similar changes in the primary somatosensory cortex as a consequence of Pavlovian conditioning.

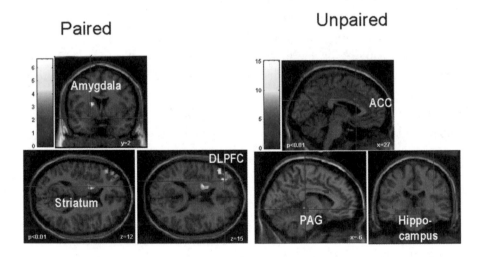

Fig. 3. Brain changes (blood-oxygenation-level-dependent group contrasts) in response to identical painful stimulation (repetitive painful electrical stimuli between pain threshold and pain tolerance) at post- minus pretraining times for two groups: (left) a group that had received 10 days of paired presentation of the visual and the painful cue, in which one visual cue (e.g., a circle) signaled the absence of pain and another (e.g., a diamond) the presence of pain in the next trial; and (right) a group that had received 10 days of unpaired stimulation (a random sequence of painful and visual stimuli). Note that the pre- and post-training painful stimulations, which are the basis of this contrast, were identical for the two groups (no visual cues were given). ACC = anterior cingulate cortex; DLPFC = dorsolateral prefrontal cortex; PAG = periaqueductal gray. Unpublished data from H. Flor et al.

Potential Mechanisms Underlying Plastic Changes of the Brain in Pain

Potential mechanisms of plasticity related to learning and memory in pain include the unmasking of previously present but inactive excitatory synapses; the growth of new connections (sprouting), which involves alterations in GABAergic inhibition; and alterations in the activity of calcium and sodium channels. Immediately after amputation, plasticity can be shown in humans, which suggests that reorganization of sensory pathways occurs very soon after amputation, potentially due to the unmasking of ordinarily silent inputs or dendritic sprouting rather than due to sprouting of new axon terminals [13,38]. Unmasking of latent excitatory synapses can be caused by increased release of excitatory neurotransmitters, increased density of postsynaptic receptors, changes in conductance of the neuronal membrane, a decrease in inhibitory inputs, or the removal of inhibition from excitatory inputs. However, the evidence to date points to the removal of inhibition from excitatory synapses as the major contributor. The crucial element in this process is the decrease in inhibition induced by gamma-aminobutyric acid (GABA). GABA is the most important inhibitory neurotransmitter in the brain, and GABAergic neurons represent about one-third of the neuronal population in the motor cortex. Alterations in GABAergic inhibition can induce rapid changes in cortical excitability. The interesting finding that drugs that enhance GABAergic inhibition increase intracortical inhibition, but do not affect motor threshold, suggests that the reduced intracortical inhibition described in that study [78] was most likely mediated by GABA, whereas changes in the motor threshold had another underlying mechanism.

As proposed by Chen et al. [11], the reduction of motor threshold might involve enhancement of cortico-cortical connections. Drugs that block voltage-gated sodium channels increase the motor threshold [12], so it is possible that the proposed enhancement in cortical connections could be mediated by these channels. In models of spinal cord injury, Waxman and Hains [74] reported a substantial calcium-channel-mediated upregulation of activity in supraspinal pathways.

In addition, structural changes, as revealed by voxel-based morphometry [17,42] and magnetic resonance spectroscopy [31,32], suggest that neuronal loss and cell death are induced in chronic pain. However, the relationship of these changes to pain severity has not yet been documented. A lack of deactivation in baseline brain activity (the default network) was reported by Baliki et al. [5], suggesting that pain may dramatically interfere with the adaptive abilities of the brain to varying demands. However, these baseline changes may also be a vulnerability factor for chronic pain.

Learning, Plasticity, and Pain: Implications for Treatment

We have shown that learning influences subjective, behavioral, neurophysiological, and biochemical aspects of pain that outlast the phase of acute pain and may contribute to an enhanced experience of chronic pain. In particular, the extinction of learned pain associations may be impaired in chronic pain patients and should be the focus of pain management. Site-specific peripheral and central changes related to pain memory processes may need to be addressed separately. It is not only the physical stimulus but also the learning history that determines the response to noxious stimulation, and thus the learning history must be assessed and addressed in treatment.

Extinction Training: A New Approach in Pain Management

Characteristics of Extinction

In contrast to the acquisition of a pain-related response, which generalizes easily across stimuli and responses, the extinction or unlearning of a pain response is specific to the stimulus and the response [56]. Therefore, training a patient to extinguish pain-related responses may be much more difficult than their acquisition. Moreover, extinction involves the learning of an inhibitory process, not just the erasure of an old memory trace. Further characteristics of extinction are that the changes in memory fade with the passage of time, whereas acquired emotional memories often become stronger over time. In addition, a change of context can reactivate the extinguished memory, a phenomenon that has been termed "renewal." In memory acquisition, generalization of stimuli and responses occurs, making the acquired response very resistant to extinction. Finally, stressful events such as a new episode of pain can function as an unconditioned stimulus and can reactivate the extinguished memory in a process known as reinstatement. This process is problematic in chronic pain patients, who are likely to experience new episodes of stress and pain. (See Table I for important characteristics of extinction.) Treatment thus requires massed practice (i.e., many sessions in a short time) in varying contexts during stressful and nonstressful conditions. Success can be achieved by specific operant-based extinction training, but also by cognitive-behavioral or respondent (biofeedback) approaches. In addition, pharmacological interventions that can enhance the extinction of a learned response may be utilized in combination with behavioral interventions. Interventions that are designed to directly alter brain plasticity and memory-related changes such as central stimulation, neurofeedback or imagery, mirror use, and virtual reality may also be effective. Moreover, chronic pain must be prevented as early as possible by pharmacological and psychological interventions in order to prevent pain memories from being established.

Behavioral Pain Extinction Training

Patients who show high levels of pain behaviors and are greatly incapacitated by their pain should profit from operant-based behavioral extinction training. The goals of such treatment are to decrease pain behaviors in an effort to extinguish aversive memories related to pain; to increase activity levels and healthy behaviors related to work, leisure time, and the family; to reduce and manage medication intake; and to change the behavior of significant others [cf. 70]. The overall goal is to reduce disability by reducing pain and increasing healthy (appetitive) behaviors. Medication is switched from a p.r.n. basis to a fixed time schedule, in which medication is given at certain times of the day to avoid negative reinforcement learning. Similar principles are applied to the enhancement of activity and the reduction of inactivity and disability. This approach has been found to be effective in patients with chronic back pain as well as in those with other pain syndromes [e.g., 69,70]. In addition, extinction training can lead to significant changes in maladaptive brain activation patterns [59]. Fig. 4 shows data on the treatment of fibromyalgia in an extinction protocol based on operant principles [69].

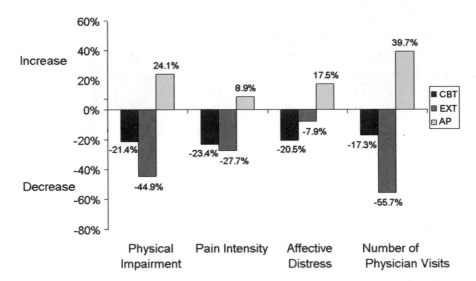

Fig. 4. Changes in three treatment groups 12 months after training compared to pretraining values (percentage change). EXT = extinction training, CBT = cognitive-behavioral training, AP = attention placebo; based on data from Thieme et al. [69]. Extinction training relied on an operant protocol that focused on video-based reduction of overt pain behaviors; increased activity; and role-playing of healthy behaviors, including social activities and work. The cognitive-behavioral training focused on education, cognitive coping skills, and problem solving. The attention placebo group involved discussions of problems around chronic pain without any specific suggestions or training by the therapists.

Cognitive-Behavioral Interventions

The cognitive-behavioral model of chronic pain emphasizes the role of cognitive, affective, and behavioral factors in the development and maintenance of chronic pain. The central tenet of cognitive-behavioral treatment is that it is important to reduce feelings of helplessness and lack of control and to establish a sense of control over pain. These results can be achieved by the modification of behaviors, cognitions, and emotions that elicit and maintain pain. The cognitive-behavioral approach teaches patients various techniques to effectively deal with episodes of pain. Pain-related cognitions are changed by cognitive restructuring and pain coping strategies such as attention diversion, use of imagery, or relaxation, which increase self-efficacy. Several studies have examined the efficacy of cognitive-behavioral pain management, which must be considered a very effective treatment of chronic pain [e.g., 72]. Both extinction training and cognitive-behavioral therapy can significantly reduce pain intensity. In addition, cognitive-behavioral therapy improves cognitive and affective variables, whereas pain extinction training yields significant improvements in physical functioning and behavioral variables [69] (see Fig. 4).

Biofeedback

Biofeedback refers to the modification of a normally nonconscious bodily process (e.g., skin temperature or muscle tension) by making the bodily process perceptible to the patient. The physiological signal is measured, amplified, and fed back to the patients by the use of a computer that translates variations in bodily processes into visual, auditory, or tactile signals. Seeing or hearing one's blood pressure or muscle tension enables individuals to self-regulate these processes. The most common type of biofeedback for chronic pain is muscle tension or electromyographic (EMG) biofeedback, which has been found effective for several chronic musculoskeletal pain syndromes. For patients with migraine headache, body temperature, blood flow in the temporal artery, or slow cortical potentials have been fed back with good results. Similar positive data are available for Raynaud's disease with respect to temperature feedback. Altering site-specific changes in physiological reactivity related to pain may also affect learning-related brain changes.

Imagery, Mirror Training, Neurofeedback, and Virtual Reality Training

The alteration of maladaptive brain plasticity is also possible by directly modifying the maladaptive learned brain response to pain by providing feedback of event-related potential components or EEG rhythms, or even blood-oxygenation-level-dependent changes in functional magnetic resonance imaging [e.g., 15,54]. Most of these methods have not yet been tested in a systematic manner, and little is known about their effects on cortical reorganization and pain-related memory processes. Alternatively, indirect methods can be used, such as imagery, mirror training, or virtual reality, which make use of the fact that the brain processes the perceived rather than the physical reality and could thus reverse maladaptive changes in pain-related memories such as phantom limb pain. For example, Moseley [55] used a three-part program for patients with CRPS.

This program contained a hand laterality recognition task (recognizing a pictured hand to be a left or right hand), imagined movements of the affected hand, and mirror therapy (adopting the hand posture shown on a picture with both hands in a mirror box while watching the reflection of the unaffected hand). After 2 weeks of treatment, pain scores were significantly reduced. McCabe et al. [52] also found a reduction in pain ratings during and after mirrored visual feedback of movement of the unaffected limb in CRPS. Recently, Chan et al. [10] reported a significant reduction of phantom limb pain with mirror treatment compared to treatment in front of a covered mirror and visualization. Significant effects on pain and brain organization were also reported in several studies that used mental imagery of phantom movements [e.g., 49]. These studies suggest that modification of input into the affected brain region may alter pain sensation, an effect that could also be achieved by virtual reality training. These methods might be able to provide "normal" input to the affected brain area and could thus inhibit prior pain-related memory traces.

Stimulation

In long-term amputees, stimulation-related procedures are also found to be effective. Intense input to the cortical amputation zone, such as by the use of a myoelectric prosthesis, can reduce both cortical reorganization and phantom limb pain [48]. Thus, extensive training with a myoelectric or sensorimotor prosthesis would seem useful in reducing phantom limb pain. In patients in whom the use of a prosthesis is not possible, sensory discrimination training might be beneficial. In one study, electrodes were closely spaced over the amputation stump in a region where their activity would excite the nerve that supplied the amputated portion of the arm. Patients then had to discriminate the frequency and the location of the stimulation in an extended training that encompassed 90 minutes per day over a 2-week period. Improvements in both two-point discrimination and phantom limb pain were substantial in these patients after training. These improvements were accompanied by changes in cortical reorganization that indicated a normalization of the shifted representation of the mouth [22].

    In some patients, cortical excitability to alleviate pain can be modulated by electrical stimulation with electrodes implanted over the motor cortex [e.g., 57]. Although positive results were reported with this method, the risk for complications limits its use. More recently, non-invasive techniques such as transcranial magnetic stimulation and transcranial direct current stimulation have been proposed as suitable alternatives to achieve this goal. Both techniques have been applied in several hundred subjects (patients and healthy volunteers) worldwide, and no significant side effects have been reported to date [e.g. 35,45,58,60]. Initial results on pain relief with these non-invasive techniques are encouraging [e.g., 27,44].

Pharmacological Interventions

Prevention of chronic pain might be possible by using pharmacological agents that are known to also prevent or reverse cortical reorganization. Among these substances, GABA agonists, NMDA-receptor antagonists, and anticholinergic substances seem to be the most promising. A double-blind, placebo-controlled study that used the NMDA-receptor antagonist memantine in the acute perioperative phase in amputations reported a decrease of the incidence of phantom limb pain from 72% to 20% 1 year after the amputation [63]. Birbaumer et al. [8] used regional anesthesia in upper-limb amputees to treat phantom limb pain and observed a rapid reversal of somatosensory cortical reorganization in those who experienced substantial pain relief, but not in those whose pain remained unchanged. This finding suggests that rapid modulation of cortical plasticity and pain is possible, even in long-term chronic pain states. However, more research is needed that takes into account that extinction is itself an active memory process that is based not on the inhibition of old memory traces but on the construction of new ones.

Combined Behavioral and Pharmacological Interventions

In the treatment of phobia, Ressler et al. [61] showed that the effects of exposure therapy related to aversive fear memories could be enhanced by combining the treatment with a partial NMDA-receptor agonist (d-cycloserine). This treatment was also found effective for social phobia [34]. Cannabinoids might also enhance the extinction of aversive memories and can be tested as enhancers of exposure [51]. Since pain seems to generally increase excitability, substances that decrease excitation such as gabapentin or pregabalin would also seem indicated as enhancers of extinction. Given that extinction is context-specific, important aspects of training are to include as many varied behaviors as possible, to train in many different environments, and to use stress and pain episodes to teach relapse prevention. In addition, cognitive and emotional aspects of pain need to be targeted, as outlined above.

Conclusion

Although recent scientific evidence has shown that chronic pain leads to changes in many brain regions, the responsiveness of pain to plastic changes also opens the door for new intervention methods, which rely on stimulation, behavioral training, or pharmacological interventions to prevent maladaptive memory formation or enhance extinction. This chapter has focused on the role of learning and memory mechanisms in the development and maintenance of chronic pain. Different psychological treatments of chronic pain have been discussed, with a focus on innovative treatments of chronic pain designed to change pain memories. Future work should investigate the combination of behavioral and pharmacological interventions. Furthermore, the role of context conditioning is virtually unexplored, and alterations in appetitive conditioning related to chronic pain require investigation.

Acknowledgments

This research was supported by the Bundesministerium für Bildung und Forschung (German Neuropathic Pain Network), the Deutsche Forschungsgemeinschaft (Research Unit Learning, Plasticity and Pain, FL156/29), and the State of Baden-Württemberg Research Prize.

References

[1]   Albanese MC, Duerden EG, Rainville P, Duncan GH. Memory traces of pain in human cortex. J Neurosci 2007;27:4612–20.
[2]   Apkarian AV. Pain perception in relation to emotional learning. Curr Opin Neurobiol 2008;18:464–8.

[3] Avenanti A, Bueti D, Galati G, Aglioti SM. Transcranial magnetic stimulation highlights the sensorimotor side of empathy for pain. Nat Neurosci 2005;8:955–60.

[4] Baliki MN, Chialvo DR, Geha PY, Levy RM, Harden RN, Parrish TB, Apkarian AV. Chronic pain and the emotional brain: specific brain activity associated with spontaneous fluctuations of intensity of chronic back pain. J Neurosci 2006;26:12165–73.

[5] Baliki MN, Geha PY, Apkarian AV, Chialvo DR. Beyond feeling: chronic pain hurts the brain, disrupting the default-mode network dynamics. J Neurosci 2008;28:1398–1403.

[6] Becerra L, Morris S, Bazes S, Gostic R, Sherman S, Gostic J, Pendse G, Moulton E, Scrivani S, Keith D, et al. Trigeminal neuropathic pain alters responses in CNS circuits to mechanical (brush) and thermal (cold and heat) stimuli. J Neurosci 2006;26:10646–57.

[7] Becker S, Kleinböhl D, Klossika I, Hölzl R. Operant conditioning of enhanced pain sensitivity by heat-pain titration. Pain 2008;140:104–14.

[8] Birbaumer N, Lutzenberger W, Montoya P, Larbig W, Unertl K, Töpfner S, Grodd W, Taub E, Flor H. Effects of regional anesthesia on phantom limb pain are mirrored in changes in cortical reorganization. J Neurosci 1997;17:5503–8.

[9] Borsook D, Becerra L, Fishman S, Edwards A, Jennings CL, Stojanovic M, Papinicolas L, Ramachandran VS, Gonzalez RG, Breiter H. Acute plasticity in the human somatosensory cortex following amputation. Neuroreport 1998;9:1013–7.

[10] Chan BL, Witt R, Charrow AP, Magee A, Howard R, Pasquina PF, Heilman KM, Tsao JW. Mirror therapy for phantom limb pain. N Engl J Med 2007;357:2206–7.

[11] Chen R, Classen J, Gerloff C, Celnik P, Wassermann EM, Hallett M, Cohen LG. Depression of motor cortex excitability by low-frequency transcranial magnetic stimulation. Neurology 1997;48:13398–403.

[12] Chen R, Cohen LG, Hallett M. Nervous system reorganization following injury. Neuroscience 2002;111:761–73.

[13] Churchill JD, Tharp JA, Wellman CL, Sengelaub DR, Garraghty PE. Morphological correlates of injury-induced reorganization in primate somatosensory cortex. BMC Neurosci 2004;5:43.

[14] Craig K. Social modeling influences on pain. In: Sternbach RA, editor. The psychology of pain. New York: Raven Press; 1978. p. 73–110.

[15] deCharms RC, Maeda F, Glover GH, Ludlow D, Pauly JM, Soneji D, Gabrieli JD, Mackey SC. Control over brain activation and pain learned by using real-time functional MRI. Proc Natl Acad Sci USA 2005;102:18626–31.

[16] Diesch E, Flor H. Alteration in the response properties of primary somatosensory cortex related to differential aversive Pavlovian conditioning. Pain 2007;131:171–80.

[17] Draganski B, Moser T, Lummel N, Gänssbauer S, Bogdahn U, Haas F, May A. Decrease of thalamic gray matter following limb amputation. Neuroimage 2006;31:951–7.

[18] Eisenberg E, Chistyakov AV, Yudashkin M, Kaplan B, Hafner H, Feinsod M. Evidence for cortical hyperexcitability of the affected limb representation area in CRPS: a psychophysical and transcranial magnetic stimulation study. Pain 2005;113:99–105.

[19] Erskine A, Morley S, Pearce S. Memory for pain: a review. Pain 1990;41:255–65.

[20] Flor H. Maladaptive plasticity, memory for pain and phantom limb pain: review and suggestions for new therapies. Expert Rev Neurother 2008;8:809–18.

[21] Flor H, Braun C, Elbert T, Birbaumer N. Extensive reorganization of primary somatosensory cortex in chronic back pain patients. Neurosci Lett 1997;224:5–8.

[22] Flor H, Denke C, Schaefer M, Grüsser S. Effect of sensory discrimination training on cortical reorganisation and phantom limb pain. Lancet 2001;375:1763–4.

[23] Flor H, Elbert T, Knecht S, Wienbruch C, Pantev C, Birbaumer N, Larbig W, Taub E. Phantom limb pain as a perceptual correlate of massive cortical reorganization in upper extremity amputees. Nature 1995;357:482–4.

[24] Flor H, Knost B, Birbaumer N. The role of operant conditioning in chronic pain: an experimental investigation. Pain 2002;95:111–8.

[25] Flor H, Nikolajsen L, Jensen T. Phantom limb pain: a case of maladaptive CNS plasticity? Nat Rev Neurosci 2006;7:873–81.

[26] Fordyce WE. Behavioral methods for chronic pain and illness. St. Louis: Mosby; 1976.

[27] Fregni F, Freedman S, Pascual-Leone A. Recent advances in the treatment of chronic pain with non-invasive brain stimulation techniques. Lancet Neurol 2007;6:188–91.

[28] Giesecke T, Gracely RH, Grant MA, Nachemson A, Petzke F, Williams DA, Clauw DJ. Evidence of augmented central pain processing in idiopathic chronic low back pain. Arthritis Rheum 2004;50:613–23.

[29] Gracely RH, Geisser ME, Giesecke T, Grant MA, Petzke F, Williams DA, Clauw DJ. Pain catastrophizing and neural responses to pain among persons with fibromyalgia. Brain 2004;127:835–43.

[30] Gracely RH, Petzke F, Wolf JM, Clauw DJ. Functional magnetic resonance imaging evidence of augmented pain processing in fibromyalgia. Arthritis Rheum 2002;46:1333–43.

[31] Grachev ID, Fredrickson BE, Apkarian AV. Abnormal brain chemistry in chronic back pain: an in vivo proton magnetic resonance spectroscopy study. Pain 2000;89:7–18.

[32] Grachev ID, Thomas PS, Ramachandran TS. Decreased levels of N-acetyl aspartate in dorsolateral prefrontal cortex in a case of intractable severe sympathetically mediated chronic pain (complex regional pain syndrome, type I). Brain Cogn 2002;49:102–13.

[33] Hermann C, Hohmeister J, Demirakca S Zohsel K, Flor H. Long-term alteration of pain sensitivity in school-aged children with early pain experiences. Pain 2006;125:278–85.

[34] Hofmann SG, Pollack MH, Otto MW. Augmentation treatment of psychotherapy for anxiety disorders with D-cycloserine. CNS Drug Rev 2006;12:208–17.

[35] Hummel F, Cohen LG. Improvement of motor function with noninvasive cortical stimulation in a patient with chronic stroke. Neurorehabil Neural Repair 2005;19:14–9.

[36] Ji RR, Kohno T, Moore KA, Woolf CJ. Central sensitization and LTP: do pain and memory share similar mechanisms? Trends Neurosci 2003;26:696–705.

[37] Juottonen K, Gockel M, Silén T, Hurri R, Hari R, Forss N. Altered central sensorimotor processing in patients with complex regional pain syndrome. Pain 2002;98:315–23.

[38] Kaas JH, Florence SL. Mechanisms of reorganization in sensory systems of primates after peripheral nerve injury. Adv Neurol 1997;73:147–58.

[39] Karl A, Birbaumer N, Lutzenberger W, Cohen LG, Flor H. Reorganization of motor and somatosensory cortex in upper extremity amputees with phantom limb pain. J Neurosci 2001;21:3609–18.

[40] Karl A, Diers M, Flor H. P300-amplitudes in upper limb amputees with and without phantom limb pain in a visual oddball paradigm. Pain 2004;110:40–8.

[41] Kleinböhl D, Hölzl R, Möltner A, Rommel C, Weber C, Osswald PM. Psychophysical measures of sensitization to tonic heat discriminate chronic pain patients. Pain 1999;81:35–43.

[42] Kuchinad A, Schweinhardt P, Seminowicz DA, Wood PB, Chizh BA, Bushnell MC. Accelerated brain gray matter loss in fibromyalgia patients: premature aging of the brain? J Neurosci 2007;27:4004–7.

[43] Larbig W, Montoya P, Flor H, Bilow H, Weller S, Birbaumer N. Evidence for a change in neural processing in phantom limb pain patients. Pain 1996;67:275–83.

[44] Lefaucheur JP. Use of repetitive transcranial magnetic stimulation in pain relief. Expert Rev Neurother 2008;8:799–808.

[45] Liebetanz D, Nitsche MA, Tergau F, Paulus W. Pharmacological approach to the mechanisms of transcranial DC-stimulation-induced after-effects of human motor cortex excitability. Brain 2002;125:2238–47.

[46] Linton SJ, Melin L, Götestam KG. Behavioral analysis of chronic pain and its management. In: Hersen M, Eisler M, editors. Progress in behavior modification. New York: Academic Press; 1985. p. 1–42.

[47] Lotze M, Flor H, Grodd W, Larbig W, Birbaumer N. Phantom movements and pain. An fMRI study in upper limb amputees. Brain 2001;124:2268–77.

[48] Lotze M, Grodd W, Birbaumer N, Erb M, Huse E, Flor H. Does use of a myoelectric prosthesis prevent cortical reorganization and phantom limb pain? Nat Neurosci 1999;2:501–2.

[49] MacIver K, Lloyd DM, Kelly S, Roberts N, Nurmikko T. Phantom limb pain, cortical reorganization and the therapeutic effect of mental imagery. Brain 2008;131:2181–91.

[50] Maihöfner C, Handwerker HO, Neundorfer B, Birklein F. Patterns of cortical reorganization in complex regional pain syndrome. Neurology 2003;61:1707–15.

[51] Marsicano G, Wotjak CT, Azad SC, Bisogno T, Rammes G, Cascio MG, Hermann H, Tang J, Hofmann C, Zieglgänsberger W, et al. The endogenous cannabinoid system controls extinction of aversive memories. Nature 2002;418:530–4.

[52] McCabe CS, Haigh RC, Ring EF, Halligan PW, Wall PD, Blake DR. A controlled pilot study of the utility of mirror visual feedback in the treatment of complex regional pain syndrome (type 1). Rheumatology (Oxford) 2003;42:97–101.

[53] McDonald RJ, Devan BD, Hong NS. Multiple memory systems: the power of interactions. Neurobiol Learn Mem 2004;82:333–46.

[54] Miltner W, Larbig W, Braun C. Biofeedback of somatosensory event-related potentials: can individual pain sensations be modified by biofeedback-induced self-control of event-related potentials? Pain 1988;35:205–13.

[55] Moseley GL. Graded motor imagery is effective for long-standing complex regional pain syndrome: a randomised controlled trial. Pain 2004;108:192–8.

[56] Myers KM, Davis M. Mechanisms of fear extinction. Mol Psychiatry 2007;12:120–50.

[57] Nguyen JP, Lefaucher JP, Le Guerinel C, Eizenbaum JF, Nakano N, Carpentier A, Brugières P, Pollin B, Rostaing S, Keravel Y. Motor cortex stimulation in the treatment of central and neuropathic pain. Arch Med Res 2000;31:263–5.

[58] Nitsche MA, Schauenburg A, Lang N, Liebetanz D, Exner C, Paulus W, Tergau F. Facilitation of implicit motor learning by weak transcranial direct current stimulation of the primary motor cortex in the human. J Cogn Neurosci 2003;15:619–26.

[59] Paquette V, Lévesque J, Mensour B, Leroux JM, Beaudoin G, Bourgouin P, Beauregard M. "Change the mind and you change the brain": effects of cognitive-behavioral therapy on the neural correlates of spider phobia. Neuroimage 2003;18:401–9.

[60] Priori A. Brain polarization in humans: a reappraisal of an old tool for prolonged non-invasive modulation of brain excitability. Clin Neurophysiol 2003;114:589–95.

[61] Ressler KJ, Rothbaum BO, Tannenbaum L, Anderson P, Graap K, Zimand E, Hodges L, Davis M. Cognitive enhancers as adjuncts to psychotherapy: use of D-cycloserine in phobic individuals to facilitate extinction of fear. Arch Gen Psychiatry 2004;61:1136–44.

[62] Sandkühler J. Learning and memory in pain pathways. Pain 2000;88:113–8.

[63] Schley M, Topfner S, Wiech K, Schaller HE, Konrad CJ, Schmelz M, Birbaumer N. Continuous brachial plexus blockade in combination with the NMDA receptor antagonist memantine prevents phantom pain in acute traumatic upper limb amputees. Eur J Pain;11:299–308.

[64] Schneider C, Palomba D, Flor H. Pavlovian conditioning of muscular responses in chronic pain patients: central and peripheral correlates. Pain 2004;112:239–47.

[65] Schweinhardt P, Glynn C, Brooks J, McQuay H, Jack T, Chessell I, Bountra C, Tracey I. An fMRI study of cerebral processing of brush-evoked allodynia in neuropathic pain patients. Neuroimage 2006;32:256–65.

[66] Schwenkreis P, Janssen F, Rommel O, Pleger B, Völker B, Hosbach I, Dertwinkel R, Maier C, Tegenthoff M. Bilateral motor cortex disinhibition in complex regional pain syndrome (CRPS) type I of the hand. Neurology 2003;61:515–9.

[67] Singer T, Seymour B, O'Doherty J, Kaube H, Dolan RJ, Frith CD. Empathy for pain involves the affective but not sensory components of pain. Science 2004;303:1157–62.

[68] Staud R, Vierck CJ, Cannon RL, Mauderli AP, Price DD. Abnormal sensitization and temporal summation of second pain (wind-up) in patients with fibromyalgia syndrome. Pain 2001;91:165–75.

[69] Thieme K, Flor H, Turk DC. Psychological pain treatment in fibromyalgia syndrome: efficacy of operant behavioural and cognitive behavioural treatments. Arthritis Res Ther 2006;8:R121.

[70] Thieme K, Gromnica-Ihle E, Flor H. Operant behavioral treatment of fibromyalgia: a controlled study. Arthritis Rheum 2003;49:314–20.

[71] Tinazzi M, Valeriani M, Moretto G, Rosso T, Nicolato A, Fiaschi A, Agliot SM. Plastic interactions between hand and face cortical representations in patients with trigeminal neuralgia: a somatosensory-evoked potentials study. Neuroscience 2004;127:769–76.

[72] Turk DC, Okifuji A. Psychological factors in chronic pain: evolution and revolution. J Consult Clin Psychol 2002;70:678–90.

[73] Vlaeyen JW, Linton SJ. Fear-avoidance and its consequences in chronic musculoskeletal pain: a state of the art. Pain 2000;85:317–32.

[74] Waxman SG, Hains BC. Fire and phantoms after spinal cord injury: Na^+ channels and central pain. Trends Neurosci 2006;29:207–15.

[75] Willoch F, Rosen G, Tölle TR, Oye I, Wester HJ, Berner N, Schwaiger M, Bartenstein P. Phantom limb pain in the human brain: unraveling neural circuitries of phantom limb sensations using positron emission tomography. Ann Neurol 2000;48:842–9.

[76] Witting N, Kupers RC, Svensson P, Jensen TS. A PET activation study of brush-evoked allodynia in patients with nerve injury pain. Pain 2006;120:145–54.

[77] Wollgarten-Hadamek I, Hohmeister J, Demirakca S, Zohsel K, Flor H, Hermann C. Do burn injuries during infancy affect pain and sensory sensitivity in later childhood? Pain 2009;141:165–72.
[78] Ziemann U, Rothwell JC, Ridding MC. Interaction between intracortical inhibition and facilitation in human motor cortex. J Physiol 1996;496:873–81.

Correspondence to: Herta Flor, PhD, Department of Cognitive and Clinical Neuroscience, Central Institute of Mental Health, University of Heidelberg, J5, 68159 Mannheim, Germany. Tel: +49-621-1703-6302; fax: +49-621-1703-6305; email: herta.flor@zi-mannheim.de.

The Relationship between "Stress" and Pain: Lessons Learned from Fibromyalgia and Related Conditions

Daniel J. Clauw[a] and Jacob N. Ablin[b]

[a]Department of Anesthesiology and Medicine, The University of Michigan, Ann Arbor, Michigan, USA;
[b]Institute of Rheumatology, Tel Aviv Medical Center, Tel Aviv, Israel

The relationship between physical pain and emotional distress has been recognized for some time. In Genesis Chapter 3, when the pain of childbirth is inflicted upon the human race, the Bible states: "In sorrow thou shalt bring forth children," indicating an interchangeable relationship between pain and sorrow. Although pain and emotional distress are inextricably linked by scientists, clinicians, and lay persons, this relationship is much more complicated than simple cause and effect. In fact, some experts question the presupposed strong link between emotional stress and pain, and there are data suggesting that other biological stressors lead to pain more predictably than emotional stress. The object of this chapter is to present the current evidence-based understanding of the relationship between stress and pain, drawing from the rapidly evolving progress made in the field of fibromyalgia and related "central pain" syndromes.

Definitions

For the purpose of the current discussion, the term "stress" will be used as the collective physiological and emotional responses to any stimulus that disturbs an individual's homeostasis. The "stress response" refers to the fairly stereotypical physiological changes in the function of the autonomic nervous system and hypothalamic-pituitary-adrenal (HPA) axis associated with exposure to stressors. "Distress" is defined as psychological stress, typically operationalized as a combination of depression and anxiety. Finally, although the term "somatization" is not a term or construct that we agree with or espouse, in the current context we will use it to refer to the tendency of an individual to have multiple somatic symptoms, or to have pain or sensory amplification. Using these definitions should enable us to avoid ambiguity throughout the discussion.

Once these definitions have been clarified, we can address the basic questions regarding the relationship between stress and pain. Simply stated, these questions may be presented as the following: Does stress cause pain? Does pain cause stress? What are the mechanisms that underlie the relationship between stress and pain? Common wisdom is that distress leads to sympathetic nervous system (SNS) and HPA axis activation, which then leads to pain. But in conditions such as fibromyalgia, there is little experimental evidence for the notion that the symptoms are simply sympathetically mediated pain. Moreover, many other factors can contribute to the observed changes in autonomic and HPA function seen in individuals with chronic pain. It is becoming clear that a variety of stressors may lead to pain, that pain may lead to stress, and that there is not a simple unidirectional relationship between changes in stress response function and pain.

Neurobiological Findings in Fibromyalgia: The Prototypical "Central Pain" Syndrome

Fibromyalgia (FM) is a common systemic disorder estimated to affect 2% to 4% of the population, second in prevalence among rheumatological conditions only to osteoarthritis [117]. While some disagreement persists regarding its etiology and diagnosis, there is increasing evidence and acceptance that FM is the prototypical "central" or "non-nociceptive" pain condition [30,58]. This evidence does not mean that peripheral or nociceptive factors play no role in FM, but rather that functional abnormalities in central nervous system (CNS) processing of pain and other sensory stimuli play prominent roles in symptom expression. In fact, there has been a parallel recognition that common somatic syndromes such as irritable bowel syndrome (IBS), tension and migraine headache, temporomandibular joint disorder (TMJD), chronic fatigue syndrome (CFS), interstitial cystitis, and Gulf War Illnesses share overlapping symptom expression and underlying mechanisms [12,15,21].

Augmented Central Pain Processing in Fibromyalgia and Related Conditions

A rapid accumulation of data over the last two decades has brought about significant insight regarding the nature of augmented pain processing in FM. Summarizing the cardinal findings, the following statements can be made:

1) FM patients cannot detect electrical, pressure, or thermal stimuli at lower levels than normal individuals, but the point at which these stimuli cause pain or unpleasantness is lower [74,91]. FM patients also have a lower noxious threshold for many types of other sensory stimuli such as noise, which suggests that in some individuals these threshold changes may represent hyperactive processing of any or all sensory stimuli, and in others, only of pain [46].

2) These findings are noted even when stimuli are presented in a random, unpredictable fashion. These observations suggest that psychological factors such as hypervigilance play only a minor role in modulating tenderness [101]. This finding is arguably the most consistent finding in FM and other "central" pain syndromes of mechanical hyperalgesia and/or allodynia [51,75]. Although skeptics sometimes question the veracity of these findings because they rely on patient self-report of pain, multiple functional neuroimaging studies that are not reliant on self-report have now corroborated this finding of augmented central pain processing in this spectrum of illness [53,97].

3) There is substantial clinical and mechanistic overlap between FM and associated regional pain syndromes such as IBS, interstitial cystitis, TMJD, and headache. It is now clear that while individuals will occasionally have only one of these "idiopathic" (sometimes referred to as "stress-related") pain syndromes over the course of their lives, they and their family members are likely to suffer from several of these conditions [7,68]. Many terms have been used to describe these coaggregating syndromes

and symptoms, including functional somatic syndromes, somatization disorders, allied spectrum conditions, chronic multisymptom illnesses, or medically unexplained symptoms [11]. A number of common features of these syndromes include: (1) Women are 1.5 to 2 times more likely to have these disorders than men, but the sex difference is much more apparent in clinical samples (especially in tertiary care) than in population-based samples [1,40]. (2) Groups of individuals with conditions such as FM, IBS, headache, and TMJD display diffuse hyperalgesia and/or allodynia [77,94]. This finding suggests that these individuals have a fundamental problem with pain or sensory processing rather than an abnormality confined to the region of the body where the pain is currently being experienced. (3) Similar types of therapies are efficacious for all of these conditions, including both pharmacological treatments (e.g., tricyclic compounds such as amitriptyline) and nonpharmacological therapies (e.g., exercise or cognitive-behavioral therapy). Conversely, individuals with these conditions typically do not respond to therapies that are effective when pain is due to damage or inflammation of tissues (e.g., nonsteroidal anti-inflammatory drugs, opioids, injections, and surgical procedures).

The advent of research methods such as experimental pain testing, functional imaging, and modern genetics has led to substantial advances in understanding several of these conditions, most notably FM, IBS, and TMJD. New evidence has led to an emerging recognition that chronic pain itself is a "disease," and that many of the underlying mechanisms operative in these heretofore "idiopathic" or "functional" pain syndromes may be similar, no matter whether that pain is present throughout the body (e.g., in FM) or localized to the low back, the bowel, or the bladder. Hence, the more contemporary terms used to describe conditions such as FM, IBS, TMD, vulvodynia, and related entities include "central," "neuropathic," or "non-nociceptive" pain [22,120]. Furthermore, most experts feel that evidence of the neurobiological underpinnings of these conditions represents the death of the somatization construct, at least insofar as the label "somatization" implies a lack of a neurobiological basis for the symptoms.

The Genetic Basis of Pain Processing

Major advances have occurred concerning the genetics of pain. Just as we know that there is tremendous variability in nociceptive sensitivity among strains of rodents, there is great variability in pain sensitivity in humans [93]. Within the past few years alone, we have learned that genes such as those responsible for catechol-O-methyltransferase (COMT), GTP cyclohydrolase 1 (GCH1), and the voltage-gated sodium channel $Na_v1.9$ exert significant control in human pain perception [5,36,108]. Therefore, many in the pain field now believe that chronic pain is itself a disease, and the location of the body where it arises may not be as relevant as an individual's genetically determined pain sensitivity, combined with neuroplastic changes that can occur in the CNS that lead to augmented pain transmission.

Evidence exists for a strong familial component in the development of FM. First-degree relatives of individuals with FM display an eightfold greater risk of developing FM than those in the general population [7]. Family members of individuals with FM are more tender than the family members of controls, irrespective of the presence of pain, and they are also much more likely to have other disorders related to FM such as IBS, TMD, headaches, and other regional pain syndromes [19,71]. This familial and personal coaggregation of conditions was originally termed affective spectrum disorder [67], and more recently central sensitivity syndromes or chronic multisymptom illnesses [45,120].

Specific genetic polymorphisms that are associated with a higher risk of developing FM are starting to emerge. To date, the serotonin 5-HT_{2A} receptor polymorphism T/T phenotype, serotonin transporter, dopamine 4 receptor, and COMT polymorphisms are seen more frequently in individuals with FM [13,17,18,98].

The Role of Catecholamines in Pain Processing in Fibromyalgia and Other Pain States

The complex interrelationship between stress response function and pain processing is probably best understood by examining the data regarding the role of catecholamines in pain processing. For example, several research groups have been central in unraveling the role played by COMT, the enzyme that degrades catecholamines, in pain transmission. Zubieta demonstrated that the $val_{158}met$ polymorphism was responsible for differential pain sensitivity in humans, working in part by modulating opioidergic activity [122]. The same $val_{158}met$ polymorphisms are more weakly associated with psychiatric disorders [65]. Diatchenko and Maixner have carried out a series of elegant studies using haplotype analyses to identify three subsets of individuals based on the findings in four single nucleotide polymorphism (SNPs), termed low (LPS), average (APS), and high pain sensitivity (HPS) groups. These subgroups are highly predictive of pain sensitivity in a variety of different experimental pain tasks [35]. Moreover, in a prospective study in which 240 pain-free individuals were phenotyped at baseline and then followed for 3 years to determine who would develop TMJD, carriers of the HPS haplotype were 3 times as likely as others to reach this endpoint [37]. In animal models, the LPS haplotype produced much higher levels of COMT enzymatic activity when compared with the APS or HPS haplotypes, while COMT inhibition resulted in a profound increase in pain sensitivity. Finally, researchers have shown that when combined into haplotypes, these synonymously coding SNPs—which would previously have been considered "junk" SNPs—led to a different RNA structure with markedly different activity [95].

As might be expected in a complex system, COMT does not act in isolation. In addition to operating in part via opioidergic effects, Diatchenko and colleagues have shown that COMT also acts by mediating effects on β_2- and β_3-adrenergic receptors [96]. Their group showed that depressed COMT activity results in enhanced mechanical and thermal pain sensitivity in rats, and that this phenomenon was completely blocked by the nonselective β-adrenergic antagonist propranolol or by the combined administration of selective β_2- and β_3-adrenergic antagonists. On the other hand, administration of β_1-adrenergic, α-adrenergic, or dopaminergic receptor antagonists failed to alter COMT-dependent pain sensitivity. These data provide direct evidence that low COMT activity leads to increased pain sensitivity via a $\beta_{2/3}$-adrenergic mechanism.

The above-mentioned studies of COMT and β_2- and β_3-adrenergic effects suggest that catecholaminergic activity increases pain. In some clinical situations such as sympathetically mediated pain, catecholamine release in the periphery is also thought to cause or exacerbate pain. But despite these observations suggesting that hyperactivity of noradrenergic pathways might cause pain, there are even more data showing that norepinephrine exerts analgesic effects at several levels. Either electrical stimulation of supraspinal origins of noradrenergic descending fibers or direct application of norepinephrine to spinal neurons produces potent analgesia in laboratory animals [92,119]. These systems are also indirectly activated by stimulation of other brain sites involved in descending analgesia such as the periaqueductal gray, and they play a role in opioid-mediated descending pain inhibition [9,20].

Reduced Descending Analgesic Activity in Fibromyalgia and Related Conditions

Recent research point towards the presence of attenuated descending analgesic pathways, mediated by both norepinephrine and serotonin, in FM and related conditions. In healthy individuals and animals, application of an intensely painful stimulus to somatic tissues produces generalized whole-body analgesia. This analgesic effect, termed "diffuse noxious inhibitory control" (DNIC), has consistently been observed to be attenuated in groups of both FM and IBS patients compared to controls [73,115]. Attenuated DNIC is not found in all FM or IBS patients, but it is considerably more common in patients than controls. Although the DNIC response in humans is felt to be mediated in part by descending opioidergic pathways and in part by descending serotonergic-noradrenergic pathways, in FM there is accumulating evidence that the defect in DNIC is due to attenuated activity in the descending serotonergic-noradrenergic systems. In fact, recent evidence suggests that the endogenous opioidergic function in FM is augmented, as would be expected in a chronic pain state. Levels of enkephalins in the cerebrospinal fluid (CSF) are roughly twice as high in patients with FM or idiopathic low back pain as in healthy controls [10]. Moreover, positron emission tomography (PET) studies have recently shown that baseline μ-opioid receptor binding is decreased in multiple pain-processing regions in the brains of FM patients, consistent with the hypothesis that increased release of endogenous μ-opioid ligands in FM leads to increased occupancy of the receptors [60]. These biochemical and imaging findings suggesting increased activity of endogenous opioidergic systems in FM are consistent with anecdotal clinical evidence that opioids are generally ineffective analgesics in patients with FM and related conditions.

In contrast, similar studies have shown the opposite for serotonergic and noradrenergic activity in FM. Studies have shown that the principal metabolite of norepinephrine, 3-methoxy-4-hydroxyphenethylene, is lower in the CSF of FM patients [105]. Similarly, there are data suggesting low serotonin in this syndrome, as manifested by reduced levels of serotonin and its precursor, L-tryptophan, in the serum of FM patients, as well as by reduced CSF levels of the principal serotonin metabolite, 5-HIAA [121].

The data indicating that descending noradrenergic and serotonergic activity is attenuated in some patients with FM are corroborated by clinical trial data suggesting that nearly any compound that raises both of these neurotransmitters will be efficacious in this condition. Drugs that have been shown to be efficacious in FM include serotonin-norepinephrine reuptake inhibitors SNRIs such as duloxetine and milnacipran, tricyclics such as amitriptyline and cyclobenzaprine, and tramadol [48]. Both animal and human studies have suggested that norepinephrine might have stronger influences than serotonin in these descending analgesic pathways, because compounds that increase norepinephrine or both norepinephrine and serotonin are more efficacious analgesics than compounds that only increase serotonin, in both animals and humans [33,62].

Additional neurotransmitters that are involved in the human stress response also play a role in the augmentation of pain by the CNS in FM. Levels of substance P are consistently found to be elevated in the CSF of FM patients [14,104]. Moreover, nerve growth factor (NGF), brain-derived neurotrophic factor (BDNF), and glutamate have all been shown to be increased in the CSF of both FM patients and chronic migraine patients [106]. It thus appears that augmented pain processing in FM involves alterations in the delicate equilibrium between facilitatory neurotransmitters (substance P, glutamate, and NGF) and inhibitory neurotransmitters (norepinephrine, serotonin, γ-aminobutyric acid [GABA], and cannabinoids), which mediate supraspinal influences on pain and sensory processing at the spinal level. From a practical perspective, understanding this matrix has resulted in the identification and development of novel medications aimed at tipping the balance back in the desired direction. This balance can be achieved not only by increasing levels of serotonin and norepinephrine, but also by inhibiting the effects of mediators such as substance P and glutamate—which appears to be one of the modes of action of calcium channel $\alpha_2\delta$-subunit ligands, such as pregabalin and gabapentin.

These neurotransmitter imbalances may be responsible for global hypersensitivity to any sensory stimuli, not just pain. Individuals with FM also appear to have heightened sensitivity to other types of stimuli applied to the skin, which are judged as being more painful or noxious. In addition to pressure stimuli, individuals with FM also display a decreased threshold to heat [46,50,100], cold [72], and electrical stimuli [8]. Decreased sensory thresholds may not be limited to tactile mechanisms in FM. Gerster and colleagues were the first to demonstrate that individuals with FM also display a low noxious threshold to auditory tones, a finding that has subsequently been replicated [49,86]. A recent study by Geisser and colleagues used a random staircase paradigm to test both the auditory threshold and pressure threshold in FM [47]. This study found that individuals with FM display low thresholds to both types of stimuli, and the shared variance between the two thresholds was high enough to suggest a common underlying mechanism. The notion that FM might represent neurobiological amplification of all sensory stimuli has some support from functional imaging studies suggesting that the insula is the most consistently hyperactive neurocortical region of the pain matrix. This region plays a critical role in sensory integration, with the posterior insula serving a more purely sensory role, and the anterior insula being associated with the emotional processing of sensations [28,29,109].

Functional Neuroimaging Insights into the Relationship between Distress and Pain

More than four decades ago the theoretical concept of a "pain matrix" was set down, hypothesizing the existence of three domains of pain processing in the CNS [90]. These included a sensory dimension, dealing with the localization and severity of pain and involving the primary and secondary somatosensory cortices, thalamus, and posterior insula; an affective dimension, dealing with the emotional valence of pain (and ascribed to the anterior cingulate cortex, amygdalae, and anterior insula); and a cognitive dimension, involving the prefrontal cortex (as well as the affective areas). Although we now know that there are no brain regions that are only involved in pain processing, and that many brain regions other than those classically thought to be in the pain matrix are activated during painful stimuli, this demarcation between sensory and affective processing (sometimes referred to as lateral versus medial brain regions) can be useful in dissecting the role of affect in pain processing.

Over recent years imaging studies, and especially functional magnetic resonance imaging (fMRI), have been particularly useful in advancing our understanding of central pain augmentation in FM. These studies have added to a significant extent to the validity of the pain matrix concept. Experiments using fMRI have demonstrated that FM patients exhibit greater activity than controls over multiple brain regions including the prefrontal, supplemental motor, insular, and anterior cingulate cortex in response to both nonpainful and painful stimuli [26]. In an experimental design first performed by Gracely et al. [57], FM patients were exposed to painful pressures during fMRI. When stimuli of equal pressure were administered, increased neural activations (i.e., increases in the blood-oxygenation-level-dependent signal) was observed in patients compared to pain-free controls. Regions of increased activity included the primary and secondary somatosensory cortex, insula, and anterior cingulate cortex. When the pain-free controls were subjected to pressures that evoked equivalent pain ratings, similar activation patterns were observed. These findings are consistent with the "leftward shift" in stimulus-response function noted with experimental pain testing; they suggest that FM patients experience an increased gain or "volume setting" in the brain's sensory processing systems. Similar results have been reported in both FM and chronic low back pain patients [52], and also in conditions such as IBS.

Functional MRI has also proven useful in determining how comorbid psychological factors influence pain processing in FM. In a study on the relationship between depression and enhanced evoked pain sensations [53], neither the level of symptoms of depression nor the presence of comorbid major depression was associated with the results of sensory testing, or with the magnitude of neuronal activation in brain areas involved in the sensory dimension of pain (primary and secondary somatosensory cortices). Clinical depression was, however, associated with the magnitude of pain-evoked neuronal activations in brain regions involved in affective pain processing (the amygdalae and contralateral anterior insula). Clinical pain intensity was associated with measures of both the sensory and the affective dimensions of pain. This intriguing study suggests the presence of parallel, independent neural pain-processing networks for sensory and affective pain elements, in accordance with the pain matrix paradigm.

Functional brain imaging has also made it possible to assess the effect of cognitive factors such as catastrophizing on the processing of pain [56], demonstrating that catastrophizing is significantly associated with increased activity in brain areas related to pain anticipation (medial frontal cortex and cerebellum), attention to pain (dorsal anterior cingulate gyrus and dorsolateral prefrontal cortex), emotional aspects of pain (the claustrum, closely connected to the amygdala), and motor control. Additional research may shed light on the role of other cognitive characteristics, such as an internal versus external locus of control, on pain processing.

Proton magnetic resonance spectroscopy, a novel imaging modality, is a noninvasive procedure used to determine the relative concentration of specific brain metabolites in vivo. With this technique it has been possible to demonstrate high glutamate levels in the insula in FM patients, as well as dynamic changes in posterior insula glutamate levels associated with improvements in clinical pain [61]. These studies show that changes in glutamate in the posterior insula are more closely related to changes in the sensory dimension of clinical pain, whereas changes in glutamate in the anterior insula are more closely related to changes in anxiety, consistent with the differential functions of the insula first suggested by Craig [27].

Taken together, imaging studies of pain processing in FM imply that distress (i.e., depression, anxiety) and pain are independently processed in the CNS. This conclusion is supported by clinical data that suggest that drugs that act as antidepressants and analgesics, such as tricyclics or SNRIs, are equally effective analgesics in FM or other pain patients with and without depression [6,44]. While these dimensions obviously interact within the matrix of pain, it is a conceptual oversimplification to consider pain as a one-to-one consequence of distress.

Does "Stress" Lead to Pain and Other Symptoms in Fibromyalgia and Related Conditions?

Despite the clear evidence of strong familial aggregation and of strong genetic underpinnings in FM, it is also clear that a host of external triggers are capable of triggering the syndrome, presumably in the genetically predisposed host. Thus, catastrophic events such as war or terrorism, and particularly manmade disasters, are well known to initiate a broad spectrum of symptoms overlapping with those of FM [23]. Motor vehicle accidents are associated with the development of FM [87], and recently a study found that even early childhood hospitalization following such an event is associated with an increased adult risk of developing widespread pain [69]. Both peripheral pain syndromes and systemic disorders, such as rheumatoid arthritis, osteoarthritis, and systemic lupus erythematosus, which lead to regional or multifocal pain, have the well-documented capacity to act as triggers for the subsequent development of widespread pain and FM [24]. Finally, there are ample data implicating a variety of infections, both viral and bacterial, as well as antimicrobial vaccinations, in the triggering of FM and related conditions [2]. Epstein-Barr virus, *Borrelia burgdorferi* (Lyme disease), *Brucella* (brucellosis), Ross River virus, *Coxiella burnetii* (Q fever), hepatitis C virus, and human immunodeficiency virus (HIV) are among the pathogens implicated.

Specific studies have been published that help us to better understand the broader mechanisms that may underlie links between stress and pain. Thus, the role of two specific types of stressors—psychological stress and infection/vaccination—are reviewed below in detail.

The Role of Psychological Distress in Triggering Fibromyalgia and Related Conditions

The role of psychological distress in triggering FM and related illnesses has been accepted almost as a dogma for some time, based on the observation of high levels of distress among these patients, the abnormalities observed in the stress response systems among these patients, and the general feeling of "stress" experienced by clinicians caring for these patients. Although this narrative seems appealing, it is simply inaccurate: the data linking psychological distress to these illnesses is somewhat tenuous, and certainly more complex than initially imagined.

For example, it is now clear that the higher rates of distress seen in many case-control studies may in fact be due to these studies having been performed in tertiary care settings, or among individuals with high health-care-seeking behaviors. Studies have clearly demonstrated that individuals with FM or IBS who are seen in tertiary care settings have significantly more psychological comorbidity than those seen in primary care settings or enrolled in population-based studies [41]. Similarly, women with either IBS or FM seen in clinical samples are much more likely to report childhood sexual or physical abuse than controls or those who met criteria for these conditions but have never been diagnosed or sought health care [42,43]. An additional inherent limitation regarding the evaluation of the link between these conditions and previous trauma relates to the reliance on self-reported recall of distant events.

These biases can be reduced or eliminated by performing studies of individuals in the general population, rather than those seeking care. A number of U.K. groups have performed population-based studies examining the psychological predictors of chronic regional or widespread pain. These studies are important because they examine the temporal and longitudinal relationship between distress and pain (which can help identify cause and effect) rather than the cross-sectional relationship (which could be identifying distress that is due to pain rather than causing pain). These studies have consistently shown that individuals with high baseline levels of psychological distress are only somewhat more likely to subsequently develop chronic regional or widespread pain (odds ratio [OR] = 1.5–2) [32,83,84,99]. Many more individuals without baseline distress develop regional or widespread pain than those with baseline distress. In contrast to a modest relationship between baseline psychological distress and subsequent pain, these studies found stronger relationships between baseline "somatization" (the number and severity of somatic symptoms) and the subsequent development of pain (OR = 3–9). Thus, the tendency to have pain or sensory amplification at baseline is a potent predictor of subsequent pain, more so than psychological factors per se.

A number of other relationships between pain and stress have been identified in these population-based studies. For example, having baseline chronic pain is a stronger factor predicting future psychological distress (OR = 3–5) than vice versa, suggesting that some of the observed clinical relationship between stress and pain is "effect" rather than cause. Again, this association seems to be mediated by the tendency to "somatize." Using similar population-derived cohorts, these groups showed that individuals born in 1958 whose medical records indicated that they were involved in a motor traffic accident, or were institutionalized, were 1.5 to 2 times more likely to have chronic widespread pain 42 years later. This is the first study that we are aware of that shows that early life trauma is in fact a risk for developing pain, even after the investigators control for psychological factors (and eliminate the potential effect for recall bias). Finally, studies by these groups have also shown that baseline function of the stress response (in this case the HPA axis) is a predictor of chronic widespread pain, independently of distress and other psychological factors [85].

An additional opportunity for investigating the effect of distress on pain arose in the wake of the catastrophic terrorist attacks of 9/11. Based on the assumption that distress is a major trigger of pain, one would have expected a major increase in the levels of pain among both FM patients and others exposed to these highly stressful events. However, studies performed immediately before and after the attacks failed to note any increase in pain or related symptoms. Thus, no increase was noted in somatic symptoms among individuals in the general population living in New York City [103], and no increase in pain or fatigue levels was found in FM patients followed from prior to the attacks to 1 month afterward in Washington, D.C. [116]. This type of acute psychological stress might not have led to the same consequences as other types of acute emotional stressors, such as daily interpersonal hassles, which do tend to increase pain and other somatic symptoms in some settings [4].

The Role of Infectious Triggers in Fibromyalgia and Related Conditions

The symptoms of FM appear to overlap considerably with those of a viral or atypical infection. Widespread myalgia, as well as fatigue, both hallmarks of FM, are symptoms of many infections, ranging from the common cold to HIV. Hence, from the inception of the FM concept, considerable effort has been directed toward identifying infectious causes. While multiple reports associated FM or CFS with chronic infection due to viral agents such as Epstein-Barr virus, attempts to demonstrate clear serological evidence of increased rates of infection in these patients have generally met with mixed results [16]. Even in chronic fatigue patients, whose clinical manifestations are arguably most reminiscent of Epstein-Barr virus infection, it is clear that this syndrome does not represent a chronic infection with this virus [114]. Lyme disease causes diffuse arthralgia, cognitive difficulties such as impaired concentration and memory, and fatigue. Serological testing for Lyme disease is complex and not conclusive in all cases, so it is not surprising that patients suffering from FM have frequently been diagnosed as cases of "chronic Lyme disease." In rigorously conducted studies, however, patients given this designation have failed to respond to antibiotic treatment directed against *Borrelia burgdorferi*, the pathogen causing Lyme disease. On the other hand, it has been demonstrated that about 8% of patients suffering from Lyme disease will go on to develop FM within 1–3 years [38].

The connection between Lyme disease and FM can be viewed as a test case for uncovering the relationship between FM and infection. Unlike many other infectious agents that have been tied to FM, effective antimicrobial treatment against Lyme disease is available. The lack of improvement of FM symptoms in patients treated with adequate antibiotic regimes for Lyme disease tends to imply that infection serves as trigger for a chain of events which, once initiated, runs its course without the necessity of ongoing infection.

Arguably the best set of studies examining the underlying mechanisms that are operative in infections triggering this spectrum of illness have analyzed the long-term consequences of infection with three different pathogens: the Ross River virus (the cause of epidemic polyarthritis), *Coxiella burnetii* (the cause of Q fever), and Epstein-Barr virus and the development of CFS [64]. In this prospective epidemiological study, patients suffering from acute infection with these disparate pathogens were recruited, followed for 12 months, and monitored for the development of fatigue, muscular pain, cognitive dysfunction, and mood disturbances.

The symptom complex developed in 12% of the patients at 12 months. Even though these infections cause markedly different acute presentations, a very stereotypical chronic syndrome (characterized by pain, fatigue, and memory difficulties) occurred at a remarkably similar rate after each infection. Demographic, psychological, or microbiological factors during the acute infection did not predict the development of this symptom complex [64,110]. None of the psychiatric measurements assessed in this study, which included the presence of a premorbid or intercurrent psychiatric disorder, the neuroticism score, and the locus of control score, were significantly predictive of the development of chronic symptoms. As with the studies of emotional stress triggering pain in the population, although distress per se did not predict chronicity of symptoms after infection, the presence and severity of somatic symptoms (i.e., the degree of "somatization") during the acute infection was closely correlated with the subsequent development of chronic fatigue (and pain).

Strikingly, the relationship between acute infection and the development of chronic regional pain and other somatic symptoms has been noted in a number of other conditions related to FM. For example, in a meta-analysis summarizing the results of eight different studies, Halvorson et al. noted that approximately 10% of individuals will develop postinfectious IBS following an episode of acute infectious gastroenteritis caused by nearly any viral or bacterial pathogen [59]. Similarly, an episode of acute urinary tract infection is evident in a proportion of women who develop interstitial cystitis/painful bladder syndrome [111].

Taken together, these results imply that various forms of acute infection are capable of triggering widespread or regional pain (in the area of the body initially affected by pan), as well as accompanying somatic symptoms such as fatigue, memory, and mood difficulties. The risk of this symptom complex occurring with different infections is consistently seen to be approximately 10%.

The reason for this consistency is not clear. There are probably strong genetic factors that predispose to this vulnerability. Evidently the inciting infection must be of sufficient severity and duration, because the increase in occurrence of chronic symptoms is not observed following common viral infections of short duration [113]. This lack of specificity regarding the trigger effect of infection might well be associated with an underlying genetic predisposition activated in a similar manner by various pathogens, and/or with a set of "maladaptive" behavioral responses that could lead to symptoms (e.g., cessation of routine exercise or sleep).

Another related trigger that might be associated with the development of FM and related symptoms has been the administration of a variety of vaccines. Rubella vaccination has been recognized as responsible for causing a spectrum of musculoskeletal symptoms ranging from FM to frank arthritis [112]. Gulf war illness, a clinical constellation characterized by chronic fatigue, general malaise, irritability, and cognitive impairment as well as musculoskeletal symptoms, clearly overlaps with FM and CFS.

Since troops deployed to the Persian Gulf during this conflict received multiple (and often simultaneous) vaccinations, the possibility of a causal relationship between these vaccinations and the development of Gulf War illness has been extensively explored. It has been demonstrated that administration of vaccines during deployment in the Gulf was associated with fatigue, psychological distress, health perception, physical functioning, and the presence of a multisymptom illness [66]. Intriguingly, the administration of these vaccines *before* deployment led to a very different outcome, characterized by the absence of the above-mentioned symptoms and an increased incidence of post-traumatic stress reactions. It thus appears that the effect of multiple vaccinations was pathogenic when combined with various other environmental triggers that acted on individuals during deployment, possibly including the distress related to deployment and the anticipation of combat.

Abnormalities in Stress Response Function in Fibromyalgia and Related Conditions Suggest that Pain Also Causes "Stress"

Many studies have identified abnormalities in the HPA axis and the sympathetic nervous system in FM and related conditions, and more broadly in chronic pain [3,31,34,102]. But although abnormalities are typically identified between mean values in groups of patients and groups of controls, there is never "abnormal" function of stress systems in patients, and there is always tremendous overlap between individuals within the patient and control groups. Even the direction of the abnormality identified is inconsistent, with some showing hypoactivity and others hyperactivity of both the HPA axis and sympathetic nervous system.

It is likely that these inconsistencies are due to several factors. First, subtle differences in psychiatric comorbidities in the patient groups may be partly responsible. For example, increasingly, early life stressors are being shown to profoundly and permanently change the function of the HPA axis, and the age at which the stress occurs may partially determine both the magnitude and direction of the perturbation [63]. In addition to early-life stress, both comorbid depression and post-traumatic stress disorder are known to markedly influence HPA axis and autonomic function.

Finally, as previously noted, pain may cause stress, and can activate the HPA axis and the autonomic nervous system.

Recent studies in FM have tended to support the notion that these comorbidities may be more potent drivers of stress response function than whether the individual has FM. For example, in two recent studies examining HPA function in FM, McLean showed that salivary cortisol levels covaried with pain levels, and that CSF levels of corticotropin-releasing hormone were more closely related to an individual's pain level or an early life history of trauma than to their status as an individual with FM or a healthy control [88]. Most previous studies of HPA and autonomic function in FM failed to control for pain levels, a previous history of trauma and post-traumatic stress, and other comorbid disorders that could affect HPA or autonomic dysfunction.

Are Fibromyalgia and Related Conditions Simply Sympathetically Mediated Pain?

Based on a number of similarities between FM and complex regional pain syndrome (CRPS, formerly known as reflex sympathetic dystrophy)—the presence of chronic pain and allodynia, onset after physical trauma, female predominance, paresthesias, vasomotor instability, and comorbid anxiety/depression—some investigators have claimed that FM is a sympathetically maintained generalized pain syndrome, i.e., a generalized form of CRPS [78]. As evidence for this relationship, proponents have cited experiments in which injection of norepinephrine caused an increased pain response among FM patients compared with healthy controls or patients suffering from rheumatoid arthritis [81]; in addition, the abnormal results obtained in heart rate variability (HRV) studies among FM patients [25,80,107] have been cited as evidence for the sympathetically mediated nature of this syndrome [79].

The link between changes in HRV and the pathophysiology of FM and related conditions needs to be critically examined. First, the studies regarding HRV in FM have in fact demonstrated considerable overlap between patients and healthy controls in many parameters, and they have been far from conclusive. In addition, a fundamental caveat relating to the interpretation of HRV changes in FM relates to the issue of deconditioning. Prolonged reduction in physical activity leads to deconditioning, which is a physiological response characterized by predictable changes, including a reduction in cardiac volume (cardiac atrophy), a reduction in plasma volume, and a marked tachycardic response to standing or upright tilting [39,76].

As recently described by Joyner et al. [70], the autonomic effects observed in conditions such as postural orthostatic tachycardia syndrome, CFS, and FM, i.e., the sustained increase in heart rate of more than 30 beats per minute with 10 minutes of upright tilting, are in fact similar to the physiological responses seen in "normal" humans after prolonged periods of bedrest, deconditioning, or space flight. These findings cast doubt on the assumption that it is an intrinsic sympathetic dysfunction that triggers both the cardiovascular manifestations associated with FM and the widespread pain that is the defining characteristic of this condition.

If deconditioning per se is sufficient in order to cause an autonomic response comparable to postural orthostatic tachycardia syndrome, it is conceivable that lack of activity (for any reason) may act as an important factor leading to the development of other characteristic features of the chronic multisymptom illness. This concept has been tested in a study in which asymptomatic, regularly exercising, healthy adults were exposed to exercise restriction for 1 week [55]. A subset of these individuals reported an increase in one or more symptoms including pain, fatigue, and mood changes. These symptomatic subjects had lower HPA axis function (baseline cortisol prior to VO_2max testing), immune function (natural killer cell responsiveness to venipuncture), and autonomic function (measured by HRV) at baseline, prior to cessation of exercise, when compared to the subjects who did not develop symptoms. In a subsequent study, among healthy individuals with regular exercise and sleep habits, disruption of the normal routine was associated with increased pain, fatigue, negative mood, and cognitive abnormalities, with sleep restriction producing more widespread and severe symptoms than exercise deprivation [54].

A different approach has been used to identify another link between baseline stress response function and the development of pain. McBeth and colleagues assessed HPA function in a large group of pain-free individuals, and found that baseline HPA function affected the likelihood of subsequently developing chronic widespread pain [82]. They measured HPA function, as expressed by both salivary cortisol and the serum cortisol reaction to stress. A comparison was made of three groups, including individuals suffering from widespread pain, controls, and a third group of individuals considered to be at risk for developing widespread pain on the basis of the presence of strong evidence of somatization. Both in the individuals with chronic pain and in those "at risk," alterations in HPA function were observed, implying that HPA axis dysfunction may precede the development of chronic pain.

Again, it is necessary to examine the "opposite" relationship between pain and stress—the possibility that pain in an activator of the stress response. In FM, levels of cortisol secretion as well as CSF levels of CRF are correlated with momentary pain levels [88,89]. Notably, in these studies the level of cortisol was not correlated with other factors such as depression, or with self-reported history of physical or sexual abuse. As pointed out in that study, there could be three possible explanations for the association between CSF levels of CRF and pain symptoms in FM patients: CRF may be altered as a consequence of chronic stress caused by pain, CRF may be involved in the generation of pain symptoms, and/or CRF may be a "third variable" that is altered because of dysfunction of other central processes directly involved in the generation of FM pain. Taken together, these results tend to support the hypothesis that HPA axis hyperactivity is at least somewhat driven by pain in FM, and that pain may be activating the autonomic nervous system and HPA axis rather than vice versa.

Summary

In conclusion, FM, the prototype of chronic central pain, is determined to a similar extent by genetic and environmental factors. Although environmental stress is a risk factor for the development of chronic pain, psychological stress is only modestly associated with triggering or exacerbating this condition. In contrast, other types of stressors such as infections, physical trauma, and war may play a larger role in causing or exacerbating these conditions than previously suspected. Similarly, although some have purported that the subtle abnormalities in the function of the autonomic and HPA systems seen in individuals with FM and other chronic pain syndromes are causing the pain, there are now data suggesting much more complex interrelationships between these systems. In some individuals with chronic pain, observable changes in autonomic or HPA tone may represent a baseline diathesis or risk factor for the subsequent development of subsequent chronic pain, or they may be due to pain or to indirect effects of pain such as deconditioning. Further progress in the genetics of pain is likely to help identify carriers of this diathesis, as well as elucidating its mechanisms. Distress (i.e., depression, anxiety) and pain are processed somewhat independently in the brain, and clinical trials of drugs that are both antidepressants and analgesics show that treating distress does not necessarily improve pain. The dramatic advance made in understanding the pathogenesis of FM has helped shed light on the biology of pain in general and on the intricate interaction between pain and stress.

Viewed together, the results described above raise the possibility that inherent vulnerability for the development of FM and related disorders is present in a certain proportion of the general population. The most evident biological abnormality in these individuals may be augmented central processing of pain or sensory amplification, manifested as multiple somatic symptoms. These individuals may be particularly susceptible to disruption of routine exercise or sleep with respect to symptoms becoming more pronounced. When confronted with an appropriate external trigger, such as an acute infection, physical trauma, or a catastrophic event, and particularly when induced to react to these insults by a pattern of reduced activity and impaired function, these individuals may start to develop the complex of symptoms culminating in chronic pain and dysfunction.

References

[1] Aaron LA, Bradley LA, Alarcon GS, Alexander RW, Triana-Alexander M, Martin MY, Alberts KR. Psychiatric diagnoses in patients with fibromyalgia are related to health care-seeking behavior rather than to illness. Arthritis Rheum 1996;39:436–45.

[2] Ablin JN, Shoenfeld Y, Buskila D. Fibromyalgia, infection and vaccination: two more parts in the etiological puzzle. J Autoimmun 2006;27:145–52.

[3] Adler GK, Kinsley BT, Hurwitz S, Mossey CJ, Goldenberg DL. Reduced hypothalamic-pituitary and sympathoadrenal responses to hypoglycemia in women with fibromyalgia syndrome. Am J Med 1999;106:534–43.

[4] Affleck G, Urrows S, Tennen H, Higgins P, Abeles M. Sequential daily relations of sleep, pain intensity, and attention to pain among women with fibromyalgia. Pain 1996;68:363–8.

[5] Amaya F, Wang H, Costigan M, Allchorne AJ, Hatcher JP, Egerton J, Stean T, Morisset V, Grose D, Gunthorpe MJ, et al. The voltage-gated sodium channel $Na_v1.9$ is an effector of peripheral inflammatory pain hypersensitivity. J Neurosci 2006;26:12852–60.

[6] Arnold LM. Duloxetine and other antidepressants in the treatment of patients with fibromyalgia. Pain Med 2007;8(Suppl 2):S63–S74.

[7] Arnold LM, Hudson JI, Hess EV, Ware AE, Fritz DA, Auchenbach MB, Starck LO, Keck PE Jr. Family study of fibromyalgia. Arthritis Rheum 2004;50:944–52.

[8]   Arroyo JF, Cohen ML. Abnormal responses to electrocutaneous stimulation in fibromyalgia. J Rheumatol 1993;20:1925–31.
[9]   Bajic D, Proudfit HK, Van Bockstaele EJ. Periaqueductal gray neurons monosynaptically innervate extranuclear noradrenergic dendrites in the rat pericoerulear region. J Comp Neurol 2000;427:649–62.
[10]   Baraniuk JN, Whalen G, Cunningham J, Clauw DJ. Cerebrospinal fluid levels of opioid peptides in fibromyalgia and chronic low back pain. BMC Musculoskelet Disord 2004;5:48.
[11]   Barsky AJ, Borus JF. Functional somatic syndromes. Ann Intern Med 1999; 130:910–921.
[12]   Bendtsen L. Central sensitization in tension-type headache: possible pathophysiological mechanisms. Cephalalgia 2000;20:486–508.
[13]   Bondy B, Spaeth M, Offenbaecher M, Glatzeder K, Stratz T, Schwarz M, de Jonge S, Krüger M, Engel RR, Färber L, et al. The T102C polymorphism of the 5-HT2A-receptor gene in fibromyalgia. Neurobiol Dis 1999;6:433–9.
[14]   Bradley LA, Alarcon GS. Is Chiari malformation associated with increased levels of substance P and clinical symptoms in persons with fibromyalgia? Arthritis Rheum 1999;42:2731–2.
[15]   Bragdon EE, Light KC, Costello NL, Sigurdsson A, Bunting S, Bhalang K, Maixner W. Group differences in pain modulation: pain-free women compared to pain-free men and to women with TMD. Pain 2002;96:227–37.
[16]   Buchwald D, Goldenberg DL, Sullivan JL, Komaroff AL. The "chronic, active Epstein-Barr virus infection" syndrome and primary fibromyalgia. Arthritis Rheum 1987;30:1132–6.
[17]   Buskila D. Genetics of chronic pain states. Best Pract Res Clin Rheumatol 2007;21:535–47.
[18]   Buskila D, Cohen H, Neumann L, Ebstein RP. An association between fibromyalgia and the dopamine D4 receptor exon III repeat polymorphism and relationship to novelty seeking personality traits. Mol Psychiatry 2004;9:730–1.
[19]   Buskila D, Neumann L, Hazanov I, Carmi R. Familial aggregation in the fibromyalgia syndrome. Semin Arthritis Rheum 1996;26:605–11.
[20]   Chang PF, Arendt-Nielsen L, Chen AC. Dynamic changes and spatial correlation of EEG activities during cold pressor test in man. Brain Res Bull 2002;57:667–75.
[21]   Chang PF, Arendt-Nielsen L, Graven-Nielsen T, Chen AC. Psychophysical and EEG responses to repeated experimental muscle pain in humans: pain intensity encodes EEG activity. Brain Res Bull 2003;59:533–43.
[22]   Clauw DJ. Fibromyalgia: update on mechanisms and management. J Clin Rheumatol 2007;13:102–9.
[23]   Clauw DJ, Engel CC Jr, Aronowitz R, Jones E, Kipen HM, Kroenke K, Ratzan S, Sharpe M, Wessely S. Unexplained symptoms after terrorism and war: an expert consensus statement. J Occup Environ Med 2003;45:1040–8.
[24]   Clauw DJ, Katz P. The overlap between fibromyalgia and inflammatory rheumatic diseases: when and why does it occur? J Clin Rheumatol 1995;1:335–41.
[25]   Cohen H, Neumann L, Shore M, Amir M, Cassuto Y, Buskila D. Autonomic dysfunction in patients with fibromyalgia: application of power spectral analysis of heart rate variability. Semin Arthritis Rheum 2000;29:217–27.
[26]   Cook DB, Lange G, Ciccone DS, Liu WC, Steffener J, Natelson BH. Functional imaging of pain in patients with primary fibromyalgia. J Rheumatol 2004;31:364–78.
[27]   Craig AD. How do you feel? Interoception: the sense of the physiological condition of the body. Nat Rev Neurosci 2002;3:655–66.
[28]   Craig AD. A new view of pain as a homeostatic emotion. Trends Neurosci 2003;26:303–7.
[29]   Craig AD. Human feelings: why are some more aware than others? Trends Cogn Sci 2004;8:239–41.
[30]   Crofford LJ, Clauw DJ. Fibromyalgia: where are we a decade after the American College of Rheumatology classification criteria were developed? Arthritis Rheum 2002;46:1136–8.
[31]   Crofford LJ, Pillemer SR, Kalogeras KT, Cash JM, Michelson D, Kling MA, Sternberg EM, Gold PW, Chrousos GP, Wilder RL. Hypothalamic-pituitary-adrenal axis perturbations in patients with fibromyalgia. Arthritis Rheum 1994;37:1583–92.
[32]   Croft P, Burt J, Schollum J, Thomas E, Macfarlane G, Silman A. More pain, more tender points: is fibromyalgia just one end of a continuous spectrum? Ann Rheum Dis 1996;55:482–5.
[33]   D'Mello R, Dickenson AH. Spinal cord mechanisms of pain. Br J Anaesth 2008;101:8–16.
[34]   Demitrack MA, Crofford LJ. Evidence for and pathophysiologic implications of hypothalamic-pituitary-adrenal axis dysregulation in fibromyalgia and chronic fatigue syndrome. Ann NY Acad Sci 1998;840:684–97.

[35] Diatchenko L, Nackley AG, Slade GD, Bhalang K, Belfer I, Max MB, Goldman D, Maixner W. Catechol-O-methyltransferase gene polymorphisms are associated with multiple pain-evoking stimuli. Pain 2006;125:216–24.

[36] Diatchenko L, Nackley AG, Tchivileva IE, Shabalina SA, Maixner W. Genetic architecture of human pain perception. Trends Genet 2007;23:605–13.

[37] Diatchenko L, Slade GD, Nackley AG, Bhalang K, Sigurdsson A, Belfer I, Goldman D, Xu K, Shabalina SA, Shagin D, et al. Genetic basis for individual variations in pain perception and the development of a chronic pain condition. Hum Mol Genet 2005;14:135–43.

[38] Dinerman H, Steere AC. Lyme disease associated with fibromyalgia. Ann Intern Med 1992;117:281–5.

[39] Dorfman TA, Levine BD, Tillery T, Peshock RM, Hastings JL, Schneider SM, Macias BR, Biolo G, Hargens AR. Cardiac atrophy in women following bed rest. J Appl Physiol 2007;103:8–16.

[40] Drossman DA, Li Z, Andruzzi E, Temple RD, Talley NJ, Thompson WG, Whitehead WE, Janssens J, Funch-Jensen P, Corazziari E, et al. U.S. householder survey of functional gastrointestinal disorders. Prevalence, sociodemography, and health impact. Dig Dis Sci 1993;38:1569–80.

[41] Drossman DA, McKee DC, Sandler RS, Mitchell CM, Cramer EM, Lowman BC, Burger AL. Psychosocial factors in the irritable bowel syndrome. A multivariate study of patients and non-patients with irritable bowel syndrome. Gastroenterology 1988;95:701–8.

[42] Drossman DA, Talley NJ, Leserman J, Olden KW, Barreiro MA. Sexual and physical abuse and gastrointestinal illness. Review and recommendations. Ann Intern Med 1995;123:782–94.

[43] Finestone HM, Stenn P, Davies F, Stalker C, Fry R, Koumanis J. Chronic pain and health care utilization in women with a history of childhood sexual abuse. Child Abuse Negl 2000;24:547–56.

[44] Fishbain D. Evidence-based data on pain relief with antidepressants. Ann Med 2000;32:305–16.

[45] Fukuda K, Nisenbaum R, Stewart G, Thompson WW, Robin L, Washko RM, Noah DL, Barrett DH, Randall B, Herwaldt BL, Mawle AC, Reeves WC. Chronic multisymptom illness affecting Air Force veterans of the Gulf War. JAMA 1998;280:981–8.

[46] Geisser ME, Casey KL, Brucksch CB, Ribbens CM, Appleton BB, Crofford LJ. Perception of noxious and innocuous heat stimulation among healthy women and women with fibromyalgia: association with mood, somatic focus, and catastrophizing. Pain 2003;102:243–50.

[47] Geisser ME, Glass JM, Rajcevska LD, Clauw DJ, Williams DA, Kileny PR, Gracely RH. A psychophysical study of auditory and pressure sensitivity in patients with fibromyalgia and healthy controls. J Pain 2008;9:417–22.

[48] Gendreau RM, Thorn MD, Gendreau JF, Kranzler JD, Ribeiro S, Gracely RH, Williams DA, Mease PJ, McLean SA, Clauw DJ. Efficacy of milnacipran in patients with fibromyalgia. J Rheumatol 2005;32:1975–85.

[49] Gerster JC, Hadj-Djilani A. Hearing and vestibular abnormalities in primary fibrositis syndrome. J Rheumatol 1984;11:678–80.

[50] Gibson SJ, Littlejohn GO, Gorman MM, Helme RD, Granges G. Altered heat pain thresholds and cerebral event-related potentials following painful CO_2 laser stimulation in subjects with fibromyalgia syndrome. Pain 1994;58:185–93.

[51] Giesecke J, Reed BD, Haefner HK, Giesecke T, Clauw DJ, Gracely RH. Quantitative sensory testing in vulvodynia patients and increased peripheral pressure pain sensitivity. Obstet Gynecol 2004;104:126–33.

[52] Giesecke T, Gracely RH, Grant MA, Nachemson A, Petzke F, Williams DA, Clauw DJ. Evidence of augmented central pain processing in idiopathic chronic low back pain. Arthritis Rheum 2004;50:613–23.

[53] Giesecke T, Gracely RH, Williams DA, Geisser ME, Petzke FW, Clauw DJ. The relationship between depression, clinical pain, and experimental pain in a chronic pain cohort. Arthritis Rheum 2005;52:1577–84.

[54] Glass JM, Lyden AK, Byrne-Dugan JC, Groner KH, Ambrose KR, Grace PJ, et al. Effects of sleep restriction and exercise deprivation on mood, pain, fatigue, somatic symptoms and cognition in healthy adults. American College of Rheumatology (ACR) 71st Annual Meeting, November 6–11, 2007, Boston. Abstract 112.

[55] Glass JM, Lyden AK, Petzke F, Stein P, Whalen G, Ambrose K, Chrousos G, Clauw DJ. The effect of brief exercise cessation on pain, fatigue, and mood symptom development in healthy, fit individuals. J Psychosom Res 2004;57:391–8.

[56] Gracely RH, Geisser ME, Giesecke T, Grant MA, Petzke F, Williams DA, Clauw DJ. Pain catastrophizing and neural responses to pain among persons with fibromyalgia. Brain 2004;127:835–43.

[57] Gracely RH, Petzke F, Wolf JM, Clauw DJ. Functional magnetic resonance imaging evidence of augmented pain processing in fibromyalgia. Arthritis Rheum 2002;46:1333–43.

[58] Hadler NM. "Fibromyalgia" and the medicalization of misery. J Rheumatol 2003;30:1668–70.

[59] Halvorson HA, Schlett CD, Riddle MS. Postinfectious irritable bowel syndrome: a meta-analysis. Am J Gastroenterol 2006;101:1894–9.

[60] Harris RE, Gracely RH, McLean SA, Williams DA, Giesecke T, Petzke F. Comparison of clinical and evoked pain measures in fibromyalgia. J Pain 2006;7:521–7.

[61] Harris RE, Sundgren PC, Pang Y, Hsu M, Petrou M, Kim SH, McLean SA, Gracely RH, Clauw DJ. Dynamic levels of glutamate within the insula are associated with improvements in multiple pain domains in fibromyalgia. Arthritis Rheum 2008;58:903–7.

[62] Harvey VL, Dickenson AH. Mechanisms of pain in nonmalignant disease. Curr Opin Support Palliat Care 2008;2:133–9.

[63] Heim C, Plotsky PM, Nemeroff CB. Importance of studying the contributions of early adverse experience to neurobiological findings in depression. Neuropsychopharmacology 2004;29:641–8.

[64] Hickie I, Davenport T, Wakefield D, Vollmer-Conna U, Cameron B, Vernon SD, Reeves WC, Lloyd A; Dubbo Infection Outcomes Study Group. Post-infective and chronic fatigue syndromes precipitated by viral and non-viral pathogens: prospective cohort study. BMJ 2006;333:575.

[65] Hosak L. Role of the COMT gene Val$_{158}$Met polymorphism in mental disorders: a review. Eur Psychiatry 2007;22:276–81.

[66] Hotopf M, David A, Hull L, Ismail K, Unwin C, Wessely S. Role of vaccinations as risk factors for ill health in veterans of the Gulf War: cross sectional study. BMJ 2000;320:1363–7.

[67] Hudson JI, Goldenberg DL, Pope HG Jr, Keck PE Jr, Schlesinger L. Comorbidity of fibromyalgia with medical and psychiatric disorders. Am J Med 1992;92:363–7.

[68] Hudson JI, Hudson MS, Pliner LF, Goldenberg DL, Pope HG Jr. Fibromyalgia and major affective disorder: a controlled phenomenology and family history study. Am J Psychiatry 1985;142:441–6.

[69] Jones GT, Power C, Macfarlane GJ. Physical adversity and poor social environment in childhood increase the risk of chronic widespread pain in adulthood: results from the 1958 British Birth Cohort Study. American College of Rheumatology; 2007.

[70] Joyner MJ, Masuki S. POTS versus deconditioning: the same or different? Clin Auton Res 2008;18:300–7.

[71] Kato K, Sullivan PF, Evengard B, Pedersen NL. Chronic widespread pain and its comorbidities: a population-based study. Arch Intern Med 2006;166:1649–54.

[72] Kosek E, Ekholm J, Hansson P. Sensory dysfunction in fibromyalgia patients with implications for pathogenic mechanisms. Pain 1996;68:375–83.

[73] Kosek E, Hansson P. Modulatory influence on somatosensory perception from vibration and heterotopic noxious conditioning stimulation (HNCS) in fibromyalgia patients and healthy subjects. Pain 1997;70:41–51.

[74] Lautenbacher S, Rollman GB, McCain GA. Multi-method assessment of experimental and clinical pain in patients with fibromyalgia. Pain 1994;59:45–53.

[75] Leffler AS, Hansson P, Kosek E. Somatosensory perception in a remote pain-free area and function of diffuse noxious inhibitory controls (DNIC) in patients suffering from long-term trapezius myalgia. Eur J Pain 2002;6:149–59.

[76] Levine BD, Zuckerman JH, Pawelczyk JA. Cardiac atrophy after bed-rest deconditioning: a nonneural mechanism for orthostatic intolerance. Circulation 1997;96:517–25.

[77] Maixner W, Fillingim R, Booker D, Sigurdsson A. Sensitivity of patients with painful temporomandibular disorders to experimentally evoked pain. Pain 1995;63:341–51.

[78] Martinez-Lavin M. Is fibromyalgia a generalized reflex sympathetic dystrophy? Clin Exp Rheumatol 2001;19:1–3.

[79] Martinez-Lavin M. Biology and therapy of fibromyalgia. Stress, the stress response system, and fibromyalgia. Arthritis Res Ther 2007;9:216.

[80] Martinez-Lavin M, Hermosillo AG, Rosas M, Soto ME. Circadian studies of autonomic nervous balance in patients with fibromyalgia: a heart rate variability analysis. Arthritis Rheum 1998;41:1966–71.

[81] Martinez-Lavin M, Vidal M, Barbosa RE, Pineda C, Casanova JM, Nava A. Norepinephrine-evoked pain in fibromyalgia. A randomized pilot study [ISRCTN70707830]. BMC Musculoskelet Disord 2002;3:2.

[82] McBeth J, Chiu YH, Silman AJ, Ray D, Morriss R, Dickens C, Gupta A, Macfarlane GJ. Hypotha-lamic-pituitary-adrenal stress axis function and the relationship with chronic widespread pain and its antecedents. Arthritis Res Ther 2005;7:R992–R1000.

[83] McBeth J, Macfarlane GJ, Benjamin S, Silman AJ. Features of somatization predict the on-set of chronic widespread pain: results of a large population-based study. Arthritis Rheum 2001;44:940–6.

[84] McBeth J, Macfarlane GJ, Silman AJ. Does chronic pain predict future psychological distress? Pain 2002;96:239–45.

[85] McBeth J, Silman AJ, Gupta A, Chiu YH, Ray D, Morriss R, Dickens C, King Y, Macfarlane GJ. Moderation of psychosocial risk factors through dysfunction of the hypothalamic-pituitary-adrenal stress axis in the onset of chronic widespread musculoskeletal pain: findings of a popu-lation-based prospective cohort study. Arthritis Rheum 2007;56:360–71.

[86] McDermid AJ, Rollman GB, McCain GA. Generalized hypervigilance in fibromyalgia: evidence of perceptual amplification. Pain 1996;66:133–44.

[87] McLean SA, Williams DA, Clauw DJ. Fibromyalgia after motor vehicle collision: evidence and implications. Traffic Inj Prev 2005;6:97–104.

[88] McLean SA, Williams DA, Harris RE, Kop WJ, Groner KH, Ambrose K, Lyden AK, Gracely RH, Crofford LJ, Geisser ME, et al. Momentary relationship between cortisol secretion and symp-toms in patients with fibromyalgia. Arthritis Rheum 2005;52:3660–9.

[89] McLean SA, Williams DA, Stein PK, Harris RE, Lyden AK, Whalen G, Park KM, Liberzon I, Sen A, Gracely RH, et al. Cerebrospinal fluid corticotropin-releasing factor concentration is associ-ated with pain but not fatigue symptoms in patients with fibromyalgia. Neuropsychopharmacol-ogy 2006;31:2776–82.

[90] Melzack R, Wall PD. Pain mechanisms: a new theory. Science 1965;150:971–9.

[91] Mense S, Hoheisel U, Reinert A. The possible role of substance P in eliciting and modulating deep somatic pain. Prog Brain Res 1996;110:125–35.

[92] Millan MJ. Descending control of pain. Prog Neurobiol 2002;66:355–474.

[93] Mogil JS, Yu L, Basbaum AI. Pain genes? Natural variation and transgenic mutants. Annu Rev Neurosci 2000;23:777–811.

[94] Moshiree B, Price DD, Robinson ME, Gaible R, Verne GN. Thermal and visceral hypersensitivity in irritable bowel syndrome patients with and without fibromyalgia. Clin J Pain 2007;23:323–30.

[95] Nackley AG, Shabalina SA, Tchivileva IE, Satterfield K, Korchynskyi O, Makarov SS, Maixner W, Diatchenko L. Human catechol-O-methyltransferase haplotypes modulate protein expression by altering mRNA secondary structure. Science 2006;314:1930–3.

[96] Nackley AG, Tan KS, Fecho K, Flood P, Diatchenko L, Maixner W. Catechol-O-methyltransfer-ase inhibition increases pain sensitivity through activation of both beta2- and beta3-adrenergic receptors. Pain 2007;128:199–208.

[97] Naliboff BD, Derbyshire SW, Munakata J, Berman S, Mandelkern M, Chang L, Mayer EA. Ce-rebral activation in patients with irritable bowel syndrome and control subjects during rectosig-moid stimulation. Psychosom Med 2001;63:365–75.

[98] Offenbaecher M, Bondy B, de Jonge S, Glatzeder K, Krüger M, Schoeps P, Ackenheil M. Possible association of fibromyalgia with a polymorphism in the serotonin transporter gene regulatory region. Arthritis Rheum 1999;42:2482–8.

[99] Papageorgiou AC, Silman AJ, Macfarlane GJ. Chronic widespread pain in the population: a seven year follow up study. Ann Rheum Dis 2002;61:1071–4.

[100] Petzke F, Clauw DJ, Ambrose K, Khine A, Gracely RH. Increased pain sensitivity in fibromyalgia: effects of stimulus type and mode of presentation. Pain 2003;105:403–13.

[101] Petzke F, Gracely RH, Khine A, Clauw DJ. Pain sensitivity in patients with fibromyalgia (FM): expectancy effects on pain measurements. Arthritis Rheum 1999;42(Suppl):S342.

[102] Qiao ZG, Vaeroy H, Morkrid L. Electrodermal and microcirculatory activity in patients with fibro-myalgia during baseline, acoustic stimulation and cold pressor tests. J Rheumatol 1991;18:1383–9.

[103] Raphael KG, Natelson BH, Janal MN, Nayak S. A community-based survey of fibromyalgia-like pain complaints following the World Trade Center terrorist attacks. Pain 2002;100:131–9.

[104] Russell IJ, Orr MD, Littman B, Vipraio GA, Alboukrek D, Michalek JE, Lopez Y, MacKillip F. Elevated cerebrospinal fluid levels of substance P in patients with the fibromyalgia syndrome. Arthritis Rheum 1994;37:1593–1601.

[105] Russell IJ, Vaeroy H, Javors M, Nyberg F. Cerebrospinal fluid biogenic amine metabolites in fibro-myalgia/fibrositis syndrome and rheumatoid arthritis. Arthritis Rheum 1992;35:550–6.

[106] Sarchielli P, Mancini ML, Floridi A, Coppola F, Rossi C, Nardi K, Acciarresi M, Pini LA, Cala-bresi P. Increased levels of neurotrophins are not specific for chronic migraine: evidence from primary fibromyalgia syndrome. J Pain 2007;8:737–45.

[107] Stein PK, Domitrovich PP, Ambrose K, Lyden A, Fine M, Gracely RH, Clauw DJ. Sex effects on heart rate variability in fibromyalgia and Gulf War illness. Arthritis Rheum 2004;51:700–8.

[108] Tegeder I, Costigan M, Griffin RS, Abele A, Belfer I, Schmidt H, Ehnert C, Nejim J, Marian C, Scholz J, et al. GTP cyclohydrolase and tetrahydrobiopterin regulate pain sensitivity and persistence. Nat Med 2006; 2:1269–77.

[109] Tracey I, Mantyh PW. The cerebral signature for pain perception and its modulation. Neuron 2007;55:377–91.

[110] Vollmer-Conna U, Cameron B, Hadzi-Pavlovic D, Singletary K, Davenport T, Vernon S, Reeves WC, Hickie I, Wakefield D, Lloyd AR; Dubbo Infective Outcomes Study Group. Postinfective fatigue syndrome is not associated with altered cytokine production. Clin Infect Dis 2007;45:732–5.

[111] Warren JW, Brown V, Jacobs S, Horne L, Langenberg P, Greenberg P. Urinary tract infection and inflammation at onset of interstitial cystitis/painful bladder syndrome. Urology 2008;71:1085–90.

[112] Weibel RE, Benor DE. Chronic arthropathy and musculoskeletal symptoms associated with rubella vaccines. A review of 124 claims submitted to the National Vaccine Injury Compensation Program. Arthritis Rheum 1996;39:1529–34.

[113] Wessely S, Chalder T, Hirsch S, Pawlikowska T, Wallace P, Wright DJ. Postinfectious fatigue: prospective cohort study in primary care. Lancet 1995;345:1333–8.

[114] Whelton CL, Salit I, Moldofsky H. Sleep, Epstein-Barr virus infection, musculoskeletal pain, and depressive symptoms in chronic fatigue syndrome. J Rheumatol 1992;19:939–43.

[115] Wilder-Smith CH, Robert-Yap J. Abnormal endogenous pain modulation and somatic and visceral hypersensitivity in female patients with irritable bowel syndrome. World J Gastroenterol 2007;13:3699–704.

[116] Williams DA, Brown SC, Clauw DJ, Gendreau RM. Self-reported symptoms before and after September 11 in patients with fibromyalgia. JAMA 2003;289:1637–8.

[117] Wolfe F. 50 years of antirheumatic therapy: the prognosis of rheumatoid arthritis. J Rheumatol Suppl 1990;22:24–32.

[118] Woolf CJ. Pain: moving from symptom control toward mechanism-specific pharmacologic management. Ann Intern Med 2004;140:441–51.

[119] Yaksh TL. Pharmacology of spinal adrenergic systems which modulate spinal nociceptive processing. Pharmacol Biochem Behav 1985;22:845–58.

[120] Yunus MB. Central sensitivity syndromes: a new paradigm and group nosology for fibromyalgia and overlapping conditions, and the related issue of disease versus illness. Semin Arthritis Rheum 2008;37:339–52.

[121] Yunus MB, Dailey JW, Aldag JC, Masi AT, Jobe PC. Plasma tryptophan and other amino acids in primary fibromyalgia: a controlled study. J Rheumatol 1992;19:90–4.

[122] Zubieta JK, Smith YR, Bueller JA, Xu Y, Kilbourn MR, Jewett DM, Meyer CR, Koeppe RA, Stohler CS. Regional mu opioid receptor regulation of sensory and affective dimensions of pain. Science 2001;293:311–5.

Correspondence to: Daniel J. Clauw, MD, Department of Anesthesiology, University of Michigan, 24 Frank Lloyd Wright Drive, Lobby M, Ann Arbor, MI 48106, USA. Tel: 1-734-998-6961; fax: 1-734-998-6900; email: dclauw@med.umich.edu.

It's a Belief. It's an Appraisal. It's Coping ... No, It's Catastrophizing

Jennifer A. Haythornthwaite

Department of Psychiatry and Behavioral Sciences, Johns Hopkins University School of Medicine, Baltimore, Maryland, USA

History of Catastrophizing Research

Pain-related catastrophizing comprises a set of negative emotional and cognitive responses to pain that include helplessness, magnification of pain, and rumination [16,68]. Historically, catastrophizing was initially conceptualized by Albert Ellis, and subsequently utilized by Aaron Beck and colleagues, to characterize dysfunctional cognitive errors as contributory factors in major depression and generalized anxiety. Beck's work in particular set the foundation for catastrophizing in chronic pain, where the concept of cognitive errors generally, and catastrophizing specifically, was first applied in Lefebvre's dissertation work demonstrating that depressed patients with low back pain made more dysphoric cognitive errors than did non-depressed low back pain patients [47]. The depressed low back pain patients also made more general cognitive errors, as well as more back-pain-specific cognitive errors. Soon afterward, Rosenstiel and Keefe published a measure of pain-specific catastrophizing—the Coping Strategies Questionnaire (CSQ [56])—as a subscale of a larger measure of both behavioral and cognitive pain coping strategies, which enabled researchers to systematically measure catastrophizing in many patient groups with chronic pain over the next decade.

Although early laboratory research focused heavily on magnification and memory for pain [62], helplessness became the focus in clinical studies of chronic pain through widespread use of the catastrophizing subscale of the CSQ [56]. In addition to establishing associations with pain severity and pain-related activity interference, experts began to debate the conceptualization of catastrophizing as a coping strategy and its measurement as potentially confounded by depression [66]. The conceptual ambiguity concerning catastrophizing's status as a pain coping strategy lead Jensen and his colleagues to exclude it from a comprehensive review of the pain coping literature published in the early 1990s [39]. Nonetheless, empirical evidence pointed to catastrophizing as a potent correlate of pain and suffering in a number of chronic pain conditions.

Continued conceptual and measurement advances occurred following the publication of the Pain Catastrophizing Scale by Sullivan and his colleagues [65]. This scale extended Rosenstiel and Keefe's [56] original helplessness subscale to include two additional dimensions: magnification and rumination. During this time an extensive literature developed establishing pain beliefs, appraisals, and coping as important factors associated with adjustment to chronic pain. As Geisser and colleagues noted in a provocative focus article [26], the "maladaptive" aspects of pain beliefs and coping strategies such as catastrophizing were well established by the late 1990s, whereas the "adaptive" qualities of alternative beliefs and coping strategies were generally elusive. The Geisser focus article [26] provoked a fervent debate (e.g., [35,42,72]) that centered on several conceptual issues challenging this burgeoning literature, including the dispute as to whether catastrophizing should be conceptualized as a belief, an appraisal, or a coping strategy and the importance of distinguishing process from outcome.

The 21st century brought with it a systematic review of two decades of work in this area, summarizing the prolific literature available at that time [68]. Catastrophizing accounts for approximately 7–31% of the variance in pain, correlates robustly with disability independently of the contribution of pain severity, and in part accounts for the frequently observed sex differences in pain and pain behavior. The review also highlighted conceptual challenges and identified competing theoretical models, one of which has since received extensive attention, with some studies supportive (e.g., [64]) and some not [3]. Turner and Aaron's editorial, published as a commentary to this review, emphasized the need to critically evaluate whether current measures of catastrophizing encompass the full domain of relevant concepts, particularly worry; whether catastrophizing has both trait-like and state-like dimensions; and whether situational factors including pain severity might influence the report of catastrophizing thoughts or behaviors. It also pointed out the need to critically evaluate the extent to which catastrophizing plays a causal role in determining pain outcomes [74].

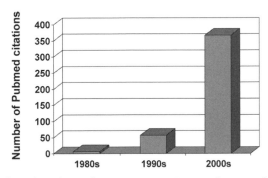

Fig. 1. Results of a PubMed search in August, 2008, using "catastrophizing" and "pain" as the search terms.

One of the more intriguing aspects of the review proposed a communal coping model in which catastrophizing is conceptualized as an interpersonal coping strategy designed to elicit proximity, support, and empathy from others [68]. The communal coping model spawned a series of investigations demonstrating that catastrophizing is associated with greater expressions of pain, particularly in the presence of another person [64], with perceptions of greater instrumental support from distressed caregivers of cancer patients [43], and with an interpersonal style that demands support and care-taking [45]. While the measurement of catastrophizing has been restricted to catastrophic thinking, conceptual work has proposed a distinction between catastrophic thinking and catastrophic behaviors in further developing the communal coping model [73].

Over two decades, catastrophizing has generally showed relationships with pain, physical functioning, and psychological functioning [68], and recently has been extended to health care utilization [75]. Given the early debates about the conceptualization and measurement of catastrophizing [66], it is of critical importance to note that studies consistently find that the relationship between catastrophizing and clinical pain is independent of the known influence of mood on pain (e.g., depression and anxiety; see [34]). However, the magnitude of the relationship between catastrophizing and pain is often small to moderate (e.g., correlations are in the range of 0.20–0.30), although the relationship with affective measures of pain is understandably stronger (e.g., [24]). Associations with physical functioning, often measured as pain-related activity interference or disability, are often in the moderate to large range (e.g., correlations in the range of 0.40–0.60). The clinical significance of catastrophizing in understanding morbidity in chronic pain is further strengthened by our own recent work demonstrating associations between catastrophizing and suicidal ideation independent of pain severity and independent of the expected relationship with depressive symptoms [20]. The fact that helplessness, a primary dimension of catastrophizing, predicts 5-year mortality in rheumatoid arthritis [7] lends further urgency to the need to understand and change this powerful cognitive and emotional process.

Catastrophizing in Pain-Free People

While most studies examine catastrophizing in clinical samples (e.g., [16]), a number of studies demonstrate that catastrophizing is an individual difference factor that varies in people who do not currently report chronic pain [5,51] and predicts pain in response to experimental noxious stimulation in healthy volunteers [17,67,69]. There is inconsistency in laboratory pain experiments on healthy volunteers, with many studies finding no relationship between catastrophizing and pain responses to cold pressor, heat pain, or ischemic pain stimulation (e.g., [18,36]). Distinguishing pain unpleasantness from intensity may reduce these inconsistencies [48], but the magnitude of the relationship between catastrophizing and experimental pain in healthy volunteers is generally small (in the range of 0.10–0.25; see [36]).

When measuring pain-specific catastrophizing among people not currently experiencing pain, the referent (i.e., "when you are in pain ...") is ambiguous: what type of pain is the respondent remembering, and from how distant in the past? Traditional measures of pain catastrophizing appear to emphasize the disposition to catastrophize more so than situational or state catastrophizing, since pain catastrophizing is quite stable over relatively long periods of time (e.g., over 6 months [40] or after resolution of acute pain [17]). Although situational catastrophizing was originally measured in the early 1990s [25], the distinction between dispositional and situational (or in vivo) catastrophizing has received more attention in recent years [70]. Studies may use different measures of situational catastrophizing, but all assess pain catastrophizing immediately after experimental noxious stimulation and refer the subject to the pain experienced during laboratory testing. Greater situational catastrophizing correlates with pain ratings [15,21,23,70] and with cold pressor tolerance [15], but not with differential modulation of spinal input as measured by the nociceptive flexion reflex [23]. In some of these studies, the traditional dispositional measurement of catastrophizing did not predict laboratory pain responses in healthy volunteers (e.g., [15,70]). Although moderate correlations have been observed between dispositional and situational measures [15], we have recently observed variability in the relationship between these measures of catastrophizing [8]. Dispositional measures of catastrophizing were uncorrelated with situational measures (reported during experimental pain) in healthy volunteers and rheumatoid arthritis patients, but they were modestly correlated in a sample of patients with temporomandibular joint disorder [8]. To add to the challenge of measuring and conceptualizing situational catastrophizing, the sole study that manipulated catastrophizing in a sample of healthy adults yielded only small increases in situational catastrophizing, and these increases were not associated with pain ratings or tolerance for the cold pressor task [58].

Catastrophizing as a Risk Factor

One of the most convincing demonstrations that catastrophizing incurs risk for pain derives from Picavet's work on pain-free community residents in the Netherlands; population-based data indicate that high levels of catastrophizing double the risk for new onset of severe and chronic back pain, as well as disability associated with low back pain [51]. These findings are crucial because the population-based selection of study participants mitigates many of the selection problems that plague research on catastrophizing, which has largely been conducted in the context of patients seeking care for persistent pain.

In clinical settings, a growing number of studies have examined the short-term, yet prospective effects of dispositional catastrophizing. One of the earliest longitudinal studies demonstrated that catastrophizing predicted pain severity, functional impairment, and depressive symptoms in rheumatoid arthritis patients over a 6-month period [40], but the effects were small and of limited clinical significance [74]. Our group has observed similar, small prospective effects of catastrophizing on pain in postherpetic neuralgia [34]. A series of recent studies have demonstrated an association between catastrophizing and postoperative outcomes, including pain during childbirth and postdelivery function [22], postamputation phantom limb pain [55], and pain following abdominal surgery [33]. This last study is of particular note, because Granot and her colleagues controlled for the well-established effects of anxiety on postoperative pain and demonstrated that these effects were in part explained by catastrophizing. Our own recent finding that catastrophizing may prolong sensitization following the resolution of an episode of acute pulpitis indirectly supports the proposition that it alters pain neuromodulatory systems [17]. Other prospective studies suggest that catastrophizing is a risk factor for unnecessary bed rest following an acute episode of back pain [80], for phantom limb pain following amputation [55], and for poor recovery from chronic shoulder pain [53] and total knee arthroplasty [63].

While the referent for measures of catastrophizing in healthy volunteers is ambiguous, dispositional catastrophizing correlates with greater reports of day-to-day pain symptoms in healthy college students [18]. This finding was further strengthened in our recent study of healthy undergraduate volunteers, some of whom reported problematic headaches [4]. Although the headache sufferers and pain-free volunteers reported comparable levels of pain-related catastrophizing, the headache group reported more depressive symptoms. Moreover, headache status moderated the relationship between catastrophizing and depressive symptoms:

catastrophizing was associated with greater depressive symptoms only in the headache group [4]. We proposed that dispositional catastrophizing acts as a latent diathesis whose negative effects on mood are activated only in the presence of pain (in this case, headache). Catastrophizing scores in these generally healthy students did not differ according to headache report and did not relate to depressive symptoms in students who did not report headaches, supporting the possibility that pain activates catastrophizing, which causes depressive symptoms. Such causal interpretations cannot derive from cross-sectional data, but require longitudinal studies of pain-free individuals who develop pain.

What Factors Are Known to Contribute to the Development of Catastrophizing?

Dispositional factors, such as temperament, personality, and beliefs play a strong role in pain-related catastrophizing, particularly the dimensions of negative affectivity, anxiety sensitivity, and fear of pain [46]. Neuroticism, or negative affectivity, is the disposition to be distressed and view challenging situations negatively, and neuroticism influences the relationship between catastrophizing and pain [31,70]. The contribution of dispositional factors such as personality to the development of catastrophizing does suggest the possibility of genetic contributions, although these studies have not yet been conducted and the evidence is inferential at best. Pain-related catastrophizing is associated with neuroticism/negative affectivity (e.g., [1]), and multiple genetic variations account for approximately 50% of the variance in cognitive and emotional responses associated with neuroticism [9]. As pain sensitivity is a complex trait and is likely to involve polymorphisms of multiple genes [14], the heritability of catastrophizing is likely to be equally complicated.

Of additional interest are recent data indicating that catastrophizing has a relationship with beliefs about the organic origins of the pain [60] and with strong beliefs about pain as a problem to be solved rather than accepted [13]. The possibility that catastrophizing contributes to perseveration about pain and its reduction gained support from recent data indicating that (a lack of) acceptance mediates the relationship between catastrophizing and mood, psychological function, and physical function [81]. Further support comes from data demonstrating that suppressing awareness of pain exaggerates lumbar paraspinal muscle responses among high catastrophizers [52], and from laboratory studies finding that catastrophizing is associated with difficulty suppressing pain-related thoughts and rumination, particularly when pain is anticipated [12,30,78,79].

Modern personality theory conceptualizes behavior as a dynamic interplay between individuals and the environment. Integrative theories of personality focus on gene-environment interactions that contribute to the neural circuitry underlying individual differences in behavior, including cognitive, affective, and social responses that both react to and shape the individual's environment [9]. Recent discussions of catastrophizing behavior [73] suggest a role for operant learning in the development of this maladaptive cognitive/emotional/behavioral response to pain, and social learning models provide a basis for expecting that the modeling of parental sick role behavior [83], which may include catastrophizing, might also shape the development of catastrophizing.

Under What Circumstances Might Catastrophizing Have Its Greatest Influence?

Personality is not only related to catastrophizing, but can moderate the negative influence of catastrophizing on pain-related outcomes. Individuals high in neuroticism who also report high levels of catastrophizing report significantly greater chronic low back pain, whereas pain and catastrophizing are not significantly related in individuals low in neuroticism [31]. The construct of negative affectivity has been incorporated as a moderator of catastrophizing in the updated fear-avoidance model of chronic musculoskeletal pain [46]; it is regarded as part of a higher-order vulnerability factor influencing anxiety sensitivity and fear of pain [44].

Although genetic studies of catastrophizing have not yet been conducted, recent data suggest an interaction between a diplotype of the catechol-O-methyltransferase (COMT) gene and catastrophizing in predicting pain following shoulder surgery [27]. No direct association between catastrophizing scores and COMT diplotype was observed, but the combination of high catastrophizing and low COMT activity (and associated with high pain sensitivity) was associated with higher pre- and postoperative pain ratings in these surgical patients.

Accumulating evidence also indicates that social environment moderates the influence of catastrophizing on key outcomes of interest in chronic pain. A single study suggests one circumstance under which catastrophizing might be associated with *better* outcomes. In patients who had undergone lower limb amputation, Jensen and his colleagues found that dispositional catastrophizing measured 1 month after amputation predicted improvements in depressive symptoms and pain-related interference 5 months later [38]. Under these circumstances, amputees reporting greater helplessness showed greater improvements early in their recuperation [38]. The authors speculated that patients who catastrophize may seek and receive greater social support during their recuperation following this major disfiguring surgery, and this support may help them modulate mood and improve their adaptation after amputation. This conclusion is in part supported by a recent diary study, which provides more detailed information on the reciprocal, transactional processes that shape catastrophizing and influence its effects over time. Data from married rheumatoid arthritis patients indicate that satisfaction with general supportive responses by the spouse on a day-to-day basis protected against later-in-the-day negative effects of catastrophizing on mood and in part on later negative effects on pain [37]. This interpretation is consistent with the communal coping model, which conceptualizes catastrophizing as a coping strategy designed to communicate and engage others in the social environment to help manage one's pain, distress, and pain-related challenges [68].

The engagement of interpersonal resources in coping with pain-related challenges may be a short-term goal that has inadvertent long-term negative consequences. While catastrophizing is associated with greater perceived solicitous responses to pain on the part of a significant other [28,43], some evidence suggests that this happens only with pain of shorter duration [3,10]. In other work, catastrophizing correlates with greater pain only among individuals living with a spouse or partner (as compared to living alone) or among those who perceived a significant other as responding to pain with support and attention (i.e., in a solicitous manner [28]). In contrast, our group [3] and others [2] have also found associations between catastrophizing and perceptions of punishing responses to pain on the part of a significant other. Not all studies of social moderators of catastrophizing are clearly conceptualized within the communal coping model, which needs to be further developed to delineate specific, testable hypotheses [73].

The Neurophysiology of Catastrophizing

Pain-related catastrophizing appears to amplify central nervous system processing of noxious input via alterations in spinal and cortical modulatory systems. Laboratory studies suggest that catastrophizing is associated with alterations in the central modulation of pain, including reductions in diffuse noxious inhibitory controls, thought to represent endogenous opioid activity [29,82], and increased temporal summation, thought to represent spinal sensitization [21]. It does not seem to be associated with measures of descending modulation of pain, such as the nociceptive flexion reflex [23,54]. Evidence supporting supraspinal modulation of pain by catastrophizing derives from studies demonstrating associations between catastrophizing and enhanced activation of higher cortical regions involved in the processing and regulation of pain [32,57]. Adding to this growing literature, our group has recently reported a relationship between situational catastrophizing and interleukin-6 reactivity to experimental pain stimulation in healthy controls [19]. In the context of current thinking about the role that endocrine and immune systems, particularly proinflammatory cytokines, play in the development, maintenance, and aggravation of chronic pain [49], these findings provide an intriguing direction for research into the neurophysiological mechanisms by which catastrophizing may shape an individual's experience of pain. Given the interdependency of the nervous, endocrine, and immune systems [11], it will be important for future research to examine the degree to which these systems additively or synergistically link catastrophizing with pain and pain-related outcomes.

Conceptual Issues

Our scientific knowledge of catastrophizing has flourished in recent years, in large part due to the generally systematic use of two interrelated measures that have been translated into many languages. The uniform use of just a few measures allows us to compare study results and amass a rich database that crosses pain conditions and countries, substantiating the broad, coherent influence of catastrophizing on adaptation to pain. Recent studies have extended these findings and adapted these commonly used tools for the situational measurement of catastrophizing in order to understand cognitive/emotional responses to known painful stimuli (e.g., [21]) or to track moment-to-moment changes in catastrophizing as patients experience their daily lives (e.g., [37,77]).

A number of conceptual issues remain in this burgeoning literature. First, the causal role of catastrophizing remains a critical issue that has not been adequately addressed. Studies that show longitudinal effects of catastrophizing (e.g., [34,40]) suffer from the potential confound of an unmeasured ("third") variable that may account for the apparent longitudinal effects. An excellent example demonstrating this potential problem comes from the prospective study by Granot and colleagues [33] in patients undergoing abdominal surgery. As has been previously shown, preoperative anxiety predicted postoperative pain in Granot's sample. Further analyses indicated that catastrophizing partially accounted for the anxiety-pain association, substantially reducing the apparent association between anxiety and postoperative pain. This is an example in which a third variable—catastrophizing—accounted for a large part of the apparent relationship between anxiety and postoperative pain. Because anxiety and catastrophizing were measured concurrently (before surgery), there is only a suggestion of mediation; demonstration of true mediation requires more frequent measurements that occur at different points in time.

The most convincing data regarding causation derive from experimental manipulation of the factor of interest—in this case, catastrophizing. A single published study specifically manipulated catastrophic thinking during experimental pain testing, showing a small (but statistically significant) increase in catastrophizing that did not influence pain during the cold pressor task [58]. As there was no difference between groups in level of catastrophizing immediately prior to cold pressor exposure, it remains uncertain as to whether this method was an adequate test of the causal role for catastrophizing in enhancing pain. In a different type of experimental manipulation, cold pressor threshold and tolerance were substantially reduced among individuals high in catastrophizing who were exposed to emotional descriptors designed to activate an affective, reactive schema

about pain [50]. These studies provide basic methodologies for experimentally manipulating catastrophizing and affective focus that deserve
continued study.

Additional causal data derive from clinical studies that demonstrate reductions in catastrophizing resulting from psychological treatments for pain [68], of which cognitive-behavioral therapy is the most
common. More detailed analyses of outcomes provide the encouraging
finding that reductions in catastrophizing mediate [61] and even precede
[6] reductions in pain and pain-related disability specific to cognitive-behavioral treatment [76].

A second related conceptual matter pertains to the extent to
which catastrophizing constitutes a *diathesis*—a latent vulnerability—that
becomes activated by pain. Pain, or the threat of pain, stimulates attentional resources and engages cognitive, emotional, and neurophysiological processes that intensify pain. Catastrophizing as a diathesis increases
the likelihood that an individual will experience pain as threatening, become worried and fearful, and have difficulty disengaging. Once aroused,
these processes, particularly the neurophysiological changes, may well
continue to enhance pain, slow injury-related healing, increase the likelihood of persistent pain, and contribute to pain-related disability. At the
present time, studies of dispositional catastrophizing lend support to the
diathesis model. However, recent findings that situational catastrophizing correlates poorly with dispositional catastrophizing in some studies
and in some patient/non-patient groups (e.g., [8]) are not consistent with
the diathesis model. Laboratory studies of situational catastrophizing in
non-patient groups may provide the strongest test of the diathesis model,
but these studies are limited in the magnitude, duration, and meaning of
painful stimulation applied. Additionally, these healthy volunteers generally show quite low levels of dispositional catastrophizing.

Third among the conceptual issues is the theoretical framework
guiding studies of catastrophizing. Many researchers have invoked a
transactional stress and coping model [35,59,68] in which beliefs, appraisal, and coping are distinguished. Catastrophizing is generally designated
as a primary and/or secondary appraisal process rather than as a coping
strategy [59]. A recent alternative formulation is the communal coping
model discussed above [68,73], which hypothesizes that catastrophizing

serves as a coping strategy with the goal not of reducing pain, but of engaging the social environment in managing distress. There is little doubt that catastrophizing is associated with heightened pain behavior [41], and recent studies are starting to illuminate the social parameters that influence the expression of communicative pain behaviors among high catastrophizers [64].

Conclusions

Our current knowledge, if placed in the context of developments in the neurosciences, support an expansion of existing conceptualizations to incorporate integrative theories of complex traits (e.g., [9]) and perspectives on psychophysiological pain "supersystems" [11] into our theoretical framework guiding future research on catastrophizing. Catastrophizing most likely poses a risk for pain and pain-related disability through biased cognitive processing of noxious input combined with alterations in central and peripheral modulation of pain. Catastrophizing develops early in life, and pain-related catastrophizing might represent a latent diathesis in the absence of ongoing clinical pain (e.g., [17]). Genetics, early life experiences, and social modeling probably contribute to the development of dispositional catastrophizing. In response to pain, cognitive processing is biased toward negative, and against positive, emotional stimuli and more strongly engages relevant neural circuits within the matrix activated during pain, particularly those circuits involved in affect, anticipation, attention, and threat appraisal. Situational catastrophizing further enhances these responses, as do dysfunctional acute psychophysiological systems (i.e., the nervous, endocrine, and/or immune systems [11]).

Despite the striking absence of longitudinal studies on catastrophizing in clinical samples, once a painful condition develops, the effects of catastrophizing become apparent [4]. In the context of ongoing pain, situational catastrophizing behavior will be shaped by social responses [71], which may contribute to the escalation of catastrophizing over time. When pain is prolonged, the psychophysiological pain systems and their interface become dysregulated, contributing to the perpetuation and enhancement of ongoing pain [11]. Immediate social responses shape the expression of pain, including catastrophic communications, as do treatments, socioeconomic factors, and culture. Such a reciprocal, transactional process approach has not yet been investigated to determine how the social environment shapes and responds to catastrophizing, how catastrophizing and its underlying neurophysiology change over time, and what factors contribute to increases—or decreases—in catastrophizing. Just as we are now discovering that the expression of genes can be altered by environmental exposures, it is critical for more work to focus on what factors change catastrophizing over time as people who are pain-free develop acute pain and transition to chronic pain.

Acknowledgments

The author would like to thank Dr. Robert Edwards for his many stimulating and critical discussions of this topic, Dr. Claudia Campbell and Dr. Phil Quartana for their critical comments on this manuscript, and grants from the National Institutes of Health that have funded the author's research on this topic (R01DE13906; K24NS002225; R21NS48593; R24AT004641).

References

[1]   Asghari A, Nicholas MK. Personality and pain-related beliefs/coping strategies: a prospective study. Clin J Pain 2006;22:10–18.
[2]   Boothby JL, Thorn BE, Overduin LY, Charles WL. Catastrophizing and perceived partner responses to pain. Pain 2004;109:500–6.
[3]   Buenaver LF, Edwards RR, Haythornthwaite JA. Pain-related catastrophizing and perceived social responses: inter-relationships in the context of chronic pain. Pain 2007;127:234–42.
[4]   Buenaver LF, Edwards RR, Smith MT, Gramling SE, Haythornthwaite JA. Catastrophizing and pain-coping in young adults: associations with depressive symptoms and headache pain. J Pain 2008;9:311–9.
[5]   Buer N, Linton SJ. Fear-avoidance beliefs and catastrophizing: occurrence and risk factor in back pain and ADL in the general population. Pain 2002;99:485–91.
[6]   Burns JW, Kubilus A, Bruehl S, Harden RN, Lofland K. Do changes in cognitive factors influence outcome following multidisciplinary treatment for chronic pain? A cross-lagged panel analysis. J Consult Clin Psychol 2003;71:81–91.
[7]   Callahan LF, Cordray DS, Wells G, Pincus T. Formal education and five-year mortality in rheumatoid arthritis: mediation by helplessness scale score. Arthritis Care Res 1996;9:463–72.
[8]   Campbell CM, Kronfli TR, Buenaver LF, Haythornthwaite JA, Smith MT, Edwards RR. In-vivo vs. standard catastrophizing in multiple pain measures among healthy, TMD and arthritis patients. J Pain 2008;9(Suppl 2):56.
[9]   Canli T. Toward a neurogenetic theory of neuroticism. Ann NY Acad Sci 2008;1129:153–74.
[10] Cano A. Pain catastrophizing and social support in married individuals with chronic pain: the moderating role of pain duration. Pain 2004;110:656–64.
[11] Chapman CR, Tuckett RP, Song CW. Pain and stress in a systems perspective: reciprocal neural, endocrine, and immune interactions. J Pain 2008;9:122–45.
[12] Crombez G, Eccleston C, Baeyens F, Eelen P. When somatic information threatens, catastrophic thinking enhances attentional interference. Pain 1998;75:187–98.

[13] Crombez G, Eccleston C, Van Hamme G, De Vlieger P. Attempting to solve the problem of pain: a questionnaire study in acute and chronic pain patients. Pain 2008;137:556–63.

[14] Diatchenko L, Nackley AG, Slade GD, Fillingim RB, Maixner W. Idiopathic pain disorders: pathways of vulnerability. Pain 2006;123:226–30.

[15] Dixon KE, Thorn BE, Ward LC. An evaluation of sex differences in psychological and physiological responses to experimentally-induced pain: a path analytic description. Pain 2004;112:188–96.

[16] Edwards RR, Bingham CO, III, Bathon J, Haythornthwaite JA. Catastrophizing and pain in arthritis, fibromyalgia, and other rheumatic diseases. Arthritis Rheum 2006;55:325–32.

[17] Edwards RR, Fillingim RB, Maixner W, Sigurdsson A, Haythornthwaite J. Catastrophizing predicts changes in thermal pain responses after resolution of acute dental pain. J Pain 2004;5:164–70.

[18] Edwards RR, Haythornthwaite JA, Sullivan MJ, Fillingim RB. Catastrophizing as a mediator of sex differences in pain: differential effects for daily pain versus laboratory-induced pain. Pain 2004;111:335–341.

[19] Edwards RR, Kronfli T, Haythornthwaite JA, Smith MT, McGuire L, Page GG. Association of catastrophizing with interleukin-6 responses to acute pain. Pain 2008;140:135–144.

[20] Edwards RR, Smith MT, Kudel I, Haythornthwaite J. Pain-related catastrophizing as a risk factor for suicidal ideation in chronic pain. Pain 2006;126:272–9.

[21] Edwards RR, Smith MT, Stonerock G, Haythornthwaite JA. Pain-related catastrophizing in healthy women is associated with greater temporal summation of and reduced habituation to thermal pain. Clin J Pain 2006;22:730–7.

[22] Flink IK, Mroczek MZ, Sullivan MJL, Linton SJ. Pain in childbirth and postpartum recovery: the role of catastrophizing. Eur J Pain 2008; Epub May 30.

[23] France CR, France JL, Al'Absi M, Ring C, McIntyre D. Catastrophizing is related to pain ratings, but not nociceptive flexion reflex threshold. Pain 2002;99:459–63.

[24] Geisser ME, Robinson ME, Keefe FJ, Weiner ML. Catastrophizing, depression and the sensory, affective and evaluative aspects of chronic pain. Pain 1994;59:79–83.

[25] Geisser ME, Robinson ME, Pickren WE. Differences in cognitive coping strategies among pain-sensitive and pain-tolerant individuals on the cold-pressor test. Behav Ther 1992;23:31–41.

[26] Geisser ME, Robinson ME, Riley JL. Pain beliefs, coping, and adjustment to chronic pain: let's focus more on the negative. Pain Forum 2008;8:161–8.

[27] George SZ, Wallace MR, Wright TW, Moser MW, Greenfield III WH, Sack BK, Herbstman DM, Fillingim RB. Evidence for a biopsychosocial influence on shoulder pain: pain catastrophizing and catechol-O-methyltransferase (COMT) diplotype predict clinical pain ratings. Pain 2008;136:53–61.

[28] Giardino ND, Jensen MP, Turner JA, Ehde DM, Cardenas DD. Social environment moderates the association between catastrophizing and pain among persons with a spinal cord injury. Pain 2003;106:19–25.

[29] Goodin BR, McGuire L, Allshouse M, Stapleton L, Haythornthwaite JA, Mayes LA, Burns N, Edwards RR. Associations between catastrophizing and endogenous pain-inhibitory processes: sex differences. J Pain; in press.

[30] Goubert L, Crombez G, Eccleston C, Devulder J. Distraction from chronic pain during a pain-inducing activity is associated with greater post-activity pain. Pain 2004;110:220–7.

[31] Goubert L, Crombez G, Van Damme S. The role of neuroticism, pain catastrophizing and pain-related fear in vigilance to pain: a structural equations approach. Pain 2004;107:234–41.

[32] Gracely RH, Geisser ME, Giesecke T, Grant MAB, Petzke F, Williams DA, Clauw DJ. Pain catastrophizing and neural responses to pain among persons with fibromyalgia. Brain 2004;127:835–43.

[33] Granot M, Ferber SG. The roles of pain catastrophizing and anxiety in the prediction of postoperative pain intensity: a prospective study. Clin J Pain 2005;21:439–45.

[34] Haythornthwaite JA, Clark MR, Pappagallo M, Raja SN. Pain coping strategies play a role in the persistence of pain in post-herpetic neuralgia. Pain 2003;106:453–60.

[35] Haythornthwaite JA, Heinberg LJ. Coping with pain: What works, under what circumstances, and in what ways? Pain Forum 1999;8:172–5.

[36] Hirsh AT, George SZ, Bialosky JE, Robinson ME. Fear of pain, pain catastrophizing, and acute pain perception: relative prediction and timing of assessment. J Pain 2008;9:806–12.

[37] Holtzman S, Delongis A. One day at a time: the impact of daily satisfaction with spouse responses on pain, negative affect and catastrophizing among individuals with rheumatoid arthritis. Pain 2007;131:202–13.

[38] Jensen MP, Ehde DM, Hoffman AJ, Patterson DR, Czerniecki JM, Robinson LR. Cognitions, coping and social environment predict adjustment to phantom limb pain. Pain 2002;95:133–42.

[39] Jensen MP, Turner JA, Romano JM, Karoly P. Coping with chronic pain: a critical review of the literature. Pain 1991;47:249–83.

[40] Keefe F, Brown G, Wallston K, Caldwell D. Coping with rheumatoid arthritis pain: catastrophizing as a maladaptive strategy. Pain 1989;37:51–6.

[41] Keefe FJ, Lefebvre JC, Egert JR, Affleck G, Sullivan MJ, Caldwell DS. The relationship of gender to pain, pain behavior, and disability in osteoarthritis patients: the role of catastrophizing. Pain 2000;87:325–34.

[42] Keefe FJ, Lefebvre JC, Smith SJ. Catastrophizing research: avoiding conceptual errors and maintaining a balanced perspective. Pain Forum 1999;8:176–80.

[43] Keefe FJ, Lipkus I, Lefebvre JC, Hurwitz H, Clipp E, Smith J, Porter L. The social context of gastrointestinal cancer pain: a preliminary study examining the relation of patient pain catastrophizing to patient perceptions of social support and caregiver stress and negative responses. Pain 2003;103:151–6.

[44] Keogh E, Asmundson GJG. Negative affectivity, catastrophizing, and anxiety sensitivity. In: Asmundson GJG, Vlaeyen JWS, Crombez G, editors. Understanding and treating fear of pain. Oxford: Oxford University Press; 2004. p. 91–116.

[45] Lackner JM, Gurtman MB. Pain catastrophizing and interpersonal problems: a circumplex analysis of the communal coping model. Pain 2004;110:597–604.

[46] Leeuw M, Goossens ME, Linton SJ, Crombez G, Boersma K, Vlaeyen JW. The fear-avoidance model of musculoskeletal pain: current state of scientific evidence. J Behav Med 2007;30:77–94.

[47] Lefebvre MF. Cognitive distortion and cognitive errors in depressed psychiatric and low back pain patients. J Consult Clin Psychol 1981;49:517–25.

[48] Lu Q, Tsao JCI, Myers CD, Kim SC, Zeltzer LK. Coping predictors of children's laboratory-induced pain tolerance, intensity, and unpleasantness. J Pain 2007;8:708–17.

[49] Marchand F, Perretti M, McMahon SB. Role of the immune system in chronic pain. Nat Rev Neurosci 2005;6:521–32.

[50] Michael ES, Burns JW. Catastrophizing and pain sensitivity among chronic pain patients: moderating effects of sensory and affect focus. Ann Behav Med 2004;27:185–94.

[51] Picavet HS, Vlaeyen JW, Schouten JS. Pain catastrophizing and kinesiophobia: predictors of chronic low back pain. Am J Epidemiol 2002;156:1028–34.

[52] Quartana PJ, Burns JW, Lofland KR. Attentional strategy moderates effects of pain catastrophizing on symptom-specific physiological responses in chronic low back pain patients. J Behav Med 2007;30:221–31.

[53] Reilingh ML, Kuijpers T, Tanja-Harfterkamp AM, van der Windt DA. Course and prognosis of shoulder symptoms in general practice. Rheumatology 2008;47:724–30.

[54] Rhudy JL, Maynard LJ, Russell JL. Does in vivo catastrophizing engage descending modulation of spinal nociception? J Pain 2006;8:325–33.

[55] Richardson C, Glenn S, Horgan M, Nurmikko T. A prospective study of factors associated with the presence of phantom limb pain six months after major lower limb amputation in patients with peripheral vascular disease. J Pain 2007;8:793–801.

[56] Rosenstiel AK, Keefe FJ. The use of coping strategies in chronic low back pain patients: relationship to patient characteristics and current adjustment. Pain 1983;17:33–44.

[57] Seminowicz DA, Mikulis DJ, Davis KD. Cognitive modulation of pain-related brain responses depends on behavioral strategy. Pain 2004;112:48–58.

[58] Severeijns R, van den Hout MA, Vlaeyen JWS. The causal status of pain catastrophizing: an experimental test with healthy participants. Eur J Pain 2005;9:257–65.

[59] Severeijns R, Vlaeyen JWS, van den Hout MA. Do we need a communal coping model of pain catastrophizing? An alternative explanation. Pain 2004;111:226–9.

[60] Sloan TJ, Gupta R, Zhang W, Walsh DA. Beliefs about the causes and consequences of pain in patients with chronic inflammatory or noninflammatory low back pain and in pain-free individuals. Spine 2008;33:966–72.

[61] Smeets RJEM, Vlaeyen JWS, Kester ADM, Knottnerus JA. Reduction of pain catastrophizing mediates the outcome of both physical and cognitive-behavioral treatment in chronic low back pain. J Pain 2006;7:261–71.

[62] Spanos NP, Stam HJ, Brazil K. The effects of suggestion and distraction on coping ideation and reported pain. J Ment Imagery 1981;5:75–90.

[63] Stephens MA, Druley JA, Zautra AJ. Older adults' recovery from surgery for osteoarthritis of the knee: psychosocial resources and constraints as predictors of outcomes. Health Psychol 2002;21:377–83.

[64] Sullivan MJ, Adams H, Sullivan ME. Communicative dimensions of pain catastrophizing: social cueing effects on pain behaviour and coping. Pain 2004;107:220–6.

[65] Sullivan MJ, Bishop SR, Pivik J. The Pain Catastrophizing Scale: development and validation. Psychol Assess 1995;7:524–32.

[66] Sullivan MJ, D'Eon JL. Relation between catastrophizing and depression in chronic pain patients. J Abnorm Psychol 1990;99:260–3.

[67] Sullivan MJ, Rodgers WM, Wilson PM, Bell GJ, Murray TC, Fraser SN. An experimental investigation of the relation between catastrophizing and activity intolerance. Pain 2002;100:47–53.

[68] Sullivan MJ, Thorn B, Haythornthwaite JA, Keefe F, Martin M, Bradley LA, Lefebvre JC. Theoretical perspectives on the relation between catastrophizing and pain. Clin J Pain 2001;17:52–64.

[69] Sullivan MJ, Thorn B, Rodgers W, Ward LC. Path model of psychological antecedents to pain experience: experimental and clinical findings. Clin J Pain 2004;20:164–73.

[70] Thorn BE, Clements KL, Ward LC, Dixon KE, Kersh BC, Boothby JL, Chaplin WF. Personality factors in the explanation of sex differences in pain catastrophizing and response to experimental pain. Clin J Pain 2004;20:275–82.

[71] Thorn BE, Keefe FJ, Anderson T. The communal coping model and interpersonal context: problems or process? Pain 2004;110:505–7.

[72] Thorn BE, Rich MA, Boothby JL. Pain beliefs and coping attempts: conceptual model building. Pain Forum 1999;8:169–71.

[73] Thorn BE, Ward LC, Sullivan MJL, Boothby JL. Communal coping model of catastrophizing: conceptual model building. Pain 2003;106:1–2.

[74] Turner JA, Aaron LA. Pain-related catastrophizing: what is it? Clin J Pain 2001;17:65–71.

[75] Turner JA, Brister H, Huggins K, Mancl L, Aaron LA, Truelove EL. Catastrophizing is associated with clinical examination findings, activity interference, and health care use among patients with temporomandibular disorders. J Orofac Pain 2005;19:291–300.

[76] Turner JA, Holtzman S, Mancl L. Mediators, moderators, and predictors of therapeutic change in cognitive-behavioral therapy for chronic pain. Pain 2007;127:276–86.

[77] Turner JA, Mancl L, Aaron LA. Pain-related catastrophizing: a daily process study. Pain 2004;110:103–11.

[78] Van Damme S, Crombez G, Eccleston C. Retarded disengagement from pain cues: the effects of pain catastrophizing and pain expectancy. Pain 2002;100:111–8.

[79] Van Damme S, Crombez G, Eccleston C. Disengagement from pain: the role of catastrophic thinking about pain. Pain 2004;107:70–76.

[80] Verbunt JA, Sieben J, Vlaeyen JWS, Portegijs P, Knottnerus J. A new episode of low back pain: Who relies on bed rest? Eur J Pain 2008;12:508–516.

[81] Vowles KE, McCracken LM, Eccleston C. Patient functioning and catastrophizing in chronic pain: The mediating effects of acceptance. Health Psychol 2008;27:S136–s143.

[82] Weissman-Fogel I, Sprecher E, Pud D. Effects of catastrophizing on pain perception and pain modulation. Exp Brain Res 2008;186:79–85.

[83] Whitehead WE, Crowell MD, Heller BR, Robinson JC, Schuster MM, Horn S. Modeling and reinforcement of the sick role during childhood predicts adult illness behavior. Psychosom Med 1994;56:541–550.

Correspondence to: Prof. Jennifer A. Haythornthwaite, PhD, 1-108 Meyer, Department of Psychiatry and Behavioral Sciences, Johns Hopkins University School of Medicine, 600 N. Wolfe Street, Baltimore, MD 21287, USA. Email: jhaytho1@jhmi.edu.

Quality Improvement and Evolving Research in Pediatric Pain Management and Palliative Care

John J. Collins,[a] Suellen M. Walker,[b] and Kirsty Campbell[a]

[a]Department of Pain Medicine and Palliative Care, The Children's Hospital at Westmead, Westmead, New South Wales, Australia; [b]Paediatric Anaesthesia and Pain Medicine, Institute of Child Health, University College London, and Great Ormond Street Hospital, London, United Kingdom

The need for improved pain management for children with acute, chronic, and cancer pain and for children receiving palliative care has been identified by clinicians as well as by children and their families. Internationally, growth has been rapid in the number of services offered to these children. Many children's hospitals throughout the world now have dedicated pain services, and specialized pediatric palliative care services have also evolved in recent years. Many such services are located in children's hospitals or in a pediatric department of a larger adult hospital, while others serve children receiving care at home or in an inpatient hospice unit. The continued advancement of these important areas of pediatric clinical practice can only be achieved by developing pediatric acute, chronic, and cancer pain and palliative care quality programs and by improving research in these areas.

Why Quality and Research Programs in Pediatric Pain and Palliative Care Service Are Needed

All stakeholders receiving and delivering clinical care are interested in the quality and safety of care. Consumers wish to know that the services they are receiving are of a certain, and preferably high, standard. Clinicians, too, wish to know that the services they provide are meeting defined standards. In addition, if clinicians aspire to attain standards of excellence in the services they deliver, a quality program will be able to identify areas for improved performance in the quest for such a goal. Administrators and policy makers also have a vested interest in the quality and the outcomes of clinical services. For example, at a governmental level, policy makers must ensure that health care monetary resources are being used well, that standards are being attained, and that problems in clinical services are identified quickly.

The implementation of a quality program is really a statement that the status quo is not good enough and that an honest appraisal of the quality of a clinical service will lead to improvement in the quest for excellence. In a similar manner, research in pediatric pain management and palliative care will inform both the standards of care and the clinical care of children and their families. It will also help transform these areas of pediatric clinical medicine into areas of practice with a substantial evidence base.

The Necessary Elements of a Pediatric Pain Management and Palliative Care Quality Program

The Quality Program of the Department of Pain Management and Palliative Care at the Children's Hospital at Westmead, Sydney, Australia, which began in 2007, is one of the first of its type in the world. The impelling forces for its development were the need to document the evidence for meeting recently established standards for pediatric acute pain management [8] and for palliative care [7,52]. The following outlines the stages in which the quality program was implemented.

Stage 1: Identify a Quality Program Manager to Lead the Program and to Create and Implement a Quality Strategic Plan

The identified need for the appointment of a nonclinical quality manager addresses several factors, including the specialized nature of the area and the lack of training in most undergraduate and postgraduate clinical education; the lack of expertise and time on the part of existing clinical personnel; and, lastly, the need for a neutral person to deal with sensitive areas of complaint that might arise in consumer satisfaction surveys. Quality management has become a specialized area with defined terminology, and it is important that the appointed person should have training, skills, and abilities in this area. It is inappropriate to appoint a clinician who simply has an interest in quality management, especially if he or she is part of the clinical program. A strategic plan must be developed for the implementation of a quality program that identifies the priorities for the department.

Stages 2, 3: Identify Defined Standards and Measure the Clinical Service against the Standards

Many countries are in the process of developing national guidelines for acute and chronic pain management and palliative care. In Australia, the National Health and Medical Research Council recently published the document "Acute pain management: scientific evidence" [8]. This document is a compilation of the highest levels of evidence relevant to acute pain management for adults and children. The clinical activities of an acute pediatric pain service should rely on evidence or on recommended best practice based on clinical experience and expert opinion. There are currently no identifiable standards for the management of chronic pain in children.

The fourth edition of the document "Standards for providing quality palliative care for all Australians" [52] is a key government document that influences both primary and specialist providers in the way care is planned and delivered. Moving away from the simplistic diagnostic basis for determining need, it focuses on establishing networks that allow patients to access the proper care when needed. The Australian and New Zealand Paediatric Palliative Care Reference Group has recommended the use of this publication for pediatric services. In tandem with this development, the Steering Committee of the European Association for Palliative Care's task force on pediatric palliative care created the document "IMPaCCT: standards for paediatric palliative care in Europe" [33]. This report describes core standards for palliative care for children and outlines their ethical and legal rights.

Once standards are identified, a review of clinical services can proceed with reference to standards. In the case of "Standards for providing quality palliative care for all Australians," service provision must be measured against 13 standards for palliative care. These standards include assessment and management, access and care coordination, communication, bereavement support, staff and volunteer education, and a commitment to quality improvement and research. A review of a clinical service against standards will present opportunities for service improvement, but to ensure its own legitimacy, the review must identify the evidence of the service meeting the standards. Clinical services should be reviewed on an ongoing basis with reference to standards.

Stage 4: Develop Measures of Quality for Acute Pain and Chronic Pain Management and for Palliative Care

Consumer Satisfaction as a Measure of the Quality of Pediatric Pain Management and Palliative Care

Consumer satisfaction surveys are frequently used in pediatric pain management and palliative care as a measure of quality. However, controversy has emerged in the literature as to their meaning and value. The use of surveys has evolved in palliative care, for example, because the traditional indicators of quality in health care—death or recovery rates—are not appropriate in this field. The controversies concerning this practice relate to the few alternatives available to indicate consumer satisfaction, the lack of a widely held definition of satisfaction, and the methodological inconsistencies across studies [5].

The term "satisfied," when used in quality evaluation, does not necessarily convey that a service was excellent, but simply that it was adequate. Likewise, "unsatisfied" may not necessarily imply that service was poor, but simply that it could have been better [5]. As such, sole reliance on consumer satisfaction surveys to determine clinical and policy changes in pediatric pain management and palliative care may not improve the quality of care. Clearly, additional data are needed to support evidence for or against quality of care.

In addition, families of children receiving palliative care, and those who are recently bereaved, are very vulnerable, and they may not feel at ease with contributing negative comments indicating inadequacies in service delivery. It is essential that families are assured of the anonymity of survey responses, that the data are collated by a nonclinical staff member, and that families have access to a contact person outside the department conducting the survey. There is no consensus in the literature about the timing of surveys for families receiving palliative care or those who are recently bereaved. In light of these issues, surveys and accompanying documents must stress the voluntary nature of participation, provide options for families to comment rather than just rate a service, and give the opportunity to select alternative care options.

Measuring Quality by Identifying or Creating Outcome Measures

Part of quality measurement involves the use of outcome measures, which may include clinical indicators (measures of clinical outcomes), process indicators (measures of clinical processes), and qualitative reflective review. Outcome measures are designed to identify the rate of occurrence (or non-occurrence) of an event, which in turn reflects the care that was (or was not) provided. Aggregated data from all patients receiving the service can highlight areas that need improving and can be used to measure the service against particular standards. Indicators can be collected over a number of settings and can be used as a way of benchmarking or comparing similar services [6]. Alternatively, with a qualitative review process, reviewers can look at individual cases to identify areas requiring improvement.

Clinical Indicators for Acute Pain Management

Traditional outcome measures for pediatric acute pain management have focused on patient and family satisfaction surveys and pain severity scores. Other important outcomes should include analgesic complications and side effects, patient education, and discharge time from hospital. A high pain severity score or repeatedly high pain scores may indicate poor pain control and the need for alternative analgesic strategies. In children, pain scores have been measured using self-report or observational pain scales. More recently, scales have been developed to measure pain in cognitively impaired children.

Self-report measures of pain in children have largely focused on the assessment of pain severity. Generally, the pediatric data support the use of visual analogue scales or numerical rating scales for children over 5 years old. Visual analogue scales have been used in the assessment of pediatric cancer pain; they frequently have anchors of "no pain" and the "worst pain possible." To use such scales, children must understand the concept of proportionality; they must be able to conceptualize their pain experience along a continuum and be able to translate that understanding to the visual representations of the line and the anchors.

Considerable research efforts have been devoted to the development of a common metric in pediatric pain measurement. The Faces Pain Scale-Revised (FPS-R) [29] has been shown to be appropriate for use in assessment of the intensity of children's acute pain from the age of 4 or 5 years, and it has the advantage of conforming closely to a linear interval scale [29]. Age is a significant predictor of children's ability to use this scale. A substantial number of young children experience difficulties using the FPS-R when rating pain in hypothetical vignettes, although the ability to use the scale does appear to improve with age [56].

A systematic review of observational (behavioral) measures of pain for children and adolescents aged 3 to 18 years was also commissioned by the Paediatric Initiative on Methods, Measurement, and Pain Assessment in Clinical Trials (PedIMMPACT) [59]. No single observational measure was broadly recommended for pain assessment across all contexts of pain—procedural pain, postoperative pain, critical care, and chronic pain.

In comparison to the measurement of pain severity, there has been comparatively little research on the measurement of other symptoms in pediatrics. A rating scale for nausea and vomiting based on verbal descriptors was used in a series of assessment studies in children with cancer aged 5–18 [36,65–67]. Child and parent ratings of children's nausea and emesis symptoms were assessed among 33 children (aged 1.7–17.5 years, median age 4.7 years) who were receiving identical chemotherapy for acute lymphoblastic leukemia [58]. While the psychometric properties of these measures were promising, they may not be appropriate measures in the context of acute pain.

Clinical Indicators for Management of Pediatric Chronic Pain and Cancer Pain

Although the desirable characteristics for pain treatment facilities caring for adults have been defined by the International Association for the Study of Pain [34], comparatively little information is available about the standards of care that are expected for children. Similarly, the evolution of quality programs for pediatric chronic pain and cancer pain management has been hampered by the fact that standards have not been defined and that measures of outcome for pediatric chronic and cancer pain management are still developing [28]. Standards and outcome measures are two major pillars of quality measurement sadly lacking in pediatric chronic pain management. One recent survey of the impact of pain management guidelines on clinical practice could not demonstrate improved pain control in the perception of children and their parents [68].

Despite the lack of standards and outcome measures, indicators can be created by consensus of clinicians based on extensive clinical experience in collaboration with their quality manager. The following points may be helpful clinical indicators for pediatric chronic and cancer pain management.

i) Access. Patients and their families want to access services in a timely manner. Timely access is not always possible, given the demand for services and the resources available. However, information about timeliness of access can be useful for reviewing booking systems, managing the frequency of patients and families who do not attend appointments, and arguing for increased resources where a demand can be demonstrated.

ii) Appropriateness. Children with chronic pain who are referred to a multidisciplinary chronic pain clinic frequently present with complex physical, psychological, social, and spiritual problems. In order to minimize repetitive assessments and questions, it is ideal to have all team members present for the initial assessment. This approach ensures that all team members are consistently informed and allows for more appropriate treatment planning.

iii) Effectiveness. Effective treatment for patients with complex pain problems requires identification of the goals of treatment. This approach allows clinicians to evaluate the effectiveness of their interventions in relation to the issues that have been identified as important by patients and their families.

iv) Patient-centered services. The patient and his or her family must be at the center of planning and implementation of care for chronic pain problems. To establish clear communication about treatment goals and plans, it is essential that health care providers give patients and family members written information. Written treatment plans provide clarity for all parties.

v) Safety. To improve the safety of medications used at home, it is important to educate children and their families about appropriate use and storage of medications.

vi) Outcome. With appropriate management and interventions, problems associated with chronic pain in children should be reduced. Outcome measures could include the demonstration of effectiveness of treatments and interventions and will help guide patient care and provide information about appropriate resources. These measures might include reduced pain, increased physical and psychological functioning, and improved school attendance. Ultimately, the achievement of the patient's own goals can be used as an overall indicator of the effectiveness of the interventions.

Clinical Indicators for Pediatric Palliative Care

Clinical indicators for pediatric palliative care currently in use cannot be identified. As such, clinical services must proceed with a consensus process in their creation. If consensus occurs, clinicians are more likely to use clinical indicators in service evaluation. Ideally, indicators should be collected at significant clinical episodes during the course of palliative care and should reflect defined standards. These episodes might include diagnosis, significant clinical episodes after diagnosis, the terminal phase and death, and bereavement.

Pediatric palliative care intervenes in the areas of physical and psychological symptom management, social support (including addressing family financial issues), spiritual and existential support, respite and bereavement support, and facilitating the hopes and expectations of the children and their families. The following may be helpful pediatric palliative care clinical indicators during the nonterminal palliative care period:

i) Equity of service provision. Respite care is seen as an important aspect of pediatric palliative care, particularly for children whose conditions are life limiting, but long-term. It can provide emotional and psychological support for families and for the children. It is important for all families to be offered respite care services to ensure equity of service provision. Recording numbers of families offered respite care will reflect the equity of service. Few offers of respite services might highlight issues of language or cultural barriers or a low profile for the respite care service.

ii) Facilitating the right location of care. Families who care for a child with a life-limiting condition often require some assistance at home. Although a pediatric palliative care service may not provide all the service directly, it is involved in establishing links with local services and acting as a resource for these services. Few offers of community services may indicate a hospital focus for care delivery and show a lack of community support to help families care for their child at home. Symptom management is a major focus of pediatric palliative care. Adequately planned and delivered palliative care will anticipate and address symptoms. Ideally, high-quality palliative care will deliver appropriate symptom management in the location of family choice, usually at or near home. A high hospital admission rate for symptom management may highlight a lack of resources and staff in palliative care or may indicate poor care planning, assessment, or care delivery.

iii) Child- and family-focused service delivery. High-quality palliative care requires service delivery by a multidisciplinary team in a variety of locations and includes the primary caregivers. A well-documented palliative care plan, which addresses issues of respite, community service, emergency plans, and symptom management, as well as identifying key team members and their contact details, will support communication among team members and provide the family with appropriate information. A high number of patients with a palliative care plan may indicate customer-focused service delivery.

End-of-Life Pediatric Palliative Care Indicators

i) Access to the right place at the right time. One of the aims of the palliative care service is to support families through the death of a child in a way that matches their hopes and expectations as closely as possible. One aspect of this goal is allowing the family/child to choose the location of death. Where possible, the palliative care team can try to assist in this process, although there may be some occasions where such assistance is not feasible. In addition, the preferred location expressed at the beginning of the terminal process may change a number of times during end-of-life care. A low number of patients dying in their preferred location may indicate poor service delivery in all aspects—poor symptom management, poor psychological support, poor spiritual support, poor nursing/medical support, poor social support—or overall inadequate communication with the family about their ongoing or changing needs and wishes.

ii) Care planning and symptom management. The management of physical symptoms is an important part of pediatric palliative care. The symptoms may be distressing for the patient or family, or both. These symptoms need to be fully assessed, and the care plan must minimize the distress being caused to the patient and family. A high number of patients whose distressing symptoms have been addressed indicates high-quality symptom assessment and care planning and implementation.

iii) Family education and social support. Social support is identified as a key part of good pediatric palliative care. If appropriate information is provided to families and caregivers, if adequate support is provided in the location of their choice, and if financial constraints do not prevent parents or family members from being with their child, then children should not be without the support of family members at the time of death. A high number of patients who did not die alone may indicate that social assessment and support were adequate to ensure that there were no barriers to caring for the dying child.

iv) Holistic care. While spiritual care is identified by the palliative care team (and the literature) as being one of the key domains of care, it is not easily provided by the health care team, nor is it necessarily appropriate for the team to play a role. We can, however, acknowledge the importance of spiritual care and offer to help patients and their families to link up with appropriate spiritual support. Satisfaction with spiritual support is a much harder aspect to measure. A high number of patients being offered spiritual support may reflect a holistic pediatric palliative care approach.

v) Admission to hospital. The pediatric palliative care service aims to provide care across several domains: home, hospice, and hospital. If the service is providing appropriate symptom management at home or in hospice, admission to the hospital should be unnecessary except at the request of the parents or patient. A high number of children being admitted to the hospital for symptom management at the end of life will reflect a poor quality of symptom management at home, because of inadequate resources/staffing, assessment or care delivery, or social support.

vi) Bereavement services. The role of the palliative care team does not end with the death of the child, and some ongoing support for the families is important. A high number of families being offered bereavement services may be an indication of thorough follow-up processes being in place. This variable could eventually be linked with the number of families accepting bereavement services, which will identify whether the services are appropriate for consumers.

Stage 5: Collate and Evaluate Data from the Quality Program and Look for Opportunities for Improvement

The reasons for collecting and evaluating data from a quality program are numerous, so a clear agreement on the aims of data collection and collation should be reached before implementation of a program. Possible aims could include:

- To ensure equity of care (making sure that all patients have access to the same opportunities).
- To identify problems with service delivery.
- To alert clinicians to aspects of care they may routinely overlook.
- To gather appropriate information for the justification of services and the debate on increases.

- To allow innovation and service improvement as a result of findings.

Data collection and collation should be an easy process with the use of clear templates and simple electronic or paper databases. Meaningful information can be gathered using descriptive statistics. Opportunities for improvement may be highlighted by collecting indicators, even after only a few months. Routinely, these data are reviewed at 6 months, but it may be worthwhile to do a review at 3 months as well. Data can be compared with similar clinical services collecting the same indicators, thus allowing benchmarking and peer review. Ultimately, the point of collecting data is to improve services. Once an opportunity for improvement has been identified, work must begin to identify how the service can be improved. Data collection for its own sake is wasted time and effort.

Stage 6: Implement Ongoing Quality Review as Part of Clinical Care

A quality program needs to be designed to be sustainable in the long term. Thus, the program needs:

- Input from all staff during development so that staff members share ownership of the program
- A data collection system that is easy and not time-consuming.
- Timely distribution of results to maximize usefulness of data and support from clinical staff for ongoing collection.
- The ability to adapt to changes in the delivery of care.
- Education for all clinical staff.

Some planning, including realistic timeframes and achievable goals, is necessary for a sustainable program. Over time, the process becomes imbedded and a normal part of the department's work. The available information can also be used to showcase the department, particularly for external review or accreditation processes. A good quality manager will eventually be out of a job, as clinicians gain skills in quality management and can continue to develop a quality program for themselves, with the support of consultation where necessary.

Research in Developmental Neurobiology and Pharmacology, Acute and Chronic Pediatric Pain Management, and Palliative Care

The care of a child in pain, regardless of the context, not only requires skills based on scientific evidence, but also demands expertise based on the art of and practice of caring for the distressed child and his or her family. A comparison of the ratio of the current scientific evidence to the art of caring makes it clear that the evidence base for pediatric acute and chronic and cancer pain is greater than that for pediatric palliative care. This research gap may be due to a multitude of reasons, including the facts that pediatric palliative care is a more recent clinical entity than pediatric pain management, that the number of subjects receiving palliative care is smaller, and that there is great heterogeneity in diagnosis across the clinical spectrum of palliative care.

Developmental Neurobiology

Nociceptive pathways are functional after birth, but postnatal changes in structure and function (including alterations in neurotransmitter levels and receptor distribution and function) can have a significant effect on the response to pain and analgesia. In addition, the enhanced plasticity of the developing nervous system can result in acute and long-term responses to injury that differ from those seen in the adult [23]. Pain processing in neonates and infants is complex and cannot be dismissed as simply a smaller version of that of an adult. Thus, data from studies conducted at older ages may not be directly applicable to early life. Laboratory studies in developmental models, such as the infant rat, allow bidirectional translation: mechanisms underlying age-related changes observed clinically can be investigated in the laboratory, and laboratory data can be used to inform clinical trials.

Developmental Pharmacology

Pharmacokinetic variables change rapidly after birth and contribute to changing analgesic dose requirements throughout postnatal development. The pharmacokinetic profile of analgesics is influenced by organ maturation, body composition, changes in protein concentration and binding, and alterations in drug elimination pathways [2]. Understanding age-related changes in pharmacokinetics has allowed refinement of dose recommendations for paracetamol (acetaminophen) [1,3] and intravenous morphine [11,35,37] in preterm and full-term neonates and infants. However, the correlation between pain score and plasma concentration is poor. This problem may relate to discrepancies between plasma and effect-site concentrations or to a large interindividual variability in kinetics [25,54,57]. Further details of analgesic use in neonates can be found in recent reviews and practice guidelines [4,10,27,57].

Developmentally regulated changes in nociceptive pathway structure and function can also have a significant impact on the response to analgesic agents. As a result, the pharmacodynamic profile of analgesic drugs can change with postnatal age, in a way that is difficult to fully evaluate in clinical studies. By enabling researchers to evaluate underlying mechanisms and quantify age-related changes, data from laboratory preclinical studies can inform and improve the design of clinical studies [9] by providing additional information on:

i) Analgesic efficacy and sensitivity to side effects, by showing dose-related effects at a range of postnatal ages in the rat pup [26,30,40,53,61,62].

ii) Changes in receptor expression and distribution that can contribute to the age-related differences in dose requirements, as shown for opioids [51].

iii) Developmental toxicity, as shown by recent data linking general anesthetics, including ketamine, with apoptosis (programmed cell death) in the developing brain [41].

Research and Pediatric Acute Pain Management

Progress in the management of acute pediatric pain management is contingent on the standardized use of observational and self-report pain severity measures in clinical trials. The use of observational scales is dependent on context, with separate measures for procedural and other brief acute pain, postoperative pain in hospital, postoperative pain at home, and critical care [59]. More recently, the PedIMMPACT group has reached a consensus on the self-report scales to be used in clinical trials in children and adolescents [42].

Recent progress in acute pain management for children includes improved management of procedural pain in infants and children (using pharmacological and/or nonpharmacological therapies), and increasing use of a range of local, regional, and systemically administered analgesics for postoperative pain. In many cases, advances have been supported by an increase in the quality and quantity of evidence-based data from pediatric trials. Further details are available in guidelines from the Australian and New Zealand College of Anaesthetists (www.anzca.edu.au) [8], the Child and Adolescent Heath Division, Royal Australasian College of Physicians (www.racp.edu.au), and the Association of Paediatric Anaesthetists of Great Britain and Ireland (www.apagbi.org.uk) [29a].

Although the pharmacokinetic and the major pharmacodynamic properties (analgesia and sedation) of most opioids have been studied in pediatrics and previously documented [64], little information is available about oral bioavailability, potency ratios, and other pharmacodynamic properties in children. There have been no controlled clinical trials of adjuvant analgesic agents in pediatrics.

Research and Pediatric Chronic Pain Management

The measurement of chronic pain in children should be multidimensional, including somatic, psychological, social, and behavioral information. The few measures that are available have varying psychometric properties [28]. These instruments include the Functional Disability Inventory [60] and the Bath Adolescent Pain Questionnaire [21]. The recently developed Pain Experience Questionnaire (PEQ) (child and parent versions) assesses the psychosocial impact of chronic pain in children [28]. It includes the subscales of pain severity, pain-related interference with activities, affective distress, and perceived social support. The parent version contains subscales for severity of the child's pain, interference with activities, and parental affective distress. Preliminary evaluation of the PEQ shows promising psychometric data.

The lack of pediatric chronic pain measures has hampered progress in this area of pain management. Although the epidemiology of chronic pain in children has been described [32], without adequate measures of outcome it is impossible to determine the effectiveness of the interventions of the pediatric chronic pain clinic.

Research and Pediatric Cancer Pain Management

The need to improve pain management in children with cancer is demonstrated by data indicating that pain is often inadequately assessed and treated in this population [63]. Improvement in pain management will be dependent not only on advances in pediatric analgesic therapeutics but also on strategies to remove the barriers to the adequate treatment of pain in these children.

The epidemiology of pain [45,47] and of intractable pain have been described in this patient population [16]. In addition, multidimensional symptom assessment scales for children with cancer have been validated [12,13]. More recent reports have described the strategy of opioid rotation [20] and discussed breakthrough pain in children with cancer [24]. Comparatively few analgesic studies have been performed in children with cancer. Although not insurmountable, there are general and specific problems related to conducting analgesic studies in these children.

The few analgesic studies performed in the setting of pediatric cancer pain have conformed to one of the following two objectives. The first is the evaluation of a drug proven efficacious in adult pain models but now targeted to the pediatric cancer pain population. For example, all the analgesic studies performed in children with cancer [43,44,46,48–50] had previously been performed in adults. Most of these studies had small numbers of subjects, and few were controlled studies. Only recently has self-report been used to measure the effectiveness of analgesia. The second objective is the evaluation of novel approaches to analgesic delivery [14,17,39] or of analgesic study design in this population [14,15].

Evolving Research in Pediatric Palliative Care

Progress in pediatric palliative care clinical research will be dependent on developing ways to measure physical and psychological symptom experience, research study designs that account for small numbers of patients in a heterogeneous population who are often extremely ill, and ways of studying social and spiritual experience in children.

To date, much of the therapeutic approach to physical symptom management in pediatric palliative care has relied on research data from adult palliative care or from acute, chronic, or cancer pain management in children. Although children with cancer account for many of those needing palliative care services, children with non-oncology diagnoses are common. Such children frequently need respite care and social support because they may survive for many years from diagnosis. Inadequate data and scientific knowledge impede efforts to deliver care, to educate clinicians to provide such care, and to design public policies that support pediatric palliative care initiatives [18].

The knowledge base for pediatric palliative care is increasing as services evolve and seek how best to care for this patient population and their families. This knowledge base is in currently in transition from an anecdotal-based practice to an evidence-based practice. This research base for pediatric palliative care now includes an understanding of the symptoms children experience at the end of life [19] and the epidemiology of their illnesses [22], as well as the nature of intractable pain in children with cancer and its causation. It also includes the content of physician communication that is valued by children and families receiving palliative care, especially prognostic information [31,38], and recognizes home as the geographical location of death for most children with chronic illnesses.

The Way Forward for Pediatric Palliative Care Research

The development of a more academic focus for pediatric palliative care can only occur with the allocation of financial resources for the establishment of pediatric palliative care academic units. The Committee on Palliative and End-of-Life Care for Children and their Families of the Institute of Medicine has prioritized research [18] looking at the effectiveness of clinical interventions including symptom management, methods of improving communication and decision making, service delivery and quality improvement, and different approaches to bereavement care. In addition, existing research networks must evolve toward national and even international collaborative approaches that prioritize these many research questions on symptom assessment and quality-of-life measures, as well as social and spiritual assessment.

Conclusion

Surveys have indicated the need for improved pain management for children with acute, chronic, and cancer pain and for children needing palliative care. Internationally, growth has been rapid in the number of services offered to these children. Many children's hospitals throughout the world have dedicated pain services and newly developed palliative care services for children. The continued advancement of these important areas of pediatric clinical practice can only be achieved through the development of pediatric acute, chronic, and cancer pain management and palliative care quality programs and through improved research output in these areas and allocation of resources to support these endeavors.

References

[1]   Allegaert K, Anderson BJ, Naulaers G, de Hoon J, Verbesselt R, Debeer A, Devlieger H, Tibboel D. Intravenous paracetamol (propacetamol) pharmacokinetics in term and preterm neonates. Eur J Clin Pharmacol 2004;60:191–7.
[2]   Anderson BJ, Holford NH. Mechanism-based concepts of size and maturity in pharmacokinetics. Annu Rev Pharmacol Toxicol 2008;48:303–32.
[3]   Anderson BJ, Meakin GH. Scaling for size: some implications for paediatric anaesthesia dosing. Paediatr Anaesth 2002;12:205–19.
[4]   Anderson BJ, Palmer GM. Recent developments in the pharmacological management of pain in children. Curr Opin Anaesthesiology 2006;19:285–92.
[5]   Aspinal F, Addington-Hall J, Hughes R, Higginson IJ. Using satisfaction to measure the quality of palliative care: a review of the literature. J Adv Nurs 2003;42:324–39.
[6]   Australian Council on Healthcare Standards. Available at: http://www.achs.org.au/ClinicalIndicators/2008.
[7]   Australian Department of Health and Ageing. Paediatric palliative care service model review. Australian Government Department of Health and Ageing; 2004.
[8]   Australian National Health and Medical Research Council. Acute pain management: scientific evidence, 2nd ed. National Health and Medical Research Council; 2005. Available at: http://www.anzca.edu.au/fpm/resources/books-and-publications.
[9]   Berde CB, Cairns B. Developmental pharmacology across species: promise and problems. Anesth Analg 2000;91:1–5.
[10] Berde CB, Jaksic T, Lynn AM, Maxwell LG, Soriano SG, Tibboel D. Anesthesia and analgesia during and after surgery in neonates. Clin Ther 2005;27:900–21.
[11] Bouwmeester NJ, Anderson BJ, Tibboel D, Holford NH. Developmental pharmacokinetics of morphine and its metabolites in neonates, infants and young children. Br J Anaesth 2004;92:208–17.
[12] Collins JJ, Byrnes ME, Dunkel IJ, Lapin J, Nadel T, Thaler HT, Polyak T, Rapkin B, Portenoy RK. The measurement of symptoms in children with cancer. J Pain Symptom Manage 2000;19:363–77.
[13] Collins JJ, Devine TB, Dick G, Johnson EA, Kilham HK. The measurement of symptoms in young children with cancer: the validation of the Memorial Symptom Assessment Scale in children aged 7–12. J Pain Symptom Manage 2002;23:10–6.
[14] Collins JJ, Dunkel IJ, Gupta SK, Inturrisi CE, Lapin J, Palmer LN, Weinstein SM, Portenoy RK. Transdermal fentanyl in children with cancer: feasibility, tolerability, and pharmacokinetic correlates. J Pediatr 1999;134:319–23.

[15] Collins JJ, Geake J, Grier HE, Houck CS, Thaler HT, Weinstein HJ, Twum-Danso NY, Berde CB. Patient-controlled analgesia for mucositis pain in children: a three-period crossover study comparing morphine and hydromorphone. J Pediatr 1996;129:722–8.

[16] Collins JJ, Grier HE, Kinney HC, Berde CB. Control of severe pain in terminal pediatric malignancy. J Pediatr 1995;126:653–7.

[17] Collins JJ, Grier HE, Sethna NF, Berde CB. Regional anesthesia for pain associated with terminal malignancy. Pain 1996;65:63–9.

[18] Committee on Palliative and End-of-Life Care for Children and their Families. In: Field MJ, Behrman RE, editors. When children die. Washington, DC: National Academies Press; 2001. p. 3.

[19] Drake R, Frost J, Collins JJ. The symptoms of dying children. J Pain Symptom Manage 2003;27:6–10.

[20] Drake R, Longworth J, Collins JJ. Opioid rotation in children with cancer. J Palliat Med 2004;7:419–22.

[21] Eccleston C, Jordan A, McCracken LM, Sleed M, Connell H, Clinch J. The Bath Adolescent Pain Questionnaire (BAPQ): development and preliminary psychometric evaluation of an instrument to assess the impact of chronic pain on adolescents. Pain 2005;118:263–70.

[22] Feudtner C, Hays RM, Haynes G, Geyer JR, Neff JM, Koepsell TD. Deaths attributed to pediatric complex chronic conditions: national trends and implications for supportive services. Pediatrics 2001;107:99.

[23] Fitzgerald M, Walker SM. Infant pain management: a developmental neurobiological approach. Nat Clin Pract Neurol. 2009;5:35–50.

[24] Friedrichsdorf S, Finney D, Bergin M, Stevens M, Collins JJ. Breakthrough pain in children with cancer. J Pain Symptom Manage 2007;34:209–16.

[25] Gibb IA, Anderson BJ. Paracetamol (acetaminophen) pharmacodynamics: interpreting the plasma concentrations. Arch Dis Child 2008;93:241–7.

[26] Gupta A, Cheng J, Wang S, Barr GA. Analgesic efficacy of ketorolac and morphine in neonatal rats. Pharmacol Biochem Behav 2001;68:635–40.

[27] Hammer GB, Golianu B. Opioid analgesia in neonates following cardiac surgery. Semin Fetal Neonatal Med 2007;11:47–58.

[28] Hermann C, Hohmeister J, Zohsel K, Tuttas ML, Flor H. The impact of chronic pain in children and adolescents: development and initial validation of a child and parent version of the Pain Experience Questionnaire. Pain 2008;135:251–61.

[29] Hicks CL, von Baeyer CL, Spafford P, van Korlaar I, Goodenough B. The Faces Pain Scale-Revised: toward a common metric in pediatric pain measurement. Pain 2001;93:173–83.

[29a] Howard R, Carter B, Curry J, Morton N, Rivett K, Rose M, Tyrrell J, Walker S, Williams G; Association of Paediatric Anaesthetists of Great Britain and Ireland. Good practice in postoperative and procedural pain management. Paediatr Anaesth 2008;18(Suppl 1):1–78.

[30] Howard RF, Hatch D, Cole TJ, Fitzgerald M. Inflammatory pain and hypersensitivity are selectively reversed by epidural bupivacaine and are developmentally regulated. Anesthesiology 2001;95:421–7.

[31] Hsiao JL, Evan EE, Zeltzer L. Parent and child perspectives on physician communication in pediatric palliative care. Palliat Support Care 2007;5:355–65.

[32] Hunfeld JAM, Perquin CW, Duivenvoorden HJ, Hazebroek-Kampschreur AA, Passchier J, van Suijlekom-Smit LW, van der Wouden JCChronic pain and its impact on quality of life in adolescents and their families. J Pediatr Psychol 2001;26:145–53.

[33] IMPaCCT. Standards for paediatric palliative care in Europe. Eur J Palliat Care 2007;14:109–14.

[34] International Association for the Study of Pain. Task Force on Guidelines for Desirable Characteristics for Pain Treatment Facilities. Desirable characteristics for pain treatment facilities. Available at: http://www.iasp-pain.org.

[35] Kart T, Christrup LL, Rasmussen M. Recommended use of morphine in neonates, infants and children based on a literature review: Part 2. Clinical use. Paediatr Anaesth 1997;7:93–101.

[36] LeBaron S, Zeltzer L. Behavioral intervention for reducing chemotherapy-related nausea and vomiting in adolescents with cancer. J Adolesc Health Care 1984;5:182.

[37] Lynn A, Nespeca MK, Bratton SL, Shen DD. Intravenous morphine in postoperative infants: intermittent bolus dosing versus targeted continuous infusions. Pain 2000;88:89–95.

[38] Mack J, Cook F, Wolfe J, Grier HE, Cleary PD, Weeks JC. Understanding prognosis among parents of children with cancer: parental optimism and the parent-physician interaction. J Clin Oncol 2007;25:1357–62.

[39] Mackie AM, Coda BC, Hill HF. Adolescents use patient controlled analgesia effectively for relief for relief from prolonged oropharyngeal mucositis pain. Pain 1991;46:265–9.

[40] Marsh D, Dickenson AH, Hatch D, Fitzgerald M. Epidural opioid analgesia in infant rats I: mechanical and heat responses. Pain 1999;82:23–32.

[41] Mellon RD, Simone AF. Use of anesthetic agents in neonates and young children. Anesth Analg 2007;104:509–20.

[42] McGrath PJ, Walco G, Turk DC, Dworkin RH, Brown MT, Davidson K, Eccleston C, Finley GA, Goldschneider K, Haverkos L, et al. Core outcome domains and measures for pediatric acute and chronic/recurrent clinical trials: PedIMMPACT recommendations. J Pain 2008;9:771–83.

[43] Miser AW, Davis DM, Hughes CS, Mulne AF, Miser JS. Continuous subcutaneous infusion of morphine in children with cancer. Am J Dis Child 1983;137:383–5.

[44] Miser AW, Dothage JA, Miser JS. Continuous intravenous fentanyl for pain control in children and young adults with cancer. Clin J Pain 1987;2:101–6.

[45] Miser AW, Dothage JA, Wesley RA, Miser JS. The prevalence of pain in a pediatric and young adult population. Pain 1987;29:265–6.

[46] Miser AW, Goh TS, Dose AM, O'Fallon JR, Niedringhaus RD, Betcher DL, Simmons P, MacKellar DJ, Arnold M, Loprinzi CL. Trial of a topically administered local anesthetic (EMLA cream) for pain relief during central venous port accesses in children with cancer. J Pain Symptom Manage 1994;9:259–64.

[47] Miser AW, McCalla J, Dothage P, Wesley M, Miser JS. Pain as a presenting symptom in children and young adults with newly diagnosed malignancy. Pain 1987;29:363–77.

[48] Miser AW, Miser JS. The use of oral methadone to control moderate and severe pain in children and young adults with malignancy. Clin J Pain 1985;1:243–8.

[49] Miser AW, Miser JS, Clark BS. Continuous intravenous infusion of morphine sulfate for control of severe pain in children with terminal malignancy. J Pediatr 1980;96:930–3.

[50] Miser AW, Moore L, Greene R. Prospective study of continuous intravenous and subcutaneous morphine infusions for therapy-related or cancer-related pain in children and young adults with cancer. Clin J Pain 1986;2:101–6.

[51] Nandi R, Fitzgerald M. Opioid analgesia in the newborn. Eur J Pain 2005;9:105–8.

[52] Palliative Care Australia. Standards for providing quality palliative care for all Australians. Palliative Care Australia; 2005. Available at: http://www.palliativecare.org.au.

[53] Sanders RD, Giobini M. Dexmedetomidine exerts dose-dependent age-independent antinociception but age-dependent hypnosis in Fischer rats. Anesth Analg 2005;100:1295–302.

[54] Scott CS. Morphine pharmacokinetics and pain assessment in premature newborns. J Pediatr 1999;135:423–9.

[55] Siden H. Quality assurance. In: Goldman A, Hain R, Liben S, editors. Oxford textbook of palliative care for children. Oxford: Oxford University Press; 2006. p. 573–93.

[56] Stanford EA, Chambers CT, Craig KD. The role of developmental factors in predicting young children's use of a self-report scale for pain. Pain 2006;120:16–23.

[57] Tibboel D, Anand KJ, van den Anker JN. The pharmacological treatment of neonatal pain. Semin Fetal Neonatal Med 2005;10:195–205.

[58] Tyc VL, Mulhern RK, Fairclough D, Ward PM, Relling MV, Longmire W. Chemotherapy induced nausea and emesis in pediatric cancer patients: external validity of child and parent ratings. Dev Behav Pediatr 1993;14:236–41.

[59] von Baeyer CL, Spagrud LJ. Systemic review of observational (behavioral) measures of pain for children and adolescents aged 3 to 18 years. Pain 2007;127:140–50.

[60] Walker LS, Greene JW. The Functional Disability Inventory: measuring a neglected dimension of child health status. J Pediatr Psychol 1991;16:39–58.

[61] Walker SM, Fitzgerald M. Characterization of spinal alpha-adrenergic modulation of nociceptive transmission and hyperalgesia throughout postnatal development in rats. Br J Pharmacol 2007;151:1334–42.

[62] Williams D, Dickenson AH, Fitzgerald M, Howard RF. Developmental regulation of codeine analgesia in the rat. Anesthesiology 2004;100:92–7.

[63] Wolfe J, Grier HE, Klar N, Wolfe J, Grier HE, Klar N. Symptoms and suffering at the end of life in children with cancer. N Engl J Med 2000;342:326–33.

[64] Yaster M, Maxwell LG. Opioid agonists and antagonists. In: Schechter NL, Berde CB, Yaster M, editors. Pain in infants, children and adolescents. 2nd ed. Baltimore: Williams and Wilkins; 2002.

[65] Zeltzer L, LeBaron S. Effects of the mechanics of administration on doxorubicin-induced side effects: a case report. Am J Pediatr Hematol Oncol 1984;6:212–5.

[66] Zeltzer L, LeBaron S, Zeltzer PM. A prospective assessment of chemotherapy related nausea and vomiting in children with cancer. Am J Pediatr Hematol Oncol 1984;6:5–16.

[67] Zeltzer L, Kellerman J, Ellenberg L, Dash J. Hypnosis for reduction of vomiting associated with chemotherapy and disease in adolescents with cancer. J Adolesc Health Care 1983;4:84.

[68] Zernikow B, Hasan C, Hechler T, Huebner B, Gordon D, Michel E. Stop the pain! A nation-wide quality improvement programme in paediatric oncology pain control. Eur J Pain 2008;12:819–33.

Correspondence to: John J. Collins, MB BS, PhD, FRACP, Department of Pain Medicine and Palliative Care, The Children's Hospital at Westmead, Sydney, NSW 2145, Australia. Email: johnc4@chw.edu.au.

16

Pain in the Developing World

M.R. Rajagopal

Pallium India; Department of Pain and Palliative Medicine, Sree Uthradam Thirunal Academy of Medical Sciences, Pattom, Trivandrum, Kerala, India

Although we lack reliable statistics, we know that there is a huge pain burden in the developing world. In the year 2000, more than 70% of the seven million deaths from cancer in the world occurred in low- and middle-income countries [13]. The American Cancer Society estimates that in the year 2007, there were 12 million new cancer cases in the world, of which 6.7 million would have been in economically developing countries [1]. About 70% of people with cancer experience pain at some time during their illness, and hence the burden of pain from cancer alone in developing countries is enormous [2]. If we take all types of chronic pain into consideration, even with a very conservative estimate of only 5% of the population having chronic pain, 250 million people in the developing world would be in pain.

In the absence of reliable data, national morphine consumption becomes a useful, although indirect, index of pain relief. However, 10 developed countries account for 75% of consumption of medical morphine in the world, indicating the appalling state of affairs in the developing world [12]. Most of the suffering is unnecessary. It has been demonstrated in the developing world that such pain can be effectively treated at low cost. What is needed is to make the latest knowledge and essential resources available to health care professionals and the public.

The Nature of Pain and Suffering in the Developing World

It is widely recognized that pain is not just a sensation; it is also an emotional experience [4]. Understandably, therefore, the pain experience is dependent on the sociocultural context in which it occurs. As an example to demonstrate this point, the following case history describes a patient treated by my team in Kerala, India.

Illustrative Case Study

Mr. K is a 42-year-old Indian plumber who felt a sudden stab of pain at work more than 3 years ago. He had excruciating pain in his back extending down to his legs. There is no effective socialized medicine in India, and the average worker has no access to health insurance. Therefore, Mr. K's medical expenses had to be paid out-of-pocket. A magnetic resonance imaging (MRI) scan (which he could ill afford) showed lumbar intervertebral disk prolapse with nerve root compression, and he was advised to have surgery. A diskectomy was performed that completely relieved his pain. Mr. K was in debt by this time. In about 9 months, the pain reappeared, and gradually it got much worse. When he was seen in our pain and palliative care clinic, he complained of pain with a score of 10 (on a 0–10 numerical scale) on the slightest movement, and a score of 7 when lying absolutely still. He was found to have intense paraspinal muscle spasm, lumbosacral radiculopathy, and severe allodynia over the surgical scar. He had seen many doctors, but they seldom brought relief. Travel costs, consultation fees, and the cost of medications had brought the family to the verge of starvation. All the doctors had advised a repeat MRI scan, and Mr. K's wife carried a burden of guilt about not being able to afford it. The most common prescriptions Mr. K received were for tramadol (the most expensive oral opioid in the country) and either gabapentin or pregabalin (the most expensive oral medications for neuropathic pain). Mr. K said he had often contemplated suicide, but the thought of his wife and children had kept him from attempting it.

Our team is supported partly by a nongovernmental organization (NGO) called Pallium India and partly by the philanthropic outreach of a private hospital (Sree Uthradam Thirunal hospital). Fortunately (and rather unusually for most of the developing world), we were at least able to offer him free outpatient care and free analgesics, but hospitalization was not possible unless he could pay for it. Further expensive investigations were out of the question. Our team offered free weekly home visits to bedridden patients, but only within a radius of 35 kilometers from our clinic. As Mr. K lived farther away, and there was no such service anywhere in his neighborhood, it was necessary to give him the best possible pain relief before we sent him home at the end of the day. This case was a pain emergency.

As was our routine practice in pain emergencies [3,6,7], after offering the patient an adequate explanation, we inserted a butterfly needle into a forearm vein (an i.v. cannula was considered needlessly expensive). We then gave the patient metoclopramide 10 mg i.v. as a prophylactic anti-emetic. This injection was followed by 1.5-mg bolus doses of i.v. morphine every 10 minutes. In this regime, the endpoint of morphine therapy was either complete pain relief or drowsiness. Mr. K had significant pain relief with 9 mg of morphine, but he became a bit drowsy. He was started on oral morphine and paracetamol (acetaminophen).

A crisis occurred when a well-meaning doctor advised Mr. K to stop taking morphine, warning him that morphine would not only make him an addict but also harm his children as they might steal his morphine and get addicted too. A very disturbed Mr. K came back to us. If we had failed to educate him about morphine in advance, he might have lost trust in us completely. Fortunately, we were able to convince him to go back on morphine.

Our NGO had to find the funds for further investigations, which showed that he did have a significant nerve root compression at a level other than the one operated on. He underwent three weekly injections of epidural triamcinolone and several injections of local anesthetic into myofascial trigger points. His pain came down, and he was weaned off oral morphine.

Mr. K still has some residual pain, but he is able to have an active life on imipramine 25 mg daily and paracetamol when necessary. He was not able to go back to plumbing, but the NGO's rehabilitation program bought him goats to rear and pays the expenses for his children's schooling.

Issues Arising out of the Case Study

Barriers to Pain Relief

Mr. K's story illustrates some of the barriers to pain relief in many parts of the developing world. Even when resources are scarce, often there is access to high-tech modalities of investigations and management, but no access to basic pharmacotherapy. There are several reasons for this situation. Pharmacotherapy, especially when drugs are inexpensive, is neither glamorous like high-tech invasive procedures, nor commercially attractive. But even when there are committed practitioners who want to provide pain management, there are several barriers. First and foremost, regulatory barriers to opioids are considerable. Opioids are often either unavailable or available under such great restrictions as to make access to them practically impossible. The medical licensing system is often complicated. Multiple licences are often needed, and they may expire before the next one can be obtained [5]. Prescription requirements are cumbersome, discouraging doctors from writing prescriptions for opioids.

In addition, fear of opioids is widespread among professionals and the public. Hence, opioids are often avoided even when available. The fear is perpetuated because pain relief is neither practiced by most doctors nor taught to medical students. Another problem is that even when it is available, pain management is usually not multidisciplinary. Thus, pain tends to be managed as a sensation rather than as an emotional experience. In the absence of a multidisciplinary approach, psychosocial issues are ignored.

A Need for Regionally Adapted Guidelines

Mr. K's story highlights several points that could be relevant to pain management in most of the developing world. First, pain management needs to be geared to local realities. If Mr. K's pain was not controlled to some extent on his first visit, it is unlikely that he would have returned, considering all the sacrifices that he had to make to come in to the clinic. The intravenous morphine titration, we believe, helped in this situation by providing quick control of the pain, by giving us an idea about the opioid sensitivity of the pain, and by giving the patient confidence that the pain was amenable to treatment. In many parts of the developing world, i.v. morphine may not be available, and even when it is available, there may not be enough manpower to perform the procedure. Therefore, research is needed on the adaptation of the World Health Organization (WHO) analgesic ladder to suit local realities. Rather than blindly copying the WHO analgesic ladder that is used in the developed world, a regional adaptation of the ladder is necessary.

Combined Pharmacotherapy and Interventional Procedures

Mr. K may need skilled pharmacotherapy for the rest of his life. Moreover, it is doubtful that the same results could have been achieved without the interventional procedures we performed. Interventional procedures should not be considered as a last resort if the pharmacotherapeutic steps of the WHO analgesic ladder should fail; they are to be used as and when they are indicated, along with pharmacotherapy.

A Need for Psychosocial Support

If the approach to the problem of pain were to be based purely on the physical domain, it is doubtful if the same results could be obtained. Counseling, screening for depression or anxiety, social support, and rehabilitation are all necessary parts of the management process.

Integrating Principles of Palliative Care into Pain Management

Unlike the situation in much of the developed world, neither pain services nor palliative care programs are widely available in the developing world. People in pain usually have other symptoms and psychosocial problems, and hence the strategy of combining pain management and palliative care principles has a major advantage in developing countries.

Lessons from Kerala, India

Mr. K's case study is a success story that took place in Kerala, a state in southern India. A community-based movement that started 15 years back in the city of Calicut has now evolved into a network of more than 125 pain and palliative care centers (Fig. 1). Most are run by NGOs and rely on trained volunteers, many of whom are trained to assess pain and are

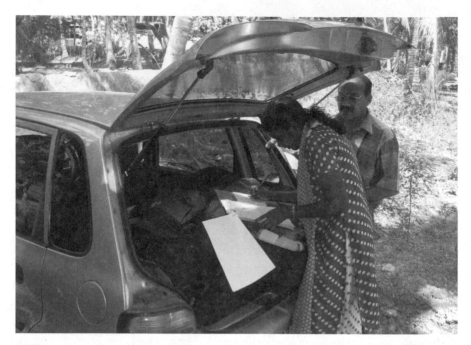

Fig. 1. A nurse dispenses morphine and other medications from the trunk of a car during a home visit in rural Kerala, South India.

taught basic counseling skills. Each center offers the services of a doctor and a nurse who have had some training in pain management and palliative care. This system now looks after thousands of patients, most of whom receive home visits if they are unable to travel to a clinic.

The movement recognizes that all three sides of a triangle (Fig. 2)—policy, education, and opioid availability—need to be addressed if such a system is to succeed. Several institutions in India now offer basic

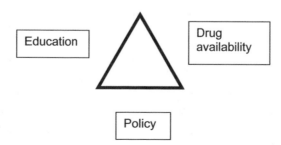

Fig. 2. All three sides of the triangle need to be satisfied for effective functioning of a pain relief program.

education in pain management and palliative care for doctors and nurses. However, progress in this area is grossly inadequate. Even today, only about six of approximately 300 medical schools in the country include systematic pain management in their curriculum.

Concurrent Work on Opioid Availability

A study was undertaken at Calicut, in which 1,723 patients received morphine over a 2-year period to demonstrate the use of morphine in the home setting. The study found no evidence of diversion or misuse [10]. This finding became an important tool in convincing skeptics about the safety of the drug. In addition, a collaborative venture between the Pain and Policy Studies Group at Madison University, Wisconsin, USA, and Indian palliative care enthusiasts has resulted in simplification of "narcotic regulations" in 13 of India's 28 states. Access to opioids has improved at least in some of them [9].

The Need for Action

Experience from Kerala [8,11] tells us that pain in the developing world can be tackled if (1) affordability is taken into consideration before pain management measures are instituted; (2) a multidisciplinary approach to pain management is adopted within the financial constraints in the region; (3) pharmacotherapy is combined with interventional procedures as and when needed; (4) access to essential medications, particularly opioids, is ensured by addressing regulatory barriers and by overcoming fear of opioids; (5) professionals are educated in the principles of pain assessment and management, and (6) public awareness about the possibilities of pain management is improved.

The international community is realizing more and more that most of the pain burden in the world is in developing countries. There may still be some lack of clarity about the action that is required. A combined approach integrating the following strategies could well be the best plan to pursue: need-based research and development of guidelines, advocacy for governmental policy and improved opioid availability, support for realistic educational programs, and support for emerging pain relief programs. Professional education on pain management, integration of principles of palliative care and psychosocial support into pain management programs, the right combination of pharmacotherapy and interventional management, overcoming regulatory barriers to opioid access, and development of guidelines suited to the local sociocultural milieu could become part of a realistic action plan for the future.

References

[1]   American Cancer Society. Global facts and figures 2007. Available at: http://www.cancer.org/docroot/STT/content/STT_1x_Global_Cancer_Facts_and_Figures_2007.asp. Accessed 16 October 2006.
[2]   Foley KM. The treatment of cancer pain. N Engl J Med 1985;313:84–95.
[3]   Harris JT, Suresh Kumar K, Rajagopal MR. Intravenous morphine for rapid control of severe cancer pain. Palliat Med 2003;17:248–56.
[4]   IASP Subcommittee on Taxonomy. Pain terms: a list with definitions and notes on usage. Pain 1980;8:249–52.
[5]   Joranson DE, Rajagopal MR, Gilson AM. Improving access to opioid analgesics for palliative care in India. J Pain Symptom Manage 2002;26:2:152–9.
[6]   Kumar KS, Rajagopal MR, Naseema AM. Intravenous morphine for emergency treatment of cancer pain. Palliat Med 2000;14:183–8.
[7]   Rajagopal MR. Cancer pain emergencies. J Pain Symptom Manage 1998;15:264–5.
[8]   Rajagopal MR. Relief from chronic pain when resources are limited. Update Anaesth 2002;15:2–6.
[9]   Rajagopal MR, Joranson DE. India: opioid availability—an update. J Pain Symptom Manage 2007;33:5:615–22.
[10] Rajagopal MR, Joranson DE, Gilson AM. Medical use, misuse and diversion of opioids in India. Lancet 2001;358:139–43.
[11] Rajagopal MR, Sureshkumar K. A model for delivery of palliative care in India: the Calicut experiment. J Palliat Care 1999;11:451–4.
[12] Salas-Herrera IG, Monestel R Costa Rica marks improvement in morphine consumption. J Pain Symptom Manage 2002;24:286–8.
[13] World Health Organization. Global burden of cancer in the year 2000: Version 1 estimates. Available at: http://www.who.int/healthinfo/statistics/bod_malignantneoplasmscancers.pdf. Accessed 16 October 2008.

Correspondence to: M.R. Rajagopal, MD, MNAMS PJRRA 65, Santhi, Pothujanam Road, Kumarapuram, Trivandrum 695011, India. Email: pallium.india@gmail.com.

Pain and Suffering Following Torture
John D. Loeser Distinguished Lecture

Inge Genefke and Bent Sørensen

International Rehabilitation Council for Torture Victims, Copenhagen, Denmark

The Definition of Torture

The Convention against Torture and Other Cruel, Inhuman or Degrading Treatment or Punishment was adopted by the United Nations General Assembly in consensus on 10 December, 1984, and went into force on June 26, 1987 [21]. By June of 2008, 145 countries (out of a possible 193) had ratified the convention.

Countries that ratify the convention are instructed to write its articles into national law. Many countries write the convention into national law directly, while others, such as Denmark, have a dualistic system. Independently of the procedure used, the provisions of the convention must be adopted into law in each individual country ratifying the convention and must be given the force of law of that country.

The legislation of the convention is a model of clarity. Article 1 gives a definition of torture. Four conditions must be met in order that an activity can be described as torture in legally binding terms. If one of the conditions is not met, the activity cannot be named torture. Those conditions are: (1) "severe pain or suffering, whether physical or mental," (2) "intentionally inflicted, " (3) "for such purposes," and (4) "inflicted by ... a public official." An analysis of these four points will illuminate why pain after torture often results in chronic pain, and will show that pain after torture differs in many ways, both physically and mentally, from pain after a disease.

1) *"severe pain"*: Our first observation is that the determination of whether or not pain is "severe" often can only be made by the victim or patient, or by a medical doctor or psychologist. Our second observation is that pain resulting from torture is nearly always both physical *and* mental. "Non-torture pain," in contrast, is often either physical *or* mental. A third observation is that "non-torture pain" is usually a serious problem if the patient does not know the reason for the pain, which creates a feeling of anxiety and fear. Patients do not know why they feel pain, or when the pain will start or stop. Could the pain be a warning sign of death? However, when the doctor has cleared up some of the problems, the pain may be considered acceptable and a part of life. Rational treatment and rehabilitation can start. In contrast, in the mind of the tortured person, there are no doubts. Torture victims know what actions have created the pain. Sometimes they understand the reasons for the pain. But they never know if or when the pain will stop.

2) *"intentionally"*: This single word holds the key to understanding the difference between pain from disease and pain resulting from torture. Torture is the only disease produced *intentionally*. All other diseases are created by cancer, bacteria, viruses, and so on. Torture pain is man-made—inflicted by a fellow human being acting in cold blood and not in anger.

3) *"for a purpose"*: The perpetrator is not an insane person acting sadistically. No, he or she serves a purpose. There is a reason for the act of torture, and a very cruel one.

4) *"a public official"*: The act is performed by a public person acting on behalf of the state. The victim understands that it is *his or her own state government that is responsible*.

When "non-torture pain" occurs, the patient perceives it as an "act of God," in a nonreligious way. The patient has a condition that is certainly painful, but with the help of professionals, the pain may be relieved. However, when pain is a result of torture, the victim realizes that the pain is produced intentionally and that it will not be relieved; on the contrary, it will continue. The perpetrators often stress the continuation of pain. It is in this way that torture-related pain stands in absolute contrast to non-torture-related pain. This is, in our opinion, the main basis for the specific aspects of pain suffered by torture victims, and it is also the reason why so many victims have pain after their release from torture, and why their pain is chronic.

Torture is the worst of all traumas because: (1) It causes unbearable physical and psychological pain. (2) It is impossible to escape. (3) You cannot fight against it. If you do, you risk death. (4) Many people die under torture. Many died under the terrible water-boarding torture, which President Bush claimed not to be torture. (5) Torture is not inflicted by a savage animal, such as a crocodile, but by a person in the shape of a human being.

One of Kipling's poems in "Just So Stories" (1902) presents a useful starting point for a discussion of torture:

> I keep six honest serving men
> (They taught me all I knew);
> Their names are *What*, and *Why*, and *When*,
> And *How*, and *Where*, and *Who*.

What is torture? The official definition of torture can be found in the Convention, article 1. Torture is the most horrible, the most disgusting, and the most perverted act.

Why torture? In dictatorships, tyrants use torture to stay in power. Torture is used to break courageous people who struggle for democracy. In wartime, torture is used to obtain information. In some democratic countries, torture is used in peacetime by the police to obtain information or confessions.

When? In wartime and in democratic countries, torture is mainly performed just after arrest, and in dictatorships it occurs not only in police stations but also in prisons.

How? We know all about the methods of torture—physical, psychological, and social.

Where? Torture is performed in more than 100 countries throughout the world. We know the names of the countries, as well as the locations within these countries, where torture is being performed.

Who? In dictatorships, torture may be directed at courageous people who are trying to obtain better conditions for the people in their country and thereby advance the cause of democracy, but dictators also torture people at random to spread anxiety and fear in the population. In armed conflict, combatants as well as civilians may suffer torture. In democratic countries, criminals (arrested for theft, fraud, rape, etc.) may undergo torture.

The Effect of Torture on Victims

Physical Sequelae

Usually, physical torture leaves symptoms and physical signs. These sequelae are often the basis for a documentation of physical torture [17]. Not least for documentary purposes, it is important to examine the victim immediately after the torture, because traces may disappear over time. Certain types of torture are related to specific symptoms and signs. Here again, it is extremely important for later documentation or for court cases to establish, if possible, a causal link between a specific form of torture and the symptoms that develop [5,13].

Chronic and late-onset physical sequelae are related to the severity of the methods used. Many torture victims coming for treatment have numerous physical complaints, and frequently they initially describe physical rather than psychological symptoms. It is therefore important to mention a few physical sequelae.

Chronic pains in the head, back, abdomen, or chest are often the major complaints; these problems may recur years after torture [3]. Such problems must be addressed, but they require physical examination and evaluation in a slower and less invasive manner than usual, and they may be a manifestation of a primary psychiatric problem. Chronic pain and tension that increase the general tension of the musculature, resulting in fibrositis, fibromyalgia, and myofascial pain, are the subject of an increasing body of research [22]. In survivors of falanga, we find smashed heels, and the rate of walking is slow and the distance limited [19].

It is characteristic that complaints related to the musculoskeletal system are the most prevalent and also the most objective medical findings. In an investigation of 50 torture survivors, Juhler and Smidt-Nielsen [11] found a discrepancy between the large number of physical complaints and the small number of objective medical findings, with the exception of musculoskeletal findings. Whereas 86% of patients expressed neurological complaints, there were objective findings in only 22% of cases. The situation was similar for cardiopulmonary and gastrointestinal complaints, where the corresponding percentages amounted to 74% versus 14% and 68% versus 24%, respectively. The survivors may feel reassured to know that their symptoms are not organically based, because they often fear that the torture has inflicted lasting damage.

Sexual torture may leave traces in the musculoskeletal system, including structural injuries, functional disturbances, and dysfunction of the pelvic joints in women and impotence in men. Women also often have low back pain and may complain about genital pain, menstrual disturbances, and sexual problems [16]. Sexual dysfunction and testicular atrophy are seen following electrical torture on the genitals [6].

Psychological Sequelae

The psychological consequences of torture are frequently persistent and incapacitating. At an early stage, the Rehabilitation and Research Centre for Torture Victims in Denmark reported that the worst sequelae of torture were psychological, as later confirmed by international studies (e.g., [12]). An increasing body of research and theory has emerged, mainly in Western countries, over the last few decades as a result of studies in torture survivors among refugees.

One of the most important questions relates to the continuing debate over the classification of trauma-related problems. After the introduction of the diagnosis of post-traumatic stress disorder (PTSD) in the *Diagnostic and Statistical Manual* (DSM-III) in 1980, a generic theory was proposed that would unify previous approaches to the long-lasting psychological effects of trauma. This theory stated that different types of trauma, such as combat experience, child abuse, sexual abuse, and torture, may provoke similar psychopathology. However, PTSD as a diagnostic category has proven inadequate to encompass the entire symptomatology of torture survivors [4,18].

Over time, terms such as "complex PTSD," "continuous training stress response" [10], and "torture syndrome" [8] have been used to denote the complexity of torture trauma. Initially, attempts to identify the key features of the effects of torture were subsumed under the heading of "torture syndrome." This proposal was based on a combination of thorough medical, including psychiatric, examinations of the short- and long-term effects of both physical and psychological torture in asylum seekers.

Primarily because of the major methodological problems that beset such research, the answers have been inconclusive. Important questions that need to be addressed include whether torture involves a specific syndrome, i.e., whether it results in a predictable phenomenology. Those in favor of this view claim that the infliction of deliberate violence on one human being by another has a decisive influence on the formation of symptoms [20]. Similarly, Gelinas [7] points to the differences between "facticity" (e.g., breaking a leg in an accident) and "agency" as causes of trauma, suggesting that the malevolent intention of the perpetrator induces the most extreme trauma.

Current knowledge has established that torture is a very important life stressor that causes numerous other stress-related events. Survivors may lose their physical, mental, and spiritual health, their work, their family, their status within their family and within society, and, if exiled, their country, language, and cultural environment [1,14].

From a psychological point of view, and as reported in a variety of settings, the prevailing manifestations include anxiety, depression, irritability, emotional instability, cognitive memory and attention problems, personality changes, behavioral disturbances, symptoms related to the autonomic nervous system (such as lack of energy), insomnia, nightmares, and sexual dysfunction [9].

Table I, based on the DSM-IV diagnostic categories from the American Psychiatric Association [2], presents the most frequent psychiatric symptoms observed by psychotherapists. Nine of the most common symptoms are encompassed by the diagnostic criteria for PTSD. It is noteworthy that the symptoms "change in personality" and "survivor's guilt" are included in the revision of PTSD in DSM-IV under the heading of associated descriptive symptoms. These symptoms are mentioned among a number of symptoms that are commonly seen in association with an interpersonal stressor.

In the World Health Organization's *International Classification of Diseases* (ICD-10) of 1992, two diagnostic categories are of importance.

Table I
The 10 most common psychological sequelae
of torture

1) Anxiety
2) Changed identity
3) Reduced self-respect
4) Feelings of guilt
5) Constant nightmares, sleep disturbances
6) Sexual problems
7) Being easily tired out
8) Reduced concentration
9) Reduced memory
10) Not wanting to talk about torture

One category is "post-traumatic stress disorder" (F43.1), and the other is "enduring personality change after catastrophic experience" (F62.0). The stress disorder should appear within 6 months of the catastrophic experience. The diagnostic guidelines for the latter category emphasize that the change should cause significant interference with daily personal functioning and must represent inflexible and maladaptive features. It must have been present for at least 2 years and should not be attributable to a preexisting personality disorder or to a mental disorder other than PTSD.

Torture as a Transgenerational Problem

In the past few years, we have begun to look very seriously at the effect of torture on children [15]. Torture is performed on children in a number of countries, sometimes for the purpose of exerting pressure on the parents, who are often forced to witness the act. In some countries, homeless children are tortured in order to force them off the streets. But often, children become victims of torture in a more indirect way. Torture endured by a parent causes great disturbance to the entire family. Parents often cannot give the necessary explanations, and their silence creates fearful fantasies and guilt in their children. Some parents become overly protective, and others cannot care for their children in an emotionally satisfactory way. Thus, torture is a transgenerational problem and should be treated as such. The effects of torture expand to the entire family. This spill-over effect magnifies the devastating results of torture.

Torture and Terror

The events of September 11, 2001 have been used throughout the world as an excuse for allowing torture as a method of investigation. In our opinion, (and according to international conventions), torture should never be allowed; that also applies to the interrogation and treatment of alleged terrorists. If we use the same methods as terrorists, we have lost our moral identity and thereby made the fight against terror meaningless. Below we list some practical reasons why torture is never appropriate.

1) Torture is prohibited according to the United Nations Convention Against Torture (UNCAT). According to UNCAT, ratified by 140 countries, torturers must be punished by national legal procedures.

2) Torture is not an adequate instrument for retrieving reliable information. Thirty years of research confirm this fact; contrary to popular belief, torture is very unreliable for such purposes, because people may say anything—truth or lies—when they are subjected to torture. However, torture is an excellent tool for destroying the personality of a human being. Thus, when political torture is exercised, the purpose is to destroy people.

3) The use of torture is a slippery slope. Once you start, there seem to be no limits to where it will end.

4) A state allowing torture ends up with a brutal, inhumane, traumatized, and uncivilized society, in which survival of the physically fittest prevails at the cost of the survival of a humane and civilized society.

5) Torture has never solved political problems; instead, it has created problems. This applies in the short term as well as over the long term.

6) Torture creates more terrorists: for each terror suspect who is tortured, 10 more terrorists will emerge. The French author Albert Camus made this claim during the Algerian war, and we can confirm that it is true.

Above, we cited the first verse of a poem by Kipling. We will end this chapter by quoting the second verse:

> I send them over land and sea,
> I send them east and west;
> But after they have worked for me,
> I give them all a rest.

References

[1] Allen K. The physiological consequences of torture. In: Peel M, Iacopino V, editors. The medical documentation of torture. London: Greenwich Medical Media; 2002. p. 117–32.

[2] American Psychiatric Association. Diagnostic and statistical manual and mental disorders. Fourth ed. Washington, DC: American Psychiatric Press; 1994. p. 427–8.

[3] Amris K. Physiotherapy for torture victims. Chronic pain in torture victims: possibly mechanism of pain. Torture 2000;10:73–6.

[4] Arcel LT, editor. War victims, trauma and the coping process. Armed conflict in Europe and survivor responses. Copenhagen: International Rehabilitation Council for Torture Victims (IRCT); 1998.

[5] Danielsen L, Rasmussen OV. Dermatological findings after alleged torture. Torture 2006;16:108–27.

[6] Daugaard G, Petersen HD, Abildgaard U, Marcussen M, Wallach M, Jess P. Sequelae to genital trauma in torture victims. Arch Androl 1983;10:245–8.

[7] Gelinas DJ. Relational patterns in incestuous families, malevolent variations, and specific interventions with the adult survivor. In: Paddison PL, editor. Treatment of adult survivors of incest. Washington, DC: American Psychiatric Press; 1993.

[8] Genefke I, Vesti P. Diagnosis of governmental torture. In: Jaranson J, Popking MK, editors. Caring for victims of torture. Washington, DC: American Psychiatric Press; 1998.

[9] Holtz TH. Refugee trauma versus torture trauma: a retrospective controlled cohort study of Tibetan refugees. J Nerv Ment Dis 1998;186:24–34.

[10] Jaranson J, Kinzie JD, Friedman M, Ortiz D, Friedman M, Southwick S, et al. Assessment, diagnosis and intervention. In: Gerrity E, Keane T, Tuma F, editors. The mental health consequences of torture. New York: Kluwer Academic/Plenum; 2001.

[11] Juhler M, Smidt-Nielsen K. Identification of torture survivors: a comparative study of medical complaints and findings in torture survivors. In: Caring for torture survivors: challenges for the medical and health professions. Abstracts: VII International Symposium on Torture, Cape Town, 1995. Available from the RCT Documentation Centre: dokumentation@rct.dk.

[12] Kordon DR, Edelman LJ, Lagos DM, Nicoletti E, Bozzolo RC, Siaky D, Hoste ML, Bonano O, Kersner D. Psychological effects of political repression. Buenos Aires: Sudamerica/Planeta; 1988.

[13] Lök V, Tunica M, Kumanlioglu K, Kapkin E, Dirik G. Bone scintigraphy as clue to previous torture. Lancet 1991;337:846–7.

[14] Mollica RF. Surviving torture. N Engl J Med 2004; 351:5–7.

[15] Montgomery E. Refugee children from the Middle East. Scand J Soc Med 1998;54 (Suppl):1–152.

[16] Musisi S, Kinyanda E, Liebling H Mayengo-Kiziri R. Posttraumatic torture disorders in Uganda. Torture 2000;10:81–7.

[17] Rasmussen OV. Medical aspects of torture. Dan Med Bull 1990;Suppl 1:1–88.

[18] Shresta NM, Sharma B, van Ommeren M, Regmi S, Makaju R, Komproe I, Shrestha GB, de Jong JT. Impact of torture on refugees displaced within the developing world. Symptomatology among Bhutanese refugees in Nepal. JAMA 1998;280:443–8.

[19] Skylv G. The physical sequelae of torture. In: Basoglu M, editor. Torture and its consequences: current treatment approaches. Cambridge: Cambridge University Press; 1992. p. 38–55.

[20] Somnier F, Vesti P, Kastrup M, Genefke I. Psychosocial consequences of torture: current knowledge and evidence. In: Basoglu M, editor. Torture and its consequences: current treatment approaches. Cambridge: Cambridge University Press; 1992.

[21] United Nations General Assembly. Convention against Torture and Other Cruel, Inhuman or Degrading Treatment or Punishment. Resolution adopted by the General Assembly, 10 December 1984.

[22] Williams AC, Amris K. Pain from torture. Pain 2007; 133:5–8.

Supplementary Bibliography

Manual on Effective Investigation and Documentation of Torture and Other Cruel, Inhuman or Degrading Treatment or Punishment. (Istanbul Protocol). United Nations; 1999.

Munczzeck DS. Short-term treatment of a central American torture survivor. Psychiatry 1998,61:318–29.

Peltzer K. A process model of ethnocultural counseling for African survivors of organized violence. Couns Psychol Q 1999;12:335–51.

Quiroga J, Jaranson J. Politically-motivated torture and its survivors: a desk study review of the literature. Torture 2005;15:1–112.

Sørensen B. The process of writing a UN report: positive outcome of Zambia. Torture 2001;11:13–16.

Tocilj-Sumunkovic G, Arcel L. Group psychotherapy with victims of torture. In: Arcel LT, editor. War victims, trauma and the coping process. Armed conflict in Europe and survivor responses. Copenhagen: International Rehabilitation Council for Torture Victims (IRCT); 1998.

Correspondence to: Inge Genefke, MD, DMSc, The International Rehabilitation Council for Torture Victims (IRCT), Borgergade 13, P.O. Box 9049, 1022 Copenhagen K, Denmark. Email: ig@irct.org.

Index

Page numbers followed by f refer to figures, and by t to tables.

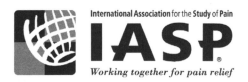